Focus on Abortion

AMERICANS SHARE THEIR STORIES

Photographs and Interviews by ROSLYN BANISH

Introduction by Daniel Grossman, MD

Skyhorse Publishing

Skyhorse Publishing books may be purchased in bulk at special discounts for sales promotion, corporate gifts, fund-raising, or educational purposes. Special editions can also be created to specifications. For details, contact the Special Sales Department, Skyhorse Publishing, 307 West 36th Street, 11th Floor, New York, NY 10018 or info@skyhorsepublishing.com.

Visit our website at www.skyhorsepublishing.com.

10 9 8 7 6 5 4 3 2 1

Library of Congress Cataloging-in-Publication Data is available on file.

Cover design by Kina Sullivan
Cover photo credit: Roslyn Banish

Print ISBN: 978-1-5107-5550-5
Ebook ISBN: 978-1-5107-6600-6

Printed in China.

With love to Paul, Andrew, Jennie, and Dave

Contents

Preface

GROWING UP IN the Midwest, my adventurous family shared lots of stories with each other, usually about other people and places. Very few of these stories were of a personal nature. Feelings were not part of the equation. We did not talk about sickness, death, loss, sadness, and things that were difficult or scary. As the middle of three girls, I remember being tempted but too inhibited to speak about these avoided subjects. I wanted to share feelings associated with my reality, but like my sisters, I didn't.

One reality that was particularly hard to share was the abortion I had when I was a college undergrad in Ann Arbor, Michigan. It was before Roe v. Wade, so the abortion was illegal and done in secrecy. Constrained by the culture of the times and my family's reluctance to speak about difficult events, I told no one except my boyfriend, a couple of friends, and my sisters. The abortion took place in Detroit, performed by someone I assumed was a doctor. In retrospect, I am not sure he was a doctor. It was a frightening experience. I was lucky to come out alive, with the capacity to have children at a future time, which fortuitously happened fourteen years later when I was ready to start a family.

It's no accident that I became a photographer. My camera allowed me to examine what was before me, to get up close, yet be safe in my own space. From the beginning, I was drawn to photographing people. It didn't take me long to question the cliché, "a picture is worth a thousand words." As soon as I realized that people's thoughts and feelings were as important as the photograph, I began incorporating interviews into my work, recording their words and presenting them alongside the photographs. This combination of words and photographs allowed me to delve more deeply into the complexities of each person who came in front of my camera.

In 2015, my friend Uta Landy shared with me over dinner her worries and despair about diminishing access to abortion in the United States. Uta is a remarkable leader in abortion services and family planning education in medical schools in the United States and abroad. We talked about the silence and stigma that cloaks abortion and agreed that trying to break through that silence by sharing personal stories could help normalize abortion.

Our conversation sat with me for almost a year while I struggled to figure out how to enlist volunteer storytellers and how to fund the project. Once in motion, I set out to document a broad sample of those who were touched by abortion: individuals who had abortions, partners, counselors, abortion care providers, and advocates. Because abortion touches all of us, it was important to include storytellers from diverse ethnic and socio-economic backgrounds, religions, generations, and from different regions in the United States. By providing a platform for these storytellers to share their experiences, my aim was to give human shape to an over-simplified, too often politicized subject. The stories told by these individuals are nuanced and the circumstances behind their decisions are complex.

Because I had previously documented individuals who were infected with the AIDS virus, I felt confident to take on a project about abortion. In *Focus on Living: Americans with HIV/AIDS,* I photographed and interviewed gay, transgender, and heterosexual adults, mothers, fathers, teenagers, a child, and drug users. These storytellers were brave, and their stories collectively gave insight into what it was like to be one of the unlucky ones who had contracted HIV/AIDS.

The sixty-two storytellers in *Focus on Abortion* are equally brave. Sometimes with trepidation, always with courage, they have found and developed their voices to speak about abortion at a time when stigma and silence still weigh heavily in our society. Together, they provide a complex and poignant picture of abortion in our country. Their narratives explore the many reasons for choosing to end a pregnancy —from fetal anomalies, to economic hardships, to abusive relationships, to mental illness, to rape, to "I just don't have the bandwidth to have one more child," to "I just don't want kids." As one doctor said, "In my mind, all reasons for choosing to have an abortion are equally valid. That is why abortion has to remain legal and accessible. . ."

Here are authentically told stories from individuals who have the deepest connections to abortion. By harnessing the power of their nuanced stories, my hope is that they will build bridges of understanding between disparate voices in the often-polarized conversations around abortion. I want these stories to move us beyond pro or con, so we can have more empathetic and effective civil discourse.

Focus on Abortion was definitely a collaboration. First and foremost were the folks who participated in the project. I am indebted to all of the storytellers who shared their complex personal stories, their images and their names, as well as the storytellers who were not included in the final edit of this book. They were thoughtful, generous, and inspiring. I am grateful for the many individuals and organizations who welcomed me into their reproductive health worlds. They educated me and introduced me to others in this dedicated and impressive network. They assisted in recruiting storytellers, coached my fundraising efforts, and cheered me on. And finally, I thank my friends, colleagues, and family who cared as much about this project as I did. All those who came on board are listed in the Acknowledgments.

I also want to pay respect to some of the early ground-breaking campaigns and platforms for abortion stories: Advocates for Youth's "Abortion Out Loud" (formerly the "1 in 3 Campaign"), "Exhale Pro-voice," "Shout Your Abortion," "The Abortion Diarist," and Renee Bracey Sherman's "We Testify." Renee generously introduced me to a number of folks who appear in this book. She has given them the support and the tools to share their stories with clarity and confidence.

Thank you all for paving the way to break the stigma and silence around abortion!

Roslyn Banish
San Francisco

Introduction by Daniel Grossman, MD

WHEN I STARTED medical school, I had no idea I would become an abortion provider. Compelled by a strong sense of social justice, I envisioned a career focused on global health, working to address disparities in health care access across countries. On my first trips to sub-Saharan Africa—to Zaire, Kenya, and Mali—I came face-to-face with the brutal inequities that contributed to unsafe abortion. I saw how patients were dying not because the diagnosis was unclear or because a cure did not exist, but because of bad public policy. It was then that I decided to work at the intersection of medicine, public health, and policy—as an abortion provider and trainer, and as a researcher focused on access to reproductive health care.

My experience working in countries where abortion is legally restricted—including living several years in Latin America—has prepared me well for the crisis in abortion access we are facing in this country. Forty-five years after abortion became legal nationwide, access to facility-based care is more precarious than ever. Similar to the disparities I saw in Africa and Latin America, people in the US are more or less likely to need and obtain an abortion depending on their income, skin color, and where they live. There are important lessons we in the US can learn from activists and providers in the Global South who have been working to ensure access to safe abortion care in restrictive settings.

The geographic barriers to abortion care in the US are extreme, especially in some parts of the country. According to the latest data from the Guttmacher Institute, 89 percent of US counties do not have an abortion provider, and 38 percent of women of reproductive age live in one of those counties. Colleagues at the University of California, San Francisco mapped the distance to the nearest abortion provider across the US and found large areas of the country were hundreds of miles from a clinic. They identified twenty-seven "deserts," which they categorized as urban centers with a population of at least 50,000 people that were located greater than one hundred miles from the nearest provider.

In addition to geographic barriers, the cost of abortion care creates a significant obstacle for people with low incomes. Since 1976, the Hyde Amendment has prohibited the use of federal funds to pay for abortion care except to save the life of the pregnant woman or in case of rape or incest. This essentially eliminates the possibility of Medicaid paying for abortion care except in the sixteen or so states that use their own funds to pay for abortion care for people with low incomes. Those who are in the military or are covered by military insurance, federal employees, and those receiving care through the Indian Health Service also face restrictions on federal funds paying for abortion care. Given that a first-trimester abortion costs a little more than $500 on average, the financial barriers to abortion care can be enormous.

It is clear that abortion is under political attack at the state level like never before. The past decade has seen a dramatic increase in the number of restrictions on abortion care enacted at the state level. Almost sixty such laws were passed in 2019. Historically, the courts have been the bulwark against legislatures passing the most extreme restrictions on abortion care, although they have not prevented the crisis of access that many in the Midwest and South currently face. But it remains to be seen whether the courts will continue to protect the right to legal abortion.

The crisis of access to abortion in the US is not affecting all people equally. Clinics are closing at an alarming rate in the South and Midwest, heightening geographic disparities. People seeking abortion are disproportionately women of color. According to the Guttmacher Institute's 2014 nationally representative survey of abortion patients, 28 percent are non-Hispanic Black, about one quarter are Hispanic, 6 percent are Asian or Pacific Islander, and 39 percent are non-Hispanic white. With regard to income, about half are living below the Federal Poverty Level (FPL), and one quarter are living between 100 percent and 200 percent of FPL. These data highlight how access to safe abortion is fundamentally an issue of racial justice and social justice more broadly.

At the same time this crisis in abortion access has evolved, a quiet revolution has been underway that is making abortion pills—a safe and effective option for ending a pregnancy on one's own—only an internet click away. When the Food and Drug Administration (FDA) approved mifepristone, also known as RU-486, for use with misoprostol for medication abortion in 2000, advocates hailed it as a revolutionary technology. The hope was that it would forever change the way American women obtain and experience abortion, moving it out of clinics and into people's homes.

Those changes have been slow in coming because of regulations that the FDA and states imposed. For example, the FDA requires that clinicians physically hand out mifepristone in their offices or hospitals; doctors cannot write a prescription to be filled at a pharmacy. Most states prohibit nurse practitioners and midwives from providing the abortion pill despite evidence demonstrating they can do it as safely as a physician. About twenty states prohibit the use of telemedicine to provide medication abortion even though rigorous research has shown the practice to be safe, effective, and well-liked by patients—and telemedicine improves access to early abortion.

Women in the Global South—initially in Brazil—were the first to realize that pills that were widely available in pharmacies for other uses could also be used to induce an abortion without seeing a doctor, a practice known as self-managed abortion. Self-managed abortion with medications has undoubtedly helped to reduce morbidity and mortality associated with unsafe abortion in Latin America and elsewhere.

As a physician, I have few medical concerns about the safety of self-managed abortion. If people know that they are ten weeks pregnant or less, if they can obtain high-quality mifepristone and misoprostol, and if they have access to back-up care if needed, medication abortion can be safely used without medical supervision. There are a few other medical conditions that might make taking the medications less safe—like if the patient also takes blood thinners that could increase bleeding—but people can self-identify these conditions.

However, I do have concerns about the legal risks people may take by attempting to self-manage their abortion. At least twenty-one people have been arrested or criminally investigated for allegedly self-inducing their abortion or for helping someone else. Not surprisingly, women of color and those living on low incomes have been disproportionately targeted for criminalization. This trend toward criminalizing women's actions during pregnancy is concerning since it may deter patients from seeking medical care when complications arise. It is also very hard to distinguish self-induced abortion from spontaneous pregnancy loss, which may lead to scrutinizing every woman with a miscarriage.

As access to facility-based abortion care becomes more constrained, it is likely that self-managed medication abortion will become more common. I believe that clinicians have a role to play in this scenario by informing patients about mifepristone and misoprostol as the safest way to self-induce an abortion and by providing needed care before and after they use the medications. This harm-reduction approach to safe abortion was spearheaded by brave clinicians and social workers in Uruguay before the abortion law there was liberalized, and their work led to a marked reduction in complications and deaths related to unsafe abortion.

The revolution in self-managed abortion will not solve all of the problems we are facing with regard to diminishing access in the US. Some patients have a strong preference for an in-clinic vacuum aspiration and do not want a medication abortion, and others may be past ten weeks and need an aspiration. Everyone should have the right to access safe abortion care in a way that respects their autonomy and allows them to receive their preferred method and model of care.

In the long term, I believe we will get to a place where these rights are respected for all. Rather than spreading as an underground practice, self-managed abortion could go mainstream by the FDA approving mifepristone and misoprostol for over-the-counter (OTC) sale. While OTC approval may take years, a growing body of evidence indicates these medications can be safely used without medical supervision. In the process of rolling out OTC medication, it will be critical to preserve access to facility-based care for those who prefer it and those needing abortion after ten weeks.

In these tumultuous times where abortion often feels like a political tool, rather than the life-saving and life-changing health care it really is, the stories of those having abortions and providing this care get lost in the rhetoric. In this moment, Roslyn Banish's beautiful photographs and the moving stories of those who collaborated with her are most welcome. Thank you for sharing your images and heartfelt narratives—they are particularly enriching as the reproductive health, rights, and justice movement faces its greatest challenges in half a century.

Portraits and Interviews

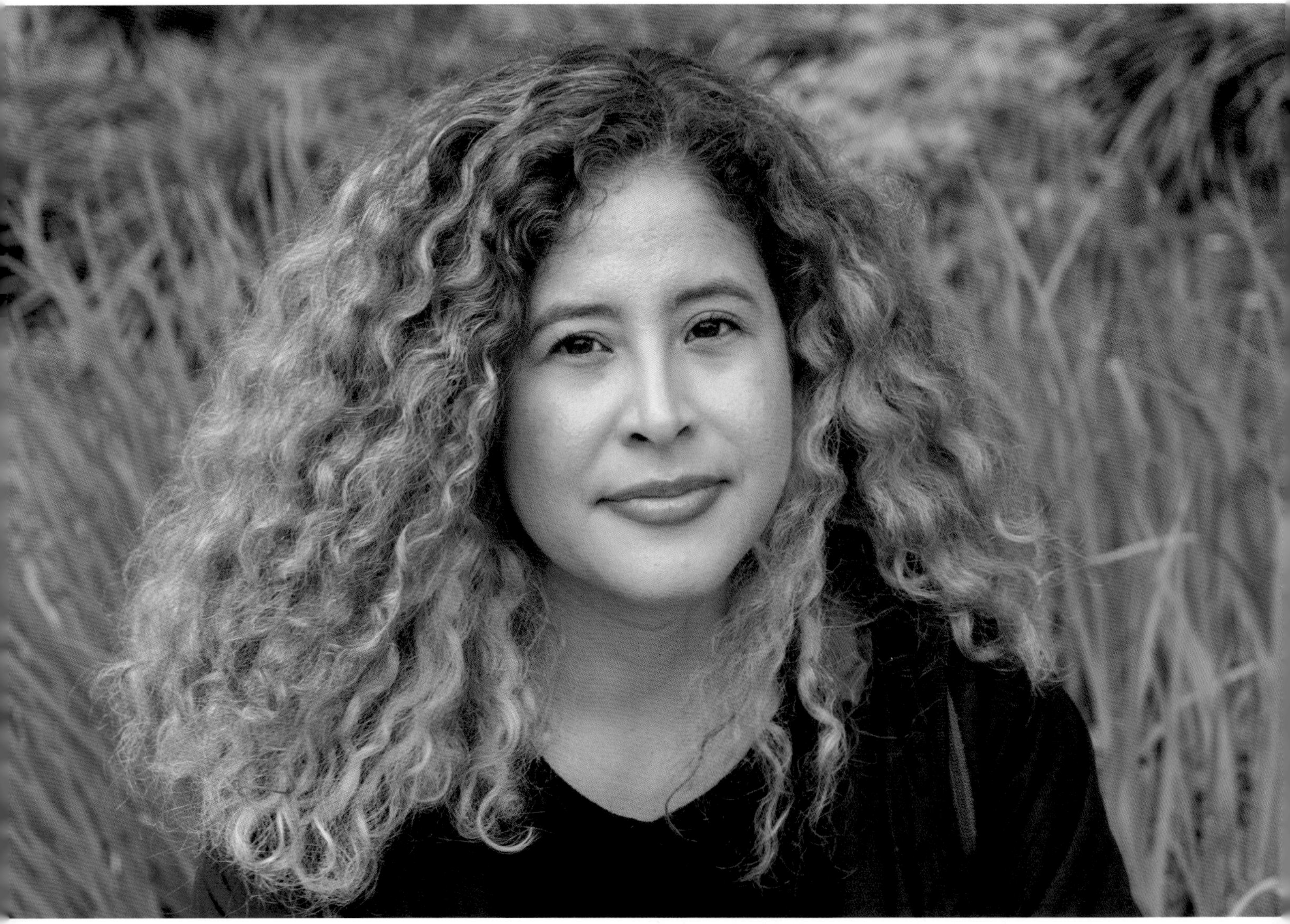

ANNA PATRICIA CASTRO ARGUETA

Anna Patricia Castro Argueta

MY MOTHER CAME to the United States to get away from the civil war in El Salvador and my father emigrated from Peru. I'm a US citizen, but I'm so much more. I'm connected to both the promise of what the United States is and also the feelings of what it is not.

I grew up in a primarily immigrant neighborhood in the San Fernando Valley in Southern California. Growing up, my mother cleaned houses, pretty much seven days a week. My dad had his own business. He did taxes, and helped fill out paperwork for people getting their citizenship.

I was the first person in my family to graduate from high school and college. I got a scholarship to Amherst College in Massachusetts. Arriving at Amherst was really tough, very alienating. But I found my home there in the Black Studies Department.

First of all, I want to say I've had multiple abortions. I think that that's important to state right off the bat because there is this stigma about multiple abortions. But it's a reality. They happen for a variety of reasons.

My first abortion happened when I was in college. I had a partner I really loved and saw a future with. Yet, the minute I found out I was pregnant, I knew I was not ready to be a parent. I had things I wanted to do. Even the decision was immediate. I could not bring myself to have a conversation about it with anybody. Even though I knew that my partner would be very supportive, I did not tell him about it until after the abortion.

I found a Planned Parenthood clinic in western Massachusetts. I was working and going to school, and the cost of the abortion—$600 or $700—was way more than I had. When I called to schedule an appointment, to my surprise I learned about an abortion fund that would contribute half the cost.

On the day of the appointment, I got up early, took a two-hour bus ride, and went there all by myself. I did tell my partner to pick me up from the appointment, and it was one of those things where he didn't ask, he just picked me up. Then I went back to school, I think the next day.

I felt like I had made the right choice by me and by my partner. It felt like an affirming thing that he and I didn't have to have the abortion conversation, even though we had talked about wanting to have children and about a future. It was affirming too, that I could choose to not have a child now, but that didn't mean that I didn't want a family in the future.

I didn't feel any stigma. I think that that probably goes back to when I was a kid having heard of people having abortions. My mother talked to me about abortions, never in a way that had any kind of like value judgment, which is interesting because my mom is a Jehovah's Witness. As a kid, I went with her, knocking on doors and spreading the good word on street corners, talking about the good word. Jehovah's Witnesses are super conservative. They don't believe in abortion, birth control, or sex before marriage.

After graduating in 2012, I accepted an executive assistant position with the ACLU of San Diego. I wanted to work in a place where I could learn about doing advocacy. A lot of my time was focused on immigrants' rights, voting rights, criminal justice, and drug policy reform. I worked there for almost five years.

After I moved to San Diego I started dating somebody new. I felt the relationship would be the one to go the distance, but really it was not a great relationship. In fact, we had pretty much broken up by the time I got pregnant. Finding out that I was pregnant was devastating. I felt ready to have a family, but I knew this was the worst possible environment that I could bring a child into. My partner said that he would resent me if I had a child. The relationship would be a breeding ground for terribleness. I thought about not telling him I was pregnant, but I also felt like this was something that we had done together and I wanted us to figure it out together.

Making the decision to have an abortion is a complex and quiet calculus. Even when it feels uncomplicated, there are nuances. With my first abortion, even though my boyfriend and I didn't talk about it, I knew he knew and understood. That was important.

As a woman of color, I grew up like with so much stigma around not being an unwed teenage mother. I knew it was wrong and should be avoided at all costs. Now that I'm older

I wonder why I got so fixated on there being only one way—married—to have kids. Now I realize that what's important is the community you're in. So much of parenting happens within a community. The women that I've been surrounded with are so amazing and so strong and a lot of them have raised children by themselves.

Community is so important in my life. In the summer of 2016, just before the election, I started working with Mi Familia Vota, a Latino civic engagement organization, where I became the national communications director. Our goal was to build power locally in communities. We encouraged people to register to vote and to stay engaged, to hold elected leaders accountable. Since September 2018, I've been consulting with organizations, and am preparing to go to law school. The work that I do is emotionally heavy. These issues—immigration, deportation—are personal to me. I have family members who are undocumented.

I FELT SO INTENSELY VULNERABLE AT THE TIME OF MY ABORTION AND THE AFTERMATH. I WAS REMINDED OF THE GRACE THAT IT TAKES TO PUT YOURSELF BACK TOGETHER AFTER FEELING SO IMMENSELY CRUSHED.

Lately I've been thinking how vulnerability is a source of power. I felt so intensely vulnerable at the time of my abortion and the aftermath. I was reminded of the grace that it takes to put yourself back together after feeling so immensely crushed. What makes you strong is the ability to acknowledge difficult moments and embrace every feeling that they give you. The awareness that those moments change you in a way that allows you to see things that you may not have seen before. I'm still working on it. It took a village of people and lots of their time but a year later, I'm still picking up all these pieces.

I've been proud to have been called a fearless woman, a powerful woman. For a long time, I created a mask that said, "I'm OK, I'm fine, I'm good. I can take all of this. I can run with it and I can succeed." This was my impenetrable shield. It was only around the time of my second abortion that I realized I was a prisoner of my own making, feeling like I had to hold myself to a different standard. If I had continued to rely on my shield and not have had this experience in which I let myself acknowledge what I was feeling, I might still be trapped behind that mask of strong. So much of the world is geared toward robbing us of feeling righteously emotional.

Now I can say that I am in pain and be public about that. I think that that's been really freeing for me. I'm in pain and I'm in progress.

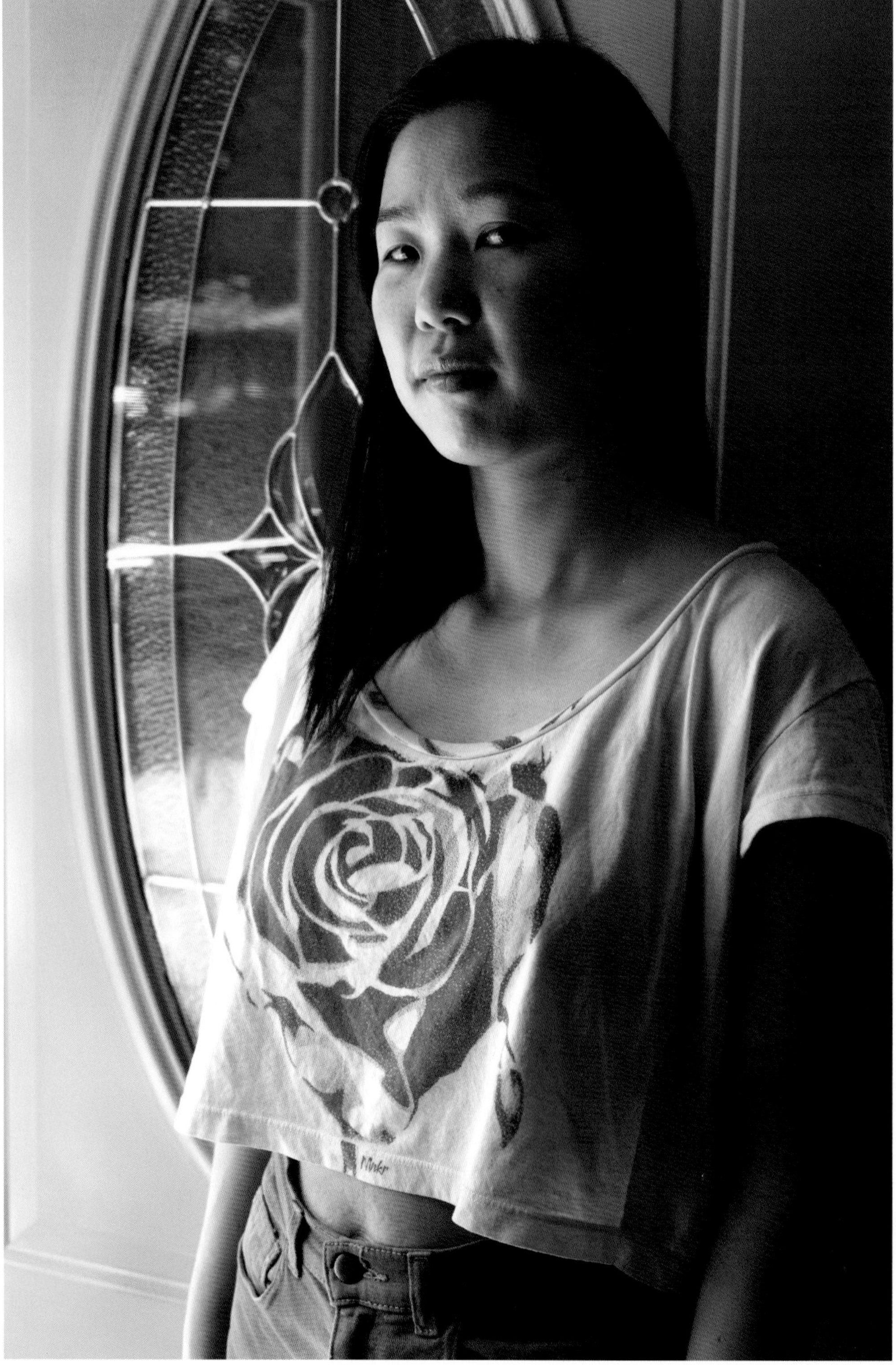

LOKYEE AU

Lokyee Au

I WAS BORN and grew up in California's San Gabriel Valley. My grandfather immigrated to California from Hong Kong in the 1970s. My biological father is still in Hong Kong. Right before my mom was about to give birth to me, she moved to California. She was a single parent but had the support of a larger community to care for me. Often my grandparents or family friends looked after me while my mom was at her job in a bank.

There was a pretty big Chinese-American community where I lived. By the time I was in high school, we lived in Arcadia, and people were fairly well off. The school was largely Asian-American. Students at my public high school pushed so hard for academic achievement and the goal was always: Don't fuck up, go to college. Even if someone did get pregnant and had an abortion, you would not talk about it.

I moved to San Diego for college and left California when I was 22 to go to graduate school in Eugene, Oregon. I've been in Oregon since. I earned two Master's, one in environmental studies and the other in urban planning. Now I am a communication strategist for a Portland City Commissioner.

My abortion happened thirteen years ago, when I was 17. It was the summer between graduation from high school and going off to college, and I was working part-time at a restaurant.

I was feeling off, not sure what was going on. Finally, I went to Planned Parenthood in Pasadena—I always want to give a shout-out to them—and I found out I was pregnant. It was far enough along where I couldn't do an at-home medication abortion, so I scheduled a procedure for about two weeks after that.

I remember very particular things about the day of my abortion. I had to go pick up my boyfriend who got me pregnant. I was running late. I was super, super stressed. At the clinic, I remember distinctly another couple there for an abortion. They were laughing and giggling. I was really moody, really closed up. My boyfriend at the time was like 'Why are you so angry? Why can't we be like that couple over there?' I was just like, 'You're shitting me, dude. Out of all this, that's what you're upset about?' Who goes to an abortion appointment and is angry that their girlfriend is moody about it?

I remember vividly the nurse who was there with the doctor. She held my hand the whole time. Just at that moment I felt the comfort that I needed for the whole day that I clearly was lacking. I don't remember the pain. I didn't completely go under, but I just remember the little pinches on my cervix that they needed for the shots to open up the cervix.

After the procedure, my boyfriend drove me home and I rested. I was really angry throughout this because he basically hadn't respected me saying no when we were having sex, and that's how I got pregnant to begin with. We had both been stressing and freaking about the pregnancy, and I just felt there was zero support for me. Then he didn't help me pay for it, so I was really angry at that. A month after that I broke up with him.

At the time of my abortion, only my boyfriend knew about it. I definitely was never going to tell my mom. I was sure that telling her would open all these doors for conversations we'd never had, like sex, like dating. I didn't want all these other doors to open. If we didn't talk about sex, and we didn't talk about relationships, how do you talk about abortion?

Thirteen years after my abortion, I now have a baby, River. On the thirteenth anniversary of my abortion, I posted my abortion story on Facebook. I wanted to post my story after a bunch of those abortion bans were happening throughout the states and I was just getting fed up. I wanted to normalize what abortion is, and who gets them. So I put out a post about it, about the circumstances, and why I did it. My mother saw it on Facebook.

She texted me something along the lines of, "It broke my heart to hear that this was happening so close to me. I can't believe that this happened. I'm going to need time to digest all the information."

When I first got that text, I was frustrated with my mom because I was feeling like she had centered herself in her feelings, telling me, "I'm so heartbroken." I texted my mom back saying she could take time to digest it, but it happened. I can't take it back. It's not a reflection on you, it's just that's where I was at. That was the end of the text conversation.

A few weeks later she reached out again because she wanted to see photos of River, my baby, her grandchild. I was like, "I'll show you photos but if you're still upset with me then I don't really want to talk to you." And she's like, "I'm calm."

It's complicated with River because River's father and I weren't married when I was pregnant. My mother had to rectify her societal expectations of my having a child out of wedlock. When I first told her I was pregnant with River I was really happy with her response. She said the way she understood these trajectories in life is that you get married and then you have a kid, but she also understood that's not what everyone wants. I appreciated that. She came to visit for a couple of weeks after I gave birth.

In my family and in Chinese culture there's a lot of expectations, and the expectations can change depending on whether you're a girl or a boy. Those expectations are rooted in a lot of patriarchy, which does so much damage. It takes so many years to unlearn and heal from that.

The expectations for me, beyond being a good kid, being a good daughter, were always listening to your family, and being very amenable to everything your family does or tells you to do. Like, if you're a girl, acting more feminine. If I were a boy they would expect me to act more masculine or maybe go into a different field in school, like the sciences.

HAVING GONE THROUGH AN ABORTION, PREGNANCY AND A MISCARRIAGE, AND THEN RIVER'S BIRTH, I WOULD NEVER, EVER WANT ANYONE TO HAVE TO GO THROUGH A PREGNANCY THAT THEY DID NOT WANT.

I just didn't want River to have to go through that. We're not gendering River. We refer to River as they/them. We've said that when they're older, and they know and decide what their gender is, they'll let us know on a functional level. After all, your genitalia don't always match your gender, right? Kids are smart. They'll take the time and will let us know when they know. We will work to give them the education and talk with them about these things and also ask them how they feel throughout.

My mother and I definitely had some hard conversations about not gendering River. It started when I was pregnant with her asking if I wanted a girl or a boy. That's when I told her we weren't going to gender the baby. I explained it in the terms of a baby's a baby and I don't want them to be treated any differently just because they're one gender or the other. I think she tries. She refers to River in Cantonese as "Little Piggy" so she can avoid gendering River. That's progress. She's trying, and she's found a way to avoid the headache and also appease me.

A baby's a baby. They have all the hopes, and dreams, and opportunities in the future they could have, so let's just do that.

I've been thinking a lot differently about my body since it's gone through all this. It makes me realize that getting an abortion at age 17 was the right decision for me. It doesn't negate any of the other experiences I've had since then.

There are so many reasons why a person needs or wants an abortion. For me, having gone through an abortion, pregnancy and a miscarriage, and then River's birth, I would never, ever want anyone to have to go through a pregnancy that they did not want. I have a deep appreciation for a person, whether they choose to get pregnant or get an abortion, because they're making whatever decision they think is best for them.

Jennifer Aubrey

I THINK MY parents wanted me to be a good homemaker. Certainly, they didn't want me to be having sex before marriage. That being said, I was the oldest virgin I knew. I was 19, which even in those times was pretty old. Sex was never discussed in our house growing up.

I grew up in New Canaan, Connecticut, in an upper middle-class family. I'm one of five children. My father commuted for forty years to New York City by train, and I never wanted for a thing. I went to Miss Porter's School, which today is still one of the only girls, boarding schools. At that time, they literally had tea pouring classes. This was '66 to '69. My mother, unbeknownst to me, had signed me up to go to a cotillion, to be a debutante. I didn't go.

At Boston University, I guess "radicalized" is appropriate. A lot of demonstrating about the Vietnam War and railing against Nixon. After being maced one too many times in Harvard Square, I dropped out and moved to Taos, New Mexico, much to my parents' dismay. I was 18 or 19. Taos was a place full of very strong women and not so strong men. I lived with a boyfriend in Taos for a couple of years.

My abortion story happened in New York City. It was probably '78 or '79, after I had left Taos for the East Coast. I got pregnant by a guy I didn't have any serious relationship with. I mean, this was certainly not a man I was going to spend the rest of my life with. And I knew that having a baby would drastically change my life. There was no question of what I was going to do.

Getting an abortion in New York wasn't difficult. That being said, I remember sitting in the hospital waiting room with a few other women and thinking it was a pretty heavy

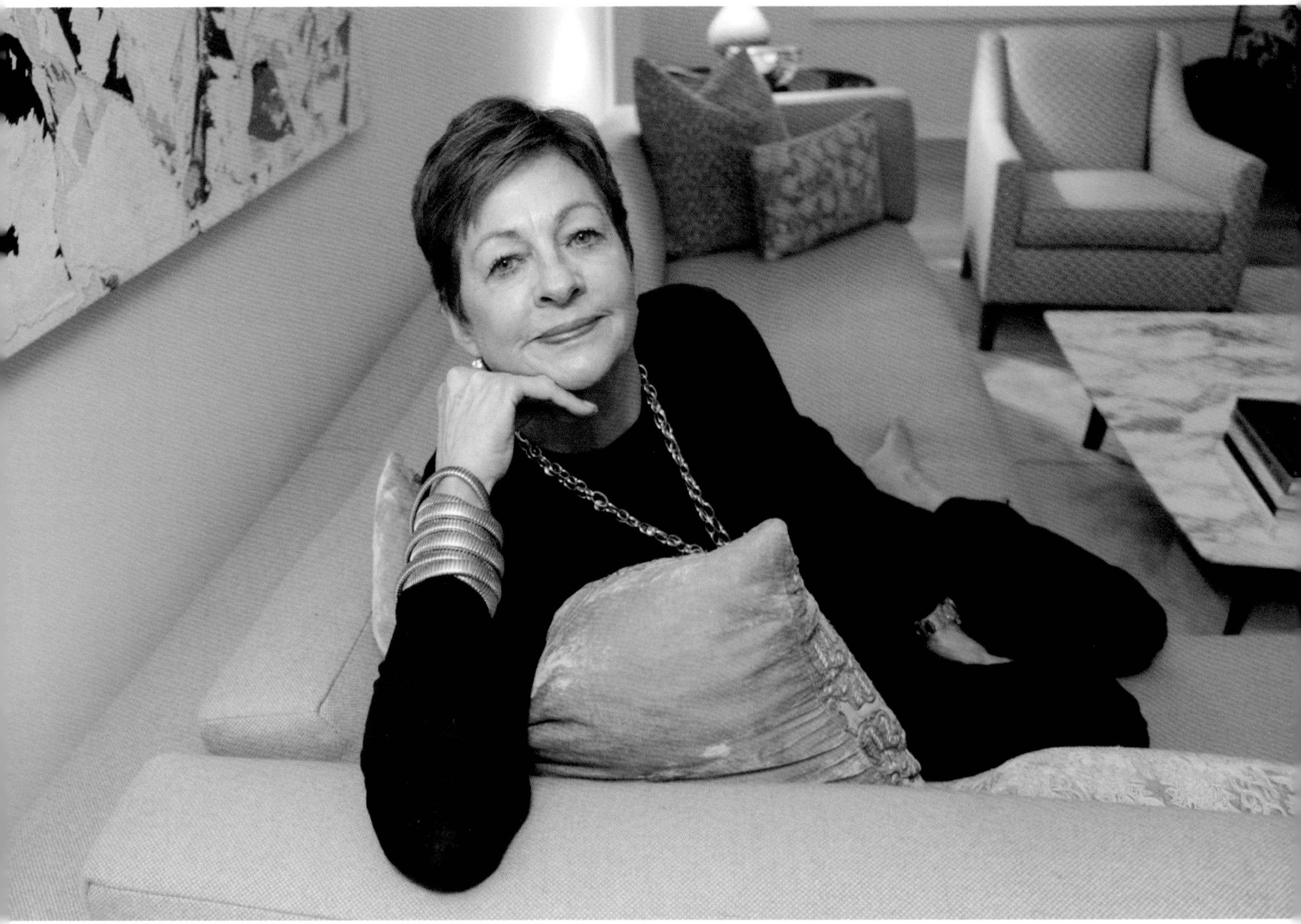

JENNIFER AUBREY

scene to be going through. Afterwards I went out with friends. I remember thinking, "Oh, sure, life goes on, and I just had an abortion." I had just done something that's life changing in either direction. I never felt guilty. I was simply glad that I had the choice to have my life go on.

Around the time of my abortion, I met the man I would marry. We had three sons together. We divorced when my youngest was 5. Now he is 27. I'm very close to my boys.

In contrast to my own experience with their father, it was very important to raise my three sons to be empathic and compassionate and always feel that their mate was going to be as important as they were and always share in that relationship. Women, girlfriends, and now their wives, have always said to me how polite and wonderful and compassionate my sons are. With the MeToo movement, I think it's wrong to just focus on girls and women. I think we need to focus on boys and how we raise boys and men.

I have never been of the opinion that abortion is a form of birth control and that young women are just stupid . . . After all, mistakes happen. That doesn't mean you have to make the whole rest of your life a mistake by having an unwanted child.

Last Thanksgiving, I had two of my three sons and one of their wives for dinner, and I decided I wanted to ask them what they thought about participating in this book project. I told them, "I'm thinking of not doing this because I really don't have a story to tell." My youngest son in particular was extremely supportive. He's the one who said, "Mom, that's your story, it could have been life-changing." He knows that this is an important issue for me. When he was 10 or 12, he traveled to Washington, D.C. with me for a pro-choice rally. Even at that age, he understood that if women did not have a choice, we were not living in a democracy.

I think what's important is to take the stigma away from abortion by showing that it's not just teenagers who get abortions, that it's all walks of life. I have never been of the opinion that abortion is a form of birth control and that young women are just stupid. I think abortion is a serious, thoughtful decision, and I can't imagine that we wouldn't have that choice or that right.

After all, mistakes happen. That doesn't mean you have to make the whole rest of your life a mistake by having an unwanted child. Nobody wants to have an abortion. It's just something that, if you have to, it should be there to happen.

I do think that young women who have never lived without access to abortion need to get on board here because I think we could seriously lose this right. If this is a democracy, we should have that right. We should have that choice. And certainly it cannot be a decision made by men sitting in courtrooms.

Pratima Gupta

I AM AN obstetrician gynecologist, and I provide the full scope of reproductive health care, everything from Pap smears to prenatal care to abortions and birth control to delivering babies. I completed my residency in 2005 in Los Angeles, and did a fellowship in family planning at University of California San Francisco. Now, in addition to my practice, I train medical students and residents in higher levels of birth control and abortion techniques.

In 2016, I took a year off from my clinical practice to do a reproductive health advocacy fellowship with Physicians for Reproductive Health. PRH is a non-profit based in New York that focuses on physician advocacy. During that year I did everything from developing curriculum related to physician advocacy to training other physicians around the country on how they can get involved. I also responded to media requests and reviewed testimony that would be given before Congress to ensure medical accuracy.

That was also the year Whole Women's Health v. Hellerstadt reached the US Supreme Court, and I had the opportunity to speak on the steps of the Supreme Court in March 2016 when the case was heard. That was probably one of the most powerful experiences of the year for me. More than 2,000 people came in support of Whole Women's Health. To speak there that day as an abortion provider and mother and to be surrounded by such a strong community of people who had travelled from around the world, who had taken buses to show their support for this case and abortion rights, was profound.

Another focus of my PRH fellowship was looking at the reproductive health angles around trans care. I work with a lot of transgender patients on their wellness and

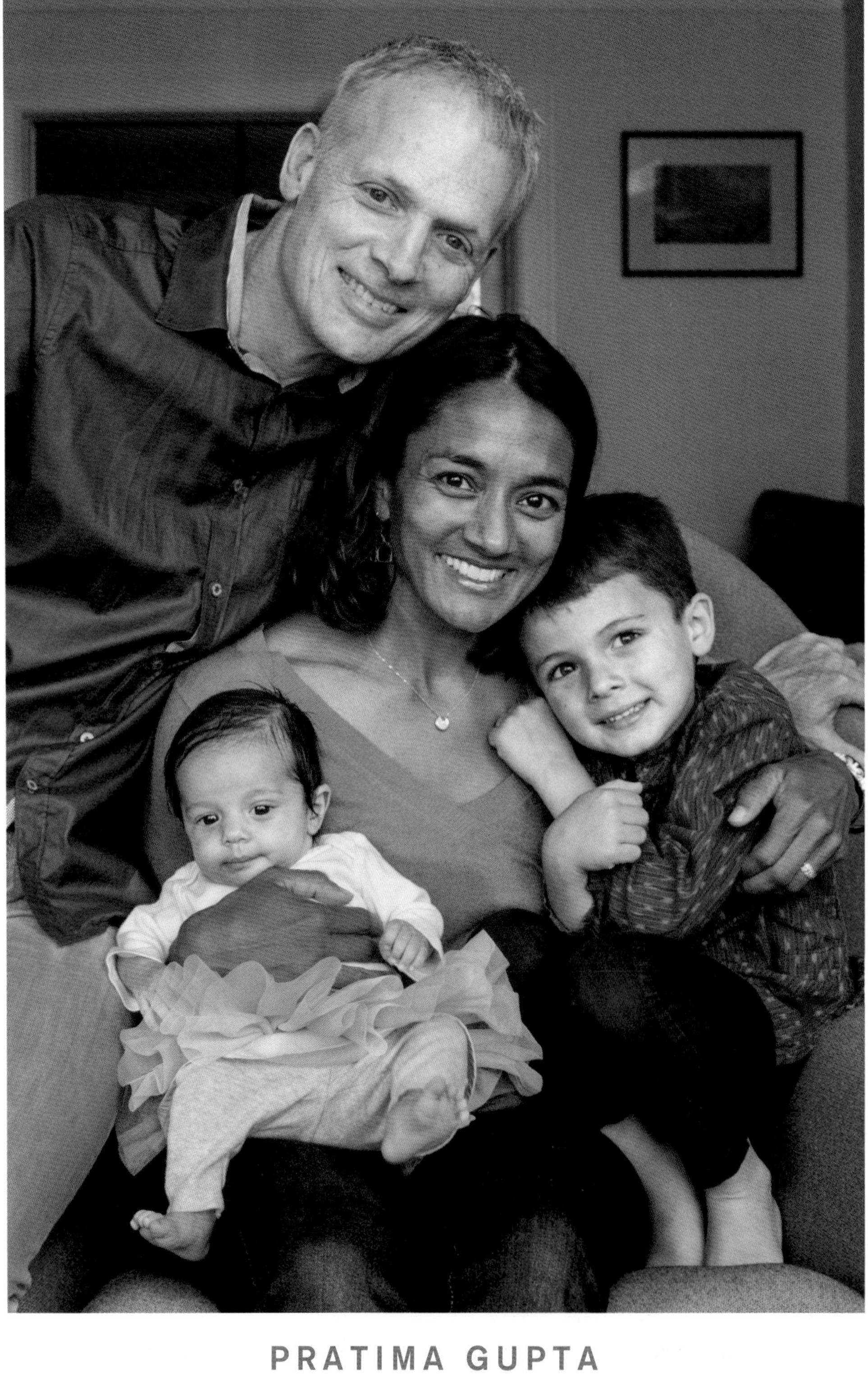

PRATIMA GUPTA

reproductive health. There are a lot of assumptions and misconceptions around people's desires and plans for individuals who identify as transgender.

I also participated in the Emerge California Program, which trains Democratic women to run for office. Although separate from the PRH fellowship, it was aligned with the advocacy aspects and using your unique voice as a physician to empower others. It was an intensive program, lasting several months, where you learn everything from fundraising to networking to campaign finance laws, how to do grassroots efforts, and how to read a voter file.

I got involved with politics because people kept asking me if I had ever thought about running for office. I hadn't because, given that I am an abortion provider, I did not believe voters would support me. It's one thing to be pro-choice and it's another thing to be the provider who actually does the abortion.

Even though I knew my chances of winning were slim, I chose to run for a seat on the Democratic County Central Committee (DCCC) here in San Francisco. There were nearly forty people running for fourteen seats. I was an unknown entity. I've never really been involved in City Hall politics. But to my surprise I was elected.

Running for office requires a lot of preparation. It is emotionally draining and financially taxing. It puts a lot of strain on your family. My target audience was women of reproductive age, and my main platform centered on me as a doctor and the mother of a young child. The perspective of having a young child is unique, along with my priorities and what's important in the city.

HOW CAN YOU SAY THAT I'M NOT PRO-LIFE WHEN I HAVE TWO CHILDREN AND I'M GIVING WOMEN THEIR LIVES BACK WHEN I AM DOING THEIR ABORTIONS?

I have a very supportive partner. We have a color-coded calendar. We plan and juggle so that we have childcare for our two children. Anyone who is considering running for office is told to have a really frank discussion with family and friends to prepare for the stress and time commitment.

As an abortion provider there's a certain dichotomy in the language used by both the people who are in favor of abortion rights and increasing access and the anti-choice side. The use of the word "choice," the word "life." These words have been taken over by the different sides. These words have become so charged. I would really like to work on taking back the word "life" because as a physician, I feel part of my responsibility is a commitment to support life. I consider myself to be pro-life. How can you say that I'm not pro-life when I have two children and I'm giving women their lives back when I am doing their abortions? I look at it as a truly pro-life stance.

When I say I am a pro-life abortion provider, it takes people a while to wrap their heads around it, until I explain it. But I think it's really about changing the terminology and not putting it in a completely separate bucket in terms of what we believe in.

In medical school, I specifically didn't think about OBGYN because my father was an OBGYN. I had memories of being at the movies with him as a child and he would get called, interrupting our father-daughter time. But I really enjoyed the continuum of women's health, that you can have a relationship with a patient through so many different phases of their life, and that it is both clinic based and procedure based. You get to build a relationship with your patients, you are utilizing your hands and your technical skills, and that it's mostly young healthy patients who are in the hospital for a relatively short and joyous reason when they have a baby.

In terms of becoming an abortion provider, I was struck by the fact that it was a separate part of OBGYN, a separate part of medicine. I perceived it as part of the whole spectrum of care that I was offering and should offer in OBGYN. In medical school, the fact that you could opt in or opt out of learning to do abortions surprised me. In my training, nobody would opt out of delivering a baby or doing a Pap smear, but abortion has become so polarized that people can choose not to get that training.

In my current practice, a lot of the high points have to do with the abortions I do. I see patients who have unplanned, undesired pregnancies, and I see patients who have fetal anomalies who are referred for termination. I am fortunate to work in a system where they have pretty good resources for patient support. My practice allows me to educate a patient about their options, and it allows me to dispel a lot of myths. I can't tell you the number of times my patients have said to me, "You are so much nicer than I was expecting." I don't know if it's the media that's projecting the abortion provider as somebody more judgmental. Surely supporting the woman and the family in whatever decision they need and either helping them continue their pregnancy and get prenatal care or terminate the pregnancy is one of the best parts of what I do.

I work with residents and medical students training the next generation of abortion providers and doctors in family planning. The residents I work with are for the most part OBGYN residents, so they have already chosen their specialty. As to the medical students, I explain to them that no matter what specialty they choose, I guarantee that they will see a woman with an unintended pregnancy at some point. Just having exposure and awareness of the fact that unintended pregnancies are very common, and making sure the students are aware of the options, whether or not they choose to offer an abortion, is another rewarding part of my job.

There is stigma both about getting an abortion and about being an abortion provider. People are reticent to talk about the fact that they had an abortion, what that experience was like for them. A lot of my patients who have miscarriages, for example, will say that once they tell one friend about their miscarriage, all of a sudden ten more friends will come out and say they had miscarriages. But nobody wants to talk about the shame or stigma around abortion.

There's a lot of work going on in social media, telling abortion stories, and removing that stigma. People tell their birth story. When you have a newborn, everybody wants to hear your birth story. When you go to a mothers' group or a playground, everybody wants to hear your birth story. Everybody has one and remembers it vividly. But there isn't that same societal acceptance around telling your abortion story and experience.

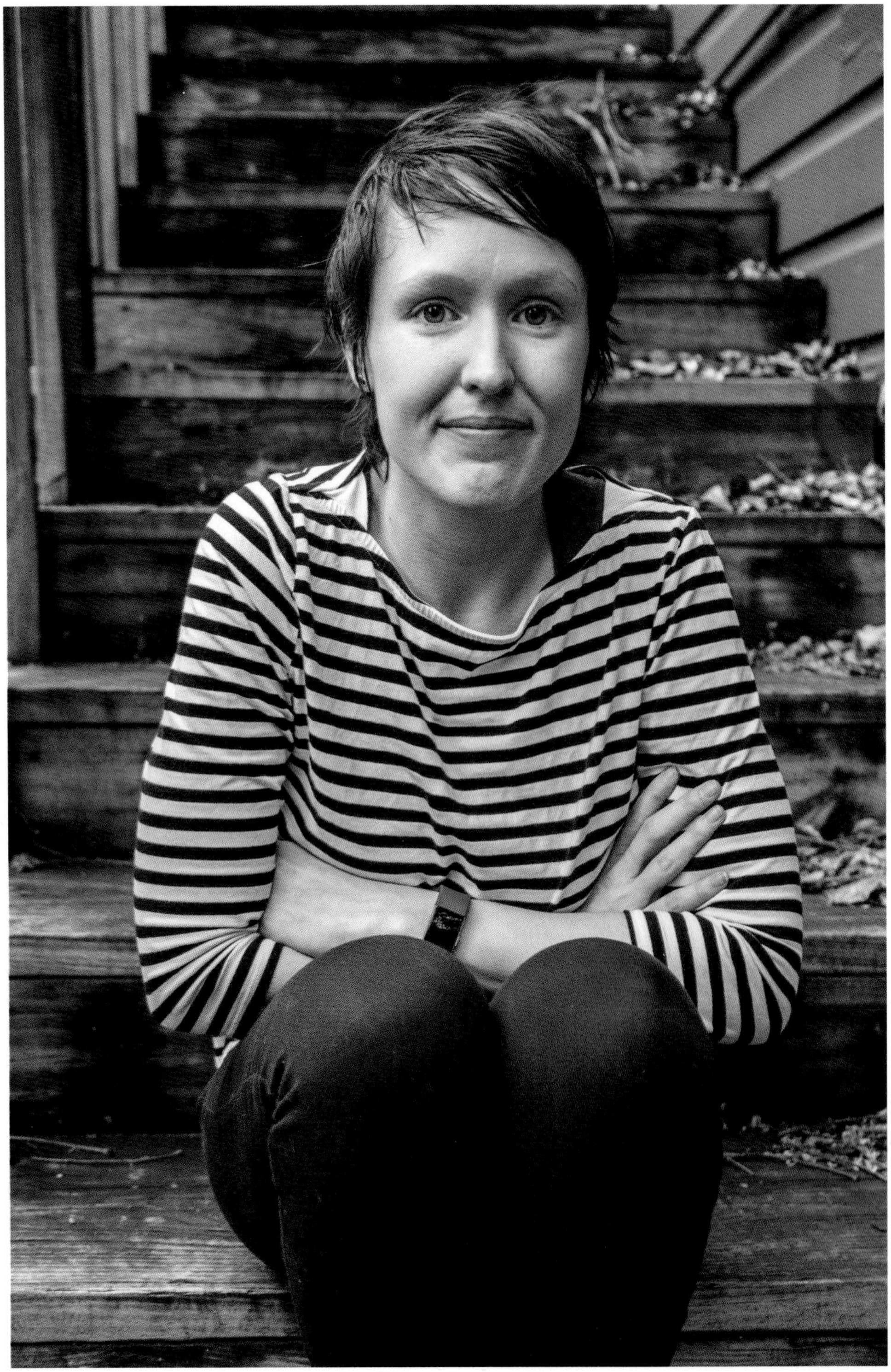

BLAIR AULT

Blair Ault

MY FIRST ABORTION was seven years ago, when I was 22. Afterwards, I didn't really know how to process it. About a year later, I decided to write my abortion story for *Story Time*. This was a theater event of a company called Boo Town. People send in stories and actors read them to an audience at a neighborhood bar in Houston.

I set up a whole Gmail account to send it in so no one would know who it came from and I left out specific details. It was really interesting to hear my story read to an audience by an actor. Nobody knew that it was my story. Up until that point, my abortion was still a secret. I hadn't really told anybody outside the people who were involved.

For the first abortion, I had immediately called my best friend and she helped me find a clinic. I told my parents and a bunch of people slowly but surely, one on one. The first time I got pregnant, I waited a really long time before finding out if I was pregnant. I was within a couple weeks of the twenty-week ban in Texas. The people at the clinic showed me the ultrasound and wanted me to get into the clinic the next day for the surgical procedure.

In the clinic waiting room were all these aquariums—did they think we were cats?—and a sign asking to keep children out of the waiting room. I guess they didn't want women to feel triggered or guilty while they're there. They gave me some medication to knock me out, which eventually it did. But before I was knocked out, I remember being in a line of women in a hallway just sitting in chairs. Each of us had a consultation with the nurse, who was really nice and understanding. She was very matter of fact. There was no bit of shaming.

It's funny because I wrote another story after my second abortion, which happened about a year and a half after the first one. I was really ashamed of the second one. I didn't admit it to my parents or even my best friend who I had told about the first one. I kept the second one under wraps.

MY IDEAL SOCIETY IS WHERE WOMEN CAN TALK ABOUT HAVING AN ABORTION WITH EACH OTHER IN FRONT OF A WATER COOLER, THE SAME WAY THAT PEOPLE LIKE TO TALK ABOUT THE TATTOO THAT THEY GOT.

The story of the second abortion came out just a couple of years ago when I went to *The Moth Story Slam*, an NPR storytelling monthly event, similar to *Story Time*. People get up in front and tell their own stories. The theme that night was pride. I was really angry because Texas had recently passed a law that would make it more difficult to get an abortion by closing a bunch of clinics. So I went up and I threw my name in the hat. I was the next one called.

I told the story of my second abortion to the entire audience, live. I even said, "Look, I've had two abortions, and I'm afraid of talking about it. That's not OK." It got really quiet when I was telling my story.

For the second abortion, I went to Planned Parenthood, and they gave me the medication and sent me home. I thought it looked as though I didn't learn anything the first time, that I had made the same exact mistakes, like not remembering to take my birth control. I had also started another medication that I've recently read might interfere with birth control, so that maybe let me off the hook a little.

When I told my abortion story on *The Moth,* that was when I felt like I was coming out of the abortion closet. "I've had two. They've happened. It's done." I got pretty open about talking about it. But still, I kept that second one under wraps for about four or five years. Even after I told the story at *The Moth*, I still was so reluctant to tell my parents. I just felt a lot of shame. Eventually, I put the radio clip on my Facebook page. That's how my parents and my co-workers found out about the second abortion. Up until then, my support team had been just me and my ex-boyfriend. Then, my therapist. And my cat.

I'm a government and economics teacher at a public charter school. In my six years of teaching, one student has found my radio clip on my YouTube. After listening to it, she came to tell me she was really proud that I was her teacher. I melted.

I have never felt judged by other people, not to my face. Except for the protestors outside the Planned Parenthood clinic. There I was publicly judged, but I didn't know them.

I have lost track of a few friends who just kind of distanced themselves from me a bit. I had a lot more people who leaned in and said, “Hey, me too” or, “I’m here for you.”

Looking back to when I shared by abortion story, I remember feeling really free as I was leaving the radio station and getting into my car. Then, when I started mini-panicking about what reactions might be like, I just remembered that whether or not people knew about my abortions, it didn’t change the fact that they happened. That was a point of strength or confidence that I could return to. This is a thing that happened to me. I would like to talk about it. I would like to be in a world where I get to talk about it.

All the time, I run into other women who have experienced the same thing. My ideal society is where women can talk about having an abortion with each other in front of a water cooler, the same way that people like to talk about the tattoo that they got.

Abortion is normal. Let’s make it something so that it’s not shocking when female comedians talk about it. I really wish we could just get over it and just move forward with how this stuff happens. And get rid of the shame and stigma.

As time goes on, my abortion story definitely becomes more humorous to me. Even when I wrote the story the first time, there were many moments in it where the audience laughed, as I intended them to. The audience was like, wait, I’m laughing and it’s about abortion.

The first time I got pregnant, I really considered having a child. Maybe I could be a young mom. That would be cool. I went all the way down that thought rabbit hole. The second time, I didn’t even consider that the family thing was going to happen.

Now that I’ve been a high school teacher for four or five years, I know what it takes to have a child be both emotionally present and healthy. I really enjoy teaching and I don’t think that I would be able to both teach and have my own child. Maybe it’s OK if I don’t have kids because I am still interacting with kids. I’m still able to be nurturing and be a coach and do all the things I would want out of being a parent.

I remember asking my mom how she would feel if I didn’t have children. She was like, “Blair, do what you want.” She almost seemed proud of me. That’s when I was OK, cool. I’m just going to have three cats. Maybe if I change my mind, I will adopt. I can definitely do that, because I’m not going to contribute to the population problem.

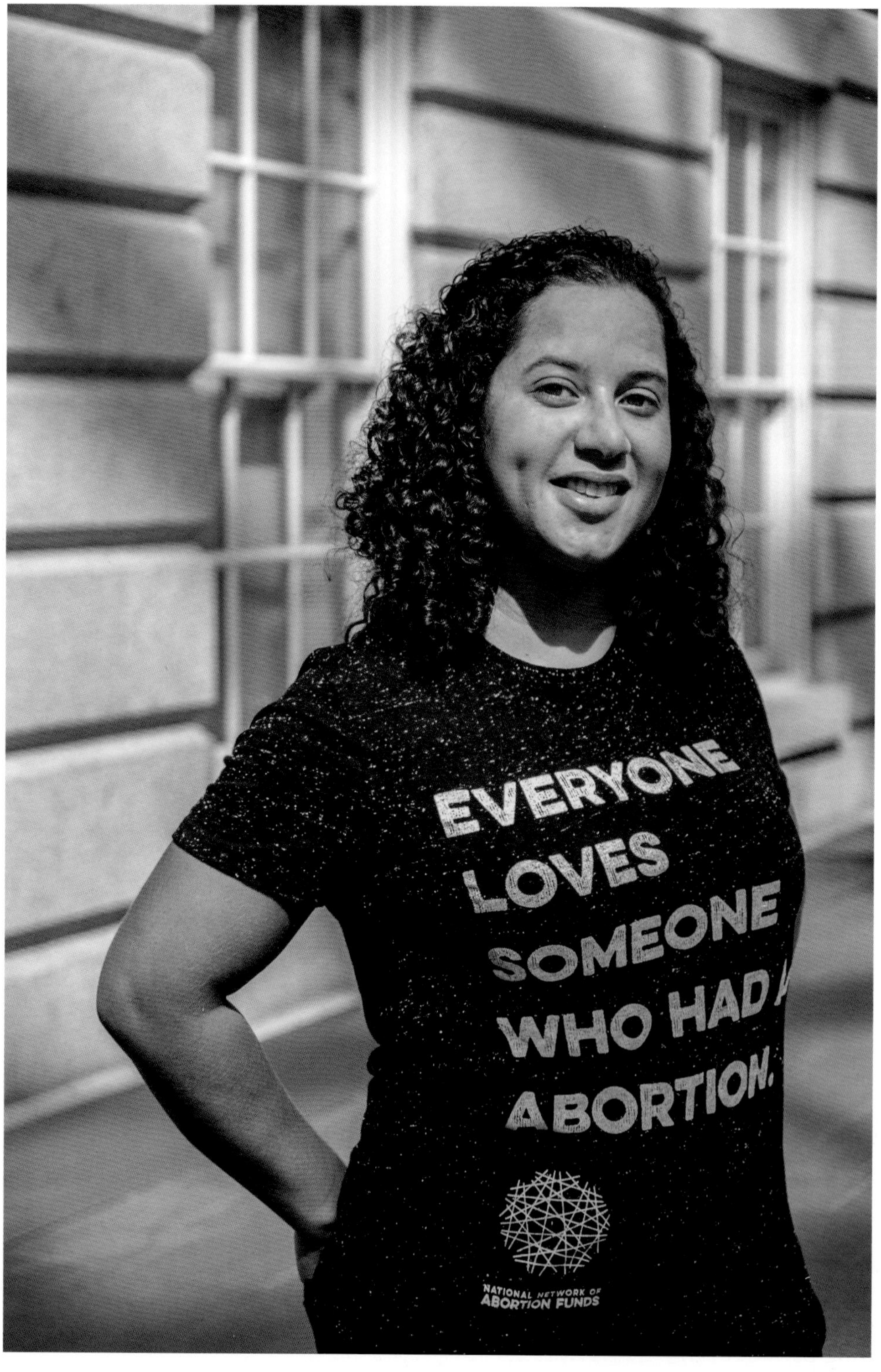

RENEE BRACEY SHERMAN

Renee Bracey Sherman

I WAS 19, living in Chicago at the time of my abortion fifteen years ago. In my public high school, we had sexual education, but it was really stigmatizing and unhelpful. When I took sexual health class freshman year, it was taught by the golf coach, who was super religious and believed in abstinence only.

One day when we were talking about HIV and AIDS, the golf teacher put on all the scrubs that a surgeon would wear, with a face mask and a hair protector. Then he took out a condom and said "A doctor wears all this," gesturing to his scrubs. "Ladies, if he is coming at you only with this condom, he really doesn't care about you. You think only this condom is going to stop HIV?" The way he talked was so stigmatizing of people who have HIV, and it was not accurate. He also created this idea that condoms don't work. They do work if you put them on correctly. His scare tactics are still very ingrained in me. Here we are fifteen years later and it's the one thing I really remember from health class.

We had a health clinic in my high school with nurse practitioners—we could get STD tests and free birth control, only if our parents signed us up. Thankfully, I got on birth control because I could pick it up monthly from the school health center. My parents are nurses. They had talked to me about sex and about abortion being an option.

After I graduated high school, I got the birth control where you take hormones for ninety days and have a week off. It was $40 a month, so every time I picked it up it was $120. I was working part-time at Victoria's Secret, where I was barely making $8 an hour. When I couldn't afford a new supply, I figured waiting a couple of days until I got paid was no big deal. My friends told me that if you have been on the pill a long time, it's harder to get pregnant because it builds up in your system. I learned later that's not how birth control works; you actually get pregnant faster.

I had been dating this guy on and off. My parents hated him. He was bad for me, but I was so deeply in love with him. After a while, I started to feel sick, throwing up a lot. I remember lying on his friend's couch, napping, and one of his friends said, "Dude, hey, she's pregnant." I thought about it and thought, yeah, maybe I am. I went to the store and picked up a pregnancy test.

I told my boyfriend I was pregnant. I knew I wanted an abortion immediately.

When my boyfriend and I talked about it, I remember him saying, "Well, you can just have it and give it to my grandma and she'll raise it." He was OK with an abortion, but absolutely not an adoption. I think adoption is really great but also you have to be willing to continue the pregnancy, and that was not something that I wanted.

THERE'S NO WAY TO DESCRIBE TO SOMEONE HOW UNBEARABLE IT IS TO BE PREGNANT WHEN YOU DON'T WANT TO BE.

I realized I needed to get out of that relationship. I felt like I was drowning. I had to save myself from my own life. I made the appointment to have an abortion. When I called the clinic, I made sure to ask that they actually did abortions because I remembered hearing that there are clinics that say they do but don't.

There's no way to describe to someone how unbearable it is to be pregnant when you don't want to be.

My boyfriend drove me to the clinic. He wouldn't come inside. He said, "I feel like you're killing a piece of us." The clinic had like this thick glass and a security camera. I didn't totally comprehend how much somebody didn't want me to have that care. When the receptionist said, "Oh, do you have insurance?" I pulled out my insurance card. She asked, "Are you the primary holder on the policy?" And I said, "No, my Dad is." She said, "It's going to show up on the explanation of the benefit. That person will know you had an abortion." I took my insurance card back and gave her a credit card. I had been told that this credit card was only to be used for emergencies, like if the car breaks down.

The abortion cost $450 including an extra $100 for sedation. I remember calculating how many hours I would have to work to pay that off. The abortion itself was pretty uneventful. I just remember so much of the kindness of the folks in the abortion clinic, including an Orthodox Jewish nurse who held my hand.

When my boyfriend picked me up from the abortion, I felt something had changed between us. Gradually I stopped seeing him. I started making sure I went to my college classes all of the time and I actually did my homework.

In my college ethics class, I skipped both days that were about abortion. I was clear with the professor that I had had an abortion and I didn't want to sit there and watch people unknowingly call me all sorts of names. When I transferred to Northeastern Illinois University, I took Sociology of HIV and AIDS, where I learned about intersectionality, the idea that there are multiple layers of impression. Like for me, I don't just experience sexism. I experience racism as well and the compounding experience of both things.

When my professor was talking about that and the stigma around sex and health care, and who's able to get access to health care, so much of it clicked for me. These are the things I care about. Then midway through the summer semester this professor disclosed that he was HIV positive. I had never known anyone who was openly HIV positive. When he finished sharing his story, there was a silence in the room. The power in his disclosure moved me. It was just seeing his vulnerability, his honesty.

Finally, six years after the fact, I talked about my abortion. I told my mom. She cried because she hadn't been there to support me. I couldn't keep the secret from her any longer. Now we are completely transparent with each other.

When I finally told my story publicly, I decided to put my name on it. There is only one Renee Bracey Sherman. It definitely crossed my mind what a potential employer might think. But then I decided that if somebody isn't going to hire me because they read on the internet that I had an abortion, that's not a place for me to be working.

Around that time I started volunteering for the local abortion fund, giving people rides to and from their abortion appointments. People needed a place to stay overnight and I invited them to stay at my home. I tried to make my house like a spa so that it was a little bit like a vacation.

That was the point at which I think I started to recognize the deep inequality of who is able to get an abortion, particularly for folks of color. I was aware of the stereotypes, especially on sex and sexuality for women of color, and Black women in particular. The thing is, by being a Black woman, my body and my existence are inherently political. For undocumented people, their existence is political. You can't erase that. That's like erasing a huge part of my story.

For three years, besides telling my own story, I tried to support other people who were sharing their stories. Then I founded We Testify, a leadership program for people who've had abortions.

We Testify specifically works with folks who have experienced financial and logistical barriers to abortion: people of color, queer-identified folks, people with disabilities, folks who live in rural communities with limited access to abortion. We want to make sure that the people speaking about abortion represent the actual demographics of who is having abortions.

The majority of people having abortions are people of color. How can we get more people of color to testify about their abortions?

We want to change the conversation around who is an expert on their own abortion experiences. People who have abortions are often shown as alone, that we're unloved, and that we don't have any family. There are a lot of us, one million people who have abortions every year. And the word "testify," to bear witness, to be an expert in, this is our experience. And we do this all as a collective. We celebrate each other. We're proud of each other.

The majority of people having abortions are people of color. How can we get more people of color to testify about their abortions? . . . What's interesting is reminding people that even if you haven't had an abortion, you know somebody who has, whether you know it or not. Everybody loves someone who had an abortion.

We Testify has supported over sixty folks who are in or have been through the program, who have attended a retreat "abortion summer camp." Here they dig deep about their own experiences. How did race, class, gender, their immigration status, play into their abortion experience? Then over the ten months we find opportunities for them to talk to reporters, share their stories in whatever medium they want to share their stories.

What's interesting is reminding people that even if you haven't had an abortion, you know somebody who has, whether you know it or not. Everybody loves someone who had an abortion. Think about the language that people use to describe us on TV, people saying awful things. They are saying that about someone you love. It's not that abstract.

No matter how you feel about it, let's talk to each other with dignity and respect. The way you vote, the way you talk about it, impacts the people you love.

Hilaria Barajas-Barragan

WHEN I WAS young, I would go to work with my mom every day. She worked as a nanny and a house cleaner for one family in San Mateo. Her working there allowed me to use that address to go to school there. My mom and I did that every single day until she passed away in 2012 during my senior year of high school.

My dad did a traditional machismo type of role, providing for the family, working all day, but not really dealing with the emotional aspect. My mom, as well as my sisters, provided more of that emotional support. My sisters were all older than me, so they were kind of like my mom, but in different ways. They would take me places with them or provide me with things that they knew my parents couldn't afford.

My family is Catholic. We went to church. I did my first communion. I did my baptism. We did all of the church stuff until high school when my mom was sick and then she didn't go as frequently. But she was still very religious. Growing up, there was a lot of emphasis on hard work, a lot of emphasis on modesty—like, don't talk unless you're spoken to—and a lot of Catholic values like waiting until you're married to have sex, or not having boyfriends, and stuff like that. I remember in high school, if I wore even like a V-neck, my mom would think it was promiscuous.

I went to UC Santa Cruz and lived with two of my best friends from high school. I definitely wanted to take full advantage of the freedom that I had. I started drinking. I tried drugs. I just wanted to do everything at once.

I studied psychology and tried to do history of consciousness as a minor, but I didn't get to finish the minor. That was when I had my abortion. It was my last

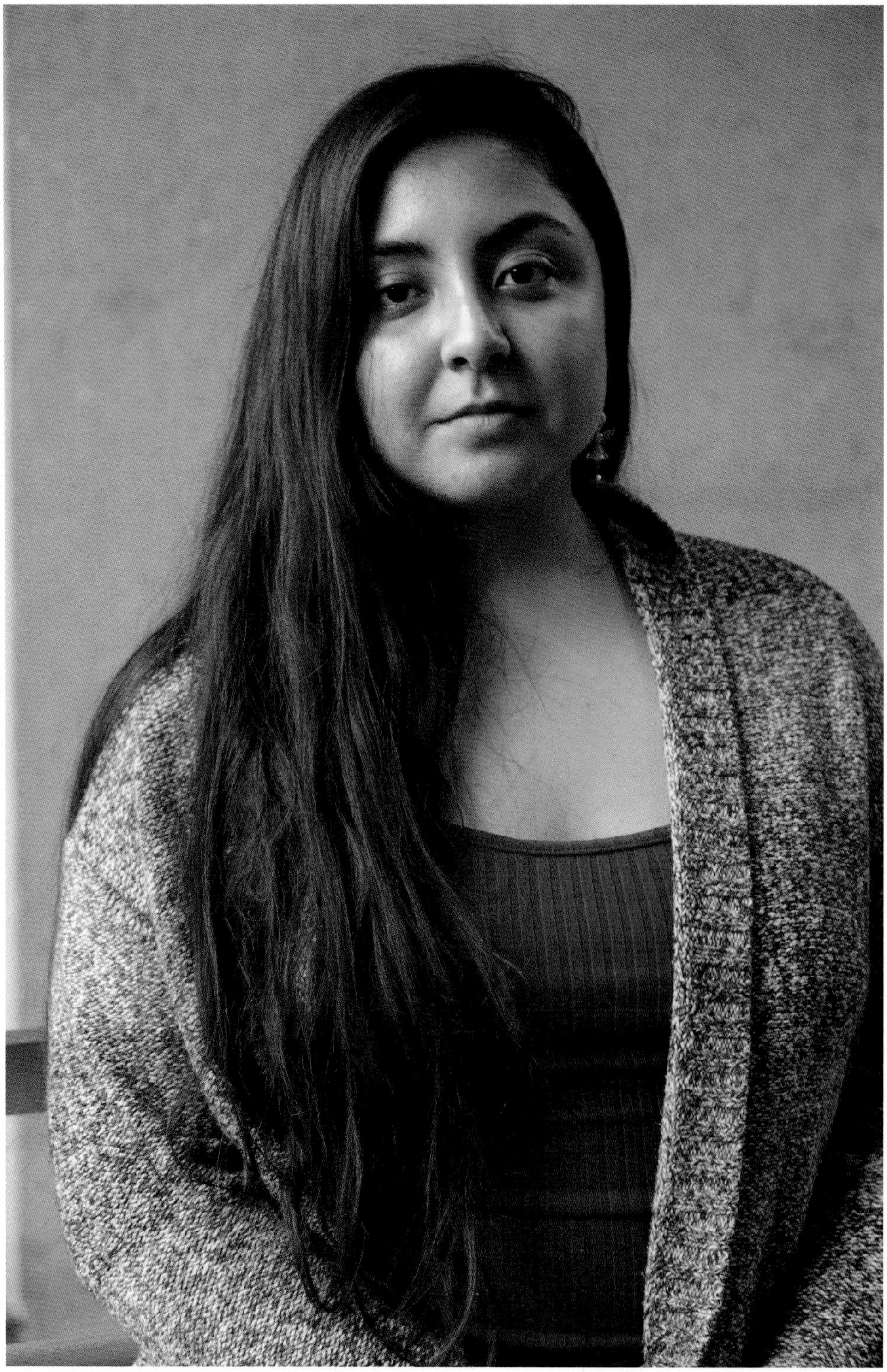

HILARIA BARAJAS-BARRAGAN

quarter at college and I was applying for graduate school. It was just a really stressful time.

My boyfriend and I had sex. I was having a lot of morning sickness and nausea, so I went to get a pregnancy test. I was super surprised that it came out positive, so I took two other tests that were positive. Then I went to the student health center on campus and did a pee test to confirm that I was pregnant.

I told my boyfriend, "I'm pregnant, but I'm not going to have the baby. I'm going to have an abortion. I'm just letting you know." He was like, "Whoa. This is a lot!" But he was really onboard and really supportive.

I knew that I couldn't afford to have a child and I didn't want one at that time. I still don't know if I really want kids. And so, I went downtown to Planned Parenthood. We set up an appointment for an ultrasound. They asked if I wanted to see the baby. And I was like, "No, I don't want to see it." They might have said fetus, I really don't remember, but they did a really crappy job of hiding the picture. At the end, when I was paying for my ultrasound, they had the picture of the ultrasound right there, so I saw it.

I went to Planned Parenthood Monterey for the abortion because they didn't offer the surgical procedure in Santa Cruz. I was, I think, seven weeks pregnant and had to wait two weeks for my appointment. My boyfriend drove me to the appointment and he paid for the procedure because the insurance I had through the university didn't cover abortion. He was really awesome to have there.

WHILE WAITING FOR MY PROCEDURE, IT WAS MY BIRTHDAY. I JUST FELT VERY LONELY. I THINK I WAS ATTACHING MY PREGNANCY TO MY MOM WHO HAD DIED FOUR YEARS EARLIER. IF SHE HAD BEEN ALIVE, I DON'T THINK I WOULD HAVE TOLD HER ABOUT MY ABORTION.

Around the time of my abortion, I had quite depressive episodes. I think that was a reflection of how I was feeling even before I found out I was pregnant. It was just intensified by the pregnancy. I was feeling really, really sad. Then, while waiting for my procedure, it was my birthday. I just felt very lonely. I think I was attaching my pregnancy to my mom who had died four years earlier.

If she had been alive, I don't think I would have told her about my abortion. Now that I am comfortable hearing other people's stories and talking about my own story, it might have been different. I know she went through a lot of her own pregnancy trauma when she had a baby boy who died when he was two weeks old. I later found out that she had several miscarriages. I just think now, knowing all that information, I would talk to her.

I told one friend I was pregnant and then she told me about her abortion story too. That was really important to me. It made me feel a lot less alone. I didn't tell any of my sisters until later, just because of the rhetoric of, "You're killing a baby." I was scared that they would put shame on me. But when I did tell three of my sisters, two of them told me that they also had had an abortion and that they went alone and they didn't tell anybody. They have told me how powerful they think the work is that I do now, and they're really proud.

My work is being an afterschool teacher for an elementary school in Oakland. I'm also an intern at Access Women's Health Justice, doing advocacy work and movement building. It's been a lot of fun. I'm waiting to start grad school soon to become a teacher full-time.

I'm a part of Youth Testify, a cohort of young people under the age of 24, who have had abortions and who would like to tell their stories. The training is awesome. We learned about practicing and shaping our stories, working together to find which parts we really want to share in our story, parts that we'll never share and will keep to ourselves, and parts that maybe we won't share now, but we're interested in sharing later. Part of the training was really gentle because it was like, "You don't have to tell your story if you don't want to, but these are tools to help you tell your story."

I have a few early memories related to abortion. One was driving down with my mom to Planned Parenthood in San Mateo and they had protesters outside who were carrying pictures of dismembered fetuses. I was just like, "what the heck is that?" And I don't even remember the answer that my mom gave me, to be honest. I just remember those vivid images.

My other memory is when one of my sisters found out she was pregnant. I was in elementary or middle school. She showed me all these pictures of the same thing, like fetuses. And now knowing what I know, I think she might have gone to a Crisis Pregnancy Center, a fake clinic, where they try to talk you out of having an abortion. My sister had her baby that time. So my thoughts about abortion were shaped by those intense images.

Sharing my story has made me feel a lot less alone. Also, it makes me feel like abortion is so normal. Something that I'm challenging myself more with this year is opening up about my abortion to more family members. I'm worried that some of them will have more negative views.

You know, there's so much anti-abortion rhetoric, and silence is not doing anything to stop that.

Heather Booth

I HAD THE great good fortune to be born into a very loving family with wonderful values. My folks believed everyone should be treated with dignity and respect, and that we had an obligation to make this a better world. I think my family helped shape who I was so that I wanted to stand up.

The history, the traditions, the values, the texts of Judaism all informed the moral view I have of the world. It was also the tradition coming out of World War II and the Holocaust. We stand up to fascism. We stand up to injustice.

In 1964, I went to Mississippi for the Freedom Summer Project. The project was designed because poor Black people in Mississippi were living in a state of terror. My mother was so frightened. In many ways, I've been scared about almost everything I ever do. I have all the insecurities that most people have, maybe even more than most: Do I know enough? Will I be good enough? Will I get in the way? Will I know what to do? I was frightened not only for myself, but for the families that I lived with. Would they be jeopardized?

My Mississippi summer taught me to trust and value the wisdom of local people who know what they want. They need to make their decisions. It also told me that sometimes there's unjust authority and you need to stand up to unjust laws and challenge them even at the risk of your own personal sacrifice. In general, in my life, imperfectly, I try to do the right thing.

I now look back and I think I was ready for the '60s and the '60s hadn't happened quite yet. I went to the University of Chicago in 1963. There, I moved quickly into activity

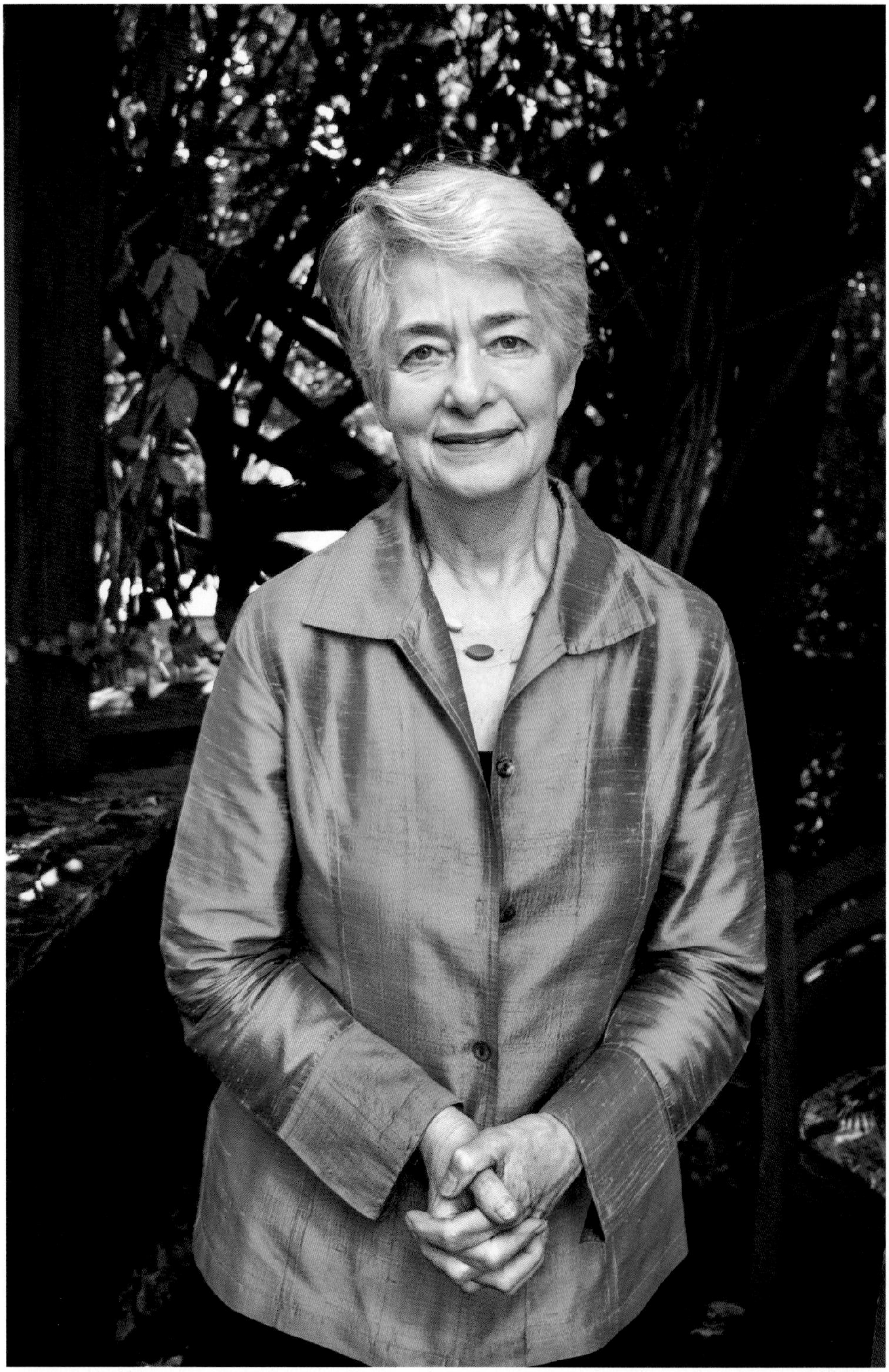

HEATHER BOOTH

with the Student Non-violent Coordinating Committee (SNCC) and became active in the Citywide Council of Community Organization (CCCO).

In 1964, there wasn't really a women's movement acknowledged in the country yet, but women were facing discriminatory practices. One example: A friend of mine was raped at night in her bed in off-campus housing and we went with her to the student health center. She was given a lecture on her promiscuity and told that student health didn't cover gynecological exams.

Against the backdrop of an emerging women's consciousness in 1965, a friend of mine said his sister, a grad student, was pregnant and nearly suicidal. She was not ready to have a baby. She wanted an abortion. I hadn't really thought about the issue. It was a more innocent time and I think I may have been a more innocent person. I'd never had to face the situation.

For my friend's sister, I found a great doctor through the Medical Committee for Human Rights, which was the medical arm of the civil rights movement. His name was Dr. T. R. M. Howard, a civil rights champion who had been a civil rights activist in Mississippi until his name appeared on a Klan death list. He was a Black doctor who set up a clinic on 63rd Street in Chicago called Friendship Clinic. I didn't learn his history until many years later.

I made the connection between the doctor and my friend and the procedure was successful. I didn't really think more about it and I didn't discuss it, but word spread. Then someone else called. And someone else called. I realized I'd better set up a system. I lived in the dormitory and when people phoned up, they were told to ask for "Jane." It was just a nondescript name. This was the beginning of the Jane Service.

I made arrangements with the doctor for how much it would cost. I came to understand what was more involved: How do I counsel the person in advance? What support do we give them? What should they be looking for? If the women had any concerns, would the doctor modify his practice to make sure that the women were well-cared for?

The abortion cost $500—at that time a great deal of money. When the volume increased, I asked if we could have a scholarship fund and we got two procedures for the price of one, and sometimes negotiated the cost. We developed a system and a relationship over a number of years. Then Dr. Howard died. People were still calling, seeking an abortion. Again, I did a search and found another provider, named Mike.

At the start of the Jane Service, all of the women getting abortions were students. Later it spread out to the greater Chicago area, well beyond Hyde Park, and then to other campuses in the Midwest. By around 1970, New York, Colorado, and Hawaii had changed their abortion laws, so if you had money, you could go there for an abortion. As the Jane population started to change, the people coming to Jane were more often poor and didn't have the money to travel to those three states.

By 1968, I had graduated. I had married in '67—I met my husband in the first campus sit-in against the war—and was expecting my first child, working full-time. I was still trying to get a graduate degree. I was very involved in other movement activities and could no longer handle the load of people coming through Jane. That's when I recruited volunteers to run Jane.

At the start of the Jane Service, all of the women getting abortions were students. Later it spread out to the greater Chicago area, well beyond Hyde Park, and then to other campuses in the Midwest . . . the women of Jane performed 11,000 abortions themselves.

After I left Jane, the volunteers set up a much more elaborate system. First of all, they were helping Mike so much that they could see what he was doing. They could learn what he was doing. There were so many women coming through, he couldn't do it alone. Mike taught these volunteers at Jane how to do abortions. Then they found out that Mike wasn't a doctor. When they realized that if Mike's not a doctor and he can do it, it demystified part of the medical profession and they said they can do it. Mike also had confidence that these women could do the procedures. During that time, the women of Jane performed 11,000 abortions themselves. These women would do the abortions in various apartments of people in the Jane Service. There was another apartment where the women would gather in advance for counseling, for intake, for support with each other. They called this place the "Front."

A study done at the University of Illinois showed that Jane had better positive outcomes than those done in the medical establishments once abortion was legal.

In '72, seven women who were involved in Jane were arrested, but no one would testify against them. We knew that the abortion laws were making their way through to the Supreme Court. The case against these seven women wasn't prosecuted and, while the women were awaiting the trial, Roe v. Wade was decided.

I don't know if the people who volunteered at Jane were fearless. I do think they were courageous. They were creative. They were dedicated. I think they felt very concerned about the lives of the women they were supporting, what would happen to them, about the medical outcomes. There were also legal concerns. But I think the fears were more about the lives of the women than for themselves.

I have wanted to stay involved and have stayed involved. The Midwest Academy, which I started in 1973, trains community organizers. We've trained about 15,000 people including people from NAACP, Planned Parenthood, the Sierra Club, and little groups you haven't heard of and all kinds of organizations.

From the Civil Rights and Women's Movement, I was involved in the movement against the war in Vietnam, in union organizing, in electoral organizing. I built an early alliance of labor and community groups on energy policy to overcome the rift between the groups built up in the McCarthy era. Later, I co-directed a large national network of statewide coalitions working on an array of consumer issues. I worked at the Democratic National Committee, first setting up a field structure, then doing outreach for the health-care campaign, and finally acting as their training director.

In 2000 the NAACP hired me to direct their advocacy arm, the NAACP National Voter Fund, a massive get-out-the-vote operation. I was strategic advisor on immigration reform efforts and I ran the campaign that passed the first Obama Budget. I directed the AFL-CIO's health-care campaign to pass the Affordable Care Act. I've done international work and ran a coalition to restore social justice to the heart of the Jewish community. I directed the campaign for Financial Reform that won the Dodd-Frank bill and created the Consumer Financial Protection Bureau. I coordinated the campaign for marriage equality around the Supreme Court decision. And I was also active on many other campaigns: tax fairness, Social Security, prescription drug prices, and more.

WHAT IT TAKES TO BE AN ORGANIZER IS YOU HAVE TO LOVE PEOPLE AND HATE INJUSTICE.

Everything I do keeps to the key lessons I learned early. If we organize we can change the world, but only if we organize. What it takes to be an organizer is you have to love people and hate injustice. Anyone can do this. The people who make change are ordinary people who do extraordinary things, not because they're more courageous, not because they're not frightened or not unsure about what's going to happen, but because they decide the goal is worth the effort.

They find the joy in standing together or sitting down together with others. They feel the inspiration of people finding their own voice, of gaining confidence. They can see that change starts to happen when we join together.

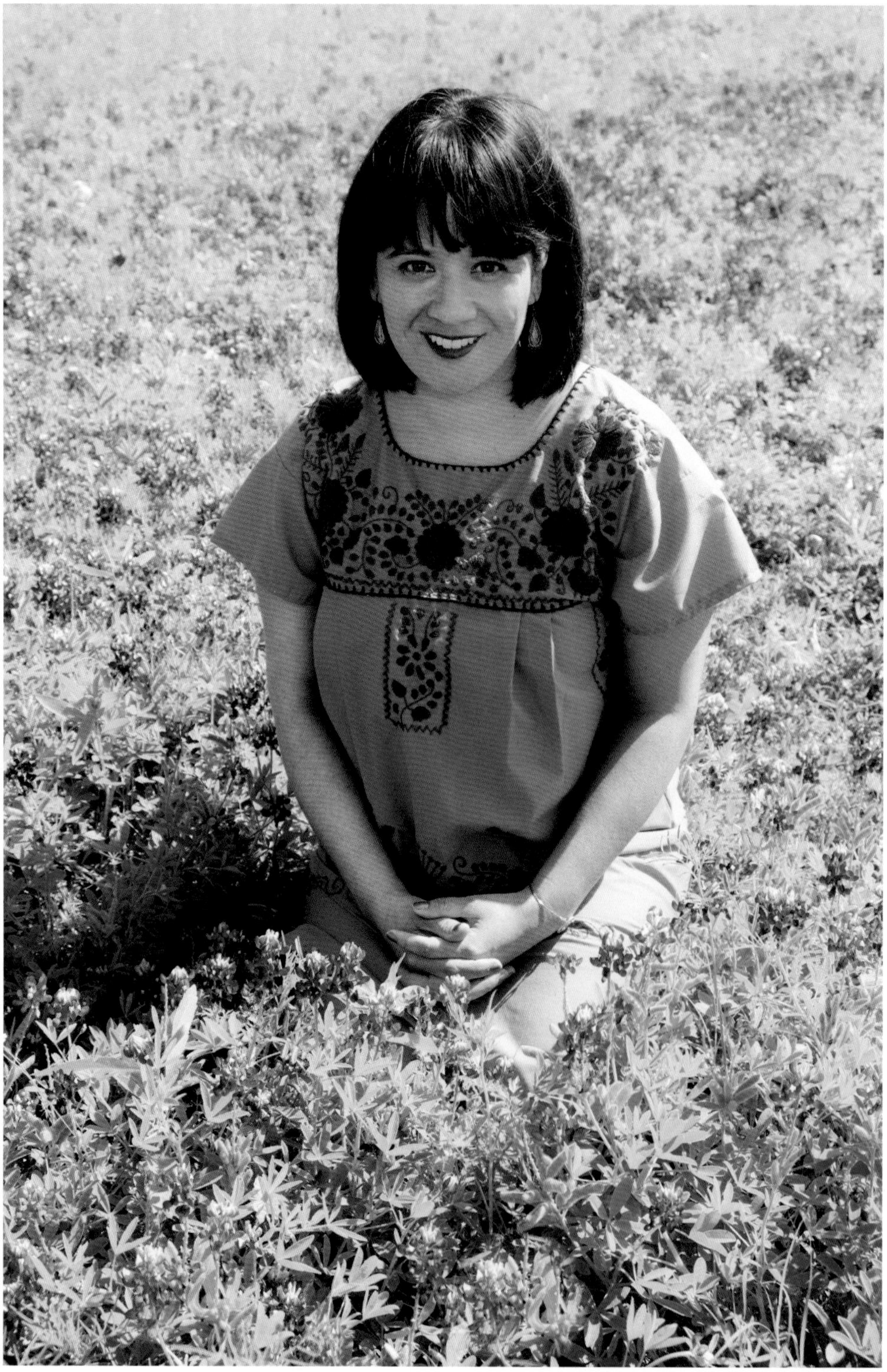

AIMEE ARRAMBIDE

Aimee Arrambide

MY MOTHER CAME from the Philippines. She was the first generation to come here, and she brought her whole family over eventually. She became a psychiatrist. My mother is one of the most independent, strong women I have ever met. My father was raised by a single mother from Mexico. He became an OBGYN.

When I was very young, probably in fifth grade, someone came up to me to tell me that my dad killed babies for a living. I said, "No, he delivers babies." I went home and asked him about what I had heard. My parents explained to me that people sometimes aren't ready to be parents. Depending upon their situation, abortion is an option that they have. I'm not sure I grasped abortion completely, but I had more empathy toward it. For better or for worse, my dad always wanted to teach me things, even if I was a little young for the lesson. And I appreciate that.

Then my dad took me to Laredo. He would fly once every other week to Laredo to do abortions and on alternative weeks he would fly to Corpus Christi to do abortions. The clinic in Laredo was in a very impoverished section of town, with the waiting room filled with people. Many people really needed this service. It just dawned on me that some of these people probably didn't have the means to raise a baby

It always seemed a little strange to me that I work in reproductive rights, that I believe in the right to abortion, that I'm unapologetically an advocate, but I would never talk about my own abortion.

What got me started on sharing my abortion story in public was when I attended the hearings in the Texas Senate in 2013. They were in the process of passing laws to restrict access to abortions. At the hearings, a woman spoke about how her mental health depended on her access to abortion. She went on to say if she were to get pregnant, she wouldn't be able to take her medication that keeps her mentally healthy.

It was the first time I'd ever heard mental health mentioned, not as the misconception that abortion causes mental illness, but rather she was saying having an abortion would allow her to stay mentally healthy. I thought, "Wow, she said this in front of a bunch of people." I was so in awe of this woman who could share that detail. So, I spent the next three years trying to gain the courage to talk about it too. I have been able to do so.

I went to a conference a couple years ago where there was a panel discussion about telling your abortion story. It was the first time I've ever been in a space where it felt safe to talk about your abortion story. There was a room full of people that had abortions. After working in this movement for quite some time, I had never told my abortion story. I guess I had never really felt safe.

THERE ARE A LOT OF FALSE NARRATIVES ABOUT ABORTION CAUSING DEPRESSION OR CAUSING MENTAL ILLNESS. WE KNOW THAT'S NOT TRUE. IN FACT, MY ABORTION HELPED ME DEAL WITH MY MENTAL HEALTH ISSUES. . . .

Then I went to D.C. and told my story on a video for the first time. It was a great experience, because I felt very supported. After that, we went to Capitol Hill to lobby Congress and shared our stories. It was very empowering.

I had kind of been cycling from high school through age 25 with these very manic and depressive phases. In high school, I had honors, I had scholarships to college, I was always on a pretty good track. At college I would take twenty-one hours of classes, have a full-time job, do internships. I would excel. But then the next semester, I would crash. I wouldn't leave my bedroom. I would spend four months in a deep depression where I didn't want to talk to anybody. Then once I hit adulthood, it was just a roller coaster.

When I found out I was pregnant, it wasn't a question of whether I was going to have an abortion. It was an absolute yes, I was going to have an abortion because I could not take care of myself. I was in no way, shape, or form able to take care of anyone else.

I had the support of my boyfriend, who is now my husband. My mother and father also supported me.

I obtained my abortion and I never looked back about the decision. Had I not had an abortion, I believe I would have hit rock bottom because there's only so much a person can handle. I was barely hanging on. Afterwards, I was able to step up and take care of my dad when he was diagnosed with a brain tumor. I was able to get better because I knew that this was something I had to do. I wanted to get better.

After I was diagnosed with bipolar disorder and treated, I've been healthy ever since. I graduated college after nine years. I married my boyfriend, whom I was dating at the time of my abortion. I moved to New York, enrolled in law school, had two children while I was in law school, and I've been able to lead a very happy life, one that I was able to dictate and choose. I like to credit my abortion with giving me the opportunity to heal myself, to find myself, and to choose the person I was going to become and the parent I am now.

I LIKE TO CREDIT MY ABORTION WITH GIVING ME THE OPPORTUNITY TO HEAL MYSELF, TO FIND MYSELF, AND TO CHOOSE THE PERSON I WAS GOING TO BECOME AND THE PARENT I AM NOW.

My abortion story was very important for me to tell because there are a lot of false narratives about abortion causing depression or causing mental illness. We know that's not true. In fact, my abortion helped me deal with my mental health issues and, because of it, I've been able to flourish and dictate my life.

There is stigma around mental illness and stigma around abortion. The first is a stigma about how you're less capable of doing things. The second is more of a moralistic stigma. Both are pretty bad. And sometimes it's a matter of self-stigmatizing.

It was stigma around mental health, not stigma around abortion, that prevented me from telling my story. I was afraid people would take me less seriously if they knew I was bipolar or on medication. My storytelling is about trying to change the narrative, trying to de-stigmatize both abortion and mental health issues. While they're connected, they're still a little separate.

I work in reproductive rights. I'm a policy person. I'm also on the board of an abortion fund. My day job is working for an organization called the Public Leadership Institute. I am the reproductive rights program manager and policy specialist.

Even working in this movement can result in stigma. When I bought my home, the woman who sold us our home promised extra money so we could repaint and fix the stuff identified in the inspection that needed work. Then she changed her mind about the money. When I talked to my realtor, who was friends with the seller's realtor, she told me it was because of what I do for a living. In the end, the buyer sold us the house but she didn't give us the money to make the repairs.

When I turned 40 recently, a switch went off that said, "I'm going to be unapologetically who I am because you can't take anything away from me even if you know I'm bipolar. Everything I've accomplished I've accomplished myself. The people that love me, love me regardless."

That's one of the lessons from the LGBTQ movement: By telling their stories, most people realized that they probably love someone who's an LGBTQ person. The same thing can be said about the one in four people you love who has had an abortion. If you loved me before you found out, you should still love me afterwards.

I recently wrote an op-ed talking about my mental health and abortion, prompted by an Indiana law that requires physicians to report any sort of physical or mental health complication associated with an abortion. It upsets me that, despite the lack of evidence of any causal effect between abortion and mental health, legislators are trying to get people to think that there's a correlation. That infuriates me, especially because every study that's ever been done shows that abortion does not cause mental health issues. It's a disservice to mental health and to abortion.

That's the impetus for me to be more vocal about my own story. I'm privileged enough to not feel threatened to talk about it. I feel like it's my duty to tell my story. I keep going because I don't want to live in a world where people don't have the rights that they should have. I'm inspired by those who are brave and young and fight for it.

Gertrude Bush

YOU SHOULD NEVER force anyone to have a kid that they don't want to have. People say, "Well, put your baby up for adoption." And I'm like, "I've been in that system." When I was five or six, I was a real skinny little girl, just like my daughter is now, and Family Services felt like my mom wasn't feeding me or she was starving me. It wasn't the case. I was just skinny, active. They snatched me out of home and put me in foster care. I think it was just a year, but I bounced between at least three or four families within that one year.

My abortion story began in 2009 while I was in high school. I was on birth control, having protected sex. I had gone for my normal three months STD testing and no pregnancy test popped up. But then one night, I threw up all over the place. They rushed me to the hospital where they told me I was almost seven months pregnant.

They pretty much told me that with all the partying I did in my last year of high school—drugs and alcohol—that the baby wouldn't survive. So, I took the initiative to stop the pregnancy. If I had continued with the pregnancy knowing the baby would not live, I'd be heartbroken.

My partner just told me whatever I decided, he would stand by me. I told him I didn't want to have this child. So, if I had kept the baby, he said he would be there. If I decided to have the abortion, he would be there. He asked me what I wanted to do and I told him I didn't want to have this child. He actually looked up all my options for me.

I went to the Preterm Clinic in Cleveland. They didn't make feel that I was a bad person by choosing myself. They walked me through the process. They dumbed everything

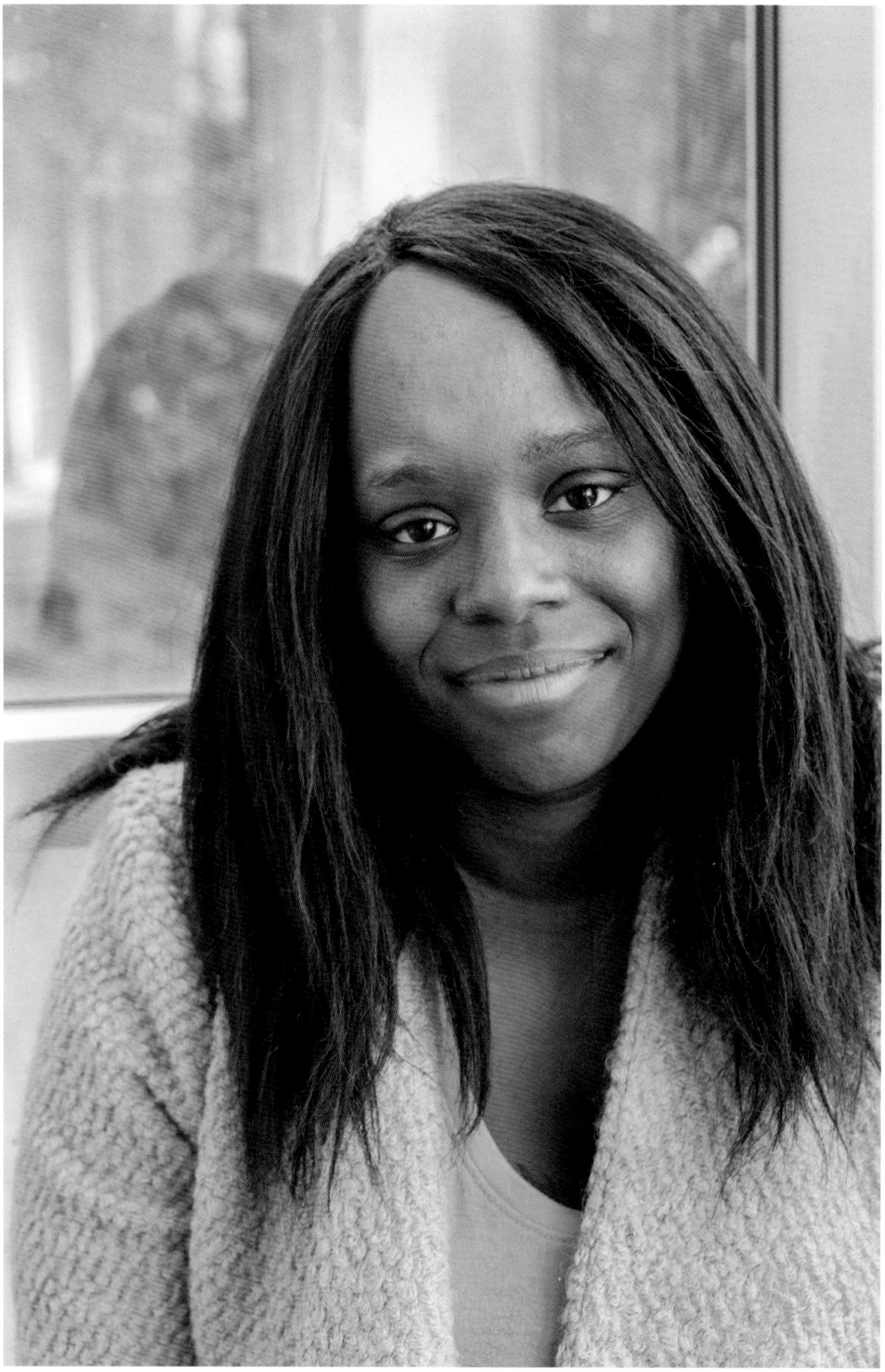

GERTRUDE BUSH

down so I could understand it. They made me feel so comfortable and didn't make me feel like I was exiled. The staff was friendly, everyone kept smiles on their faces. It didn't have that awkward feeling like you're going to kill yourself or that you're this horrible person just because you walked through the door. They understand that people make life decisions and some people know that they're not ready to have more children.

Preterm has a program to help you pay, but you have to come up with an initial $115. Between my partner and me, we had the $115. But if it wasn't for that program, I'd be stuck.

When I had the abortion, it was a delivery. I had the baby. My first visit, they gave me an ultrasound, asked me if I wanted to hear the baby's heartbeat and all that. On my second visit, they gave me a shot in my stomach to stop the baby's heartbeat and then they sent me home. The plan had been for me to come back to the clinic before I had the baby, but while I was at home, after a couple of hours, I pushed the baby out. I believe it was a boy. My boyfriend helped me. He put the baby in a bag, took me and the baby up to the clinic and gave them the bag.

The clinic took care of me, checked me out, made sure I wasn't catching an infection or anything like that. I was perfectly fine. It took me a while to get over it because delivering at home kind of freaked me out.

My abortion was a step in my life. Would I change it? No. But at the time I felt like it was a big shame. I was the token kid to my family. I was the one doing all the sports in school, I had good grades, all my cousins looked up to me. My mom and my grandma had high expectations of me. I felt like telling them about my abortion would be the biggest downfall; they would look down on me. So I never talked to anyone about it. Outside of the guy that I had got pregnant by, no one else knew. I didn't feel comfortable talking to others.

I've realized since I had the abortion that a lot of people in my family had abortions. When my favorite aunty died, me and my mom were just laughing and joking one night, reminiscing, and she's like, "Yeah, your grandmother would've had about twelve kids by now. She's only got six." I said, "What?" She's like, "Yeah. Your grandma had a couple abortions. One of them was a life-or-death situation and then the other ones, she was just like, "I'm not ready yet." When she finally decided to have kids, she had six.

Five or so years after my abortion, my mother died. I got meningitis, and was in the hospital for a while. I was in this depression state. I felt alone. My mom wasn't around. I found out I was pregnant again. I dreamt that it was a girl and it looked just like my mom.

This time everything just came back to life. I felt like that was my mom letting me know that she was not leaving me.

When my daughter was born, I was ready to have a child. I'm raising my beautiful three-year-old daughter by myself. I'm working as a field marketer, which means I go door to door and get people to sign up for quotes for windows, sliding doors, roofs, like that. And I'm going to school for massage therapy. I also have my brother here and some cousins and one aunty. My mom is no longer living, my grandparents no longer living. Very simple life.

FIVE OR SO YEARS AFTER THE ABORTION, MY MOTHER DIED . . . I FOUND OUT I WAS PREGNANT AGAIN. I DREAMT THAT IT WAS A GIRL AND IT LOOKED JUST LIKE MY MOM. THIS TIME EVERYTHING JUST CAME BACK TO LIFE . . . WHEN MY DAUGHTER WAS BORN, I WAS READY TO HAVE A CHILD.

My mom was a goofball, my daughter's a goofball. Honestly, I couldn't imagine having two kids right now, especially the way the world is turning. I'm glad I only have one right now because she's a handful. When I'm at home with her, I spend time teaching her ABCs or her numbers or colors, anything I can think of to make sure she knows stuff. After that, I let her run wild and free in the house, which is really bad, let me tell you.

For my daughter I want a world where she's free to do as she pleases with her body as long as it doesn't harm her. Let her be as educated as she wants, experiment life as much as she wants. She can say yes or no to something.

I want people reading my story to know that you're not alone. There's definitely other people out there who have had abortions and just because it's not talked about, doesn't mean it hasn't happened to someone you know. A lot of times, it's the ones closest to you that have been through the same situation or the same struggle and they just felt like they didn't have anyone to talk to about it. So, stay comfortable, and be yourself in your skin. Don't let your decision of whether or not to have an abortion change who you are.

I believe that you should keep talking about your abortion. Just have no worry or doubt when you have the conversation. Be as confident as you are in yourself, as you are in this conversation. Talking about your abortion should be just as normal as having a conversation about what are we eating for lunch. Just like sex. You see it everywhere but no one talks about it. Just like an abortion clinic. You will walk past it, you see it, but no one talks to you about it and all you hear is the negative. You need to hear more of the positive and to let people know that it's not as bad as you think it is.

Samantha Gladu

I GREW UP in Colorado with my mom's side of my family. I was with my grandparents from before I have memory to my late teenage years. My grandma had something like eleven or thirteen pregnancies and seven kids. My mom was the only daughter. My grandparents were super-involved in their local Catholic parish. Sometimes my grandma wore gold baby feet on her lapel or had a magnet on the fridge with infant pictures who weren't infants in our family and quotes that I had no frame of reference for. I recognized later, after I'd had an abortion, that those were anti-choice materials. I didn't think about it when I was growing up though.

My uncles and mom were into music, especially contemporary punk stuff, also Billy Idol, Blondie, David Bowie. My mom was a fierce feminist. She wanted people, and women in particular, to feel like we could do whatever. She was a musician, a singer in a punk band. She had a European tour booked at the time that she found out she was pregnant with me.

My mom stopped playing when I was in third grade and her band broke up. She was trying to get her life together for a lot of my early years. I moved in with her during middle school and the beginning of high school. When her relationship blew up, we moved back in with my grandparents.

High school felt like a weird world. Going to a very wealthy high school where kids would get $20 for lunch and drive fancy cars was surreal. I didn't have much in common with them, and I was looking for a way out of my family's house, trying to be on my own.

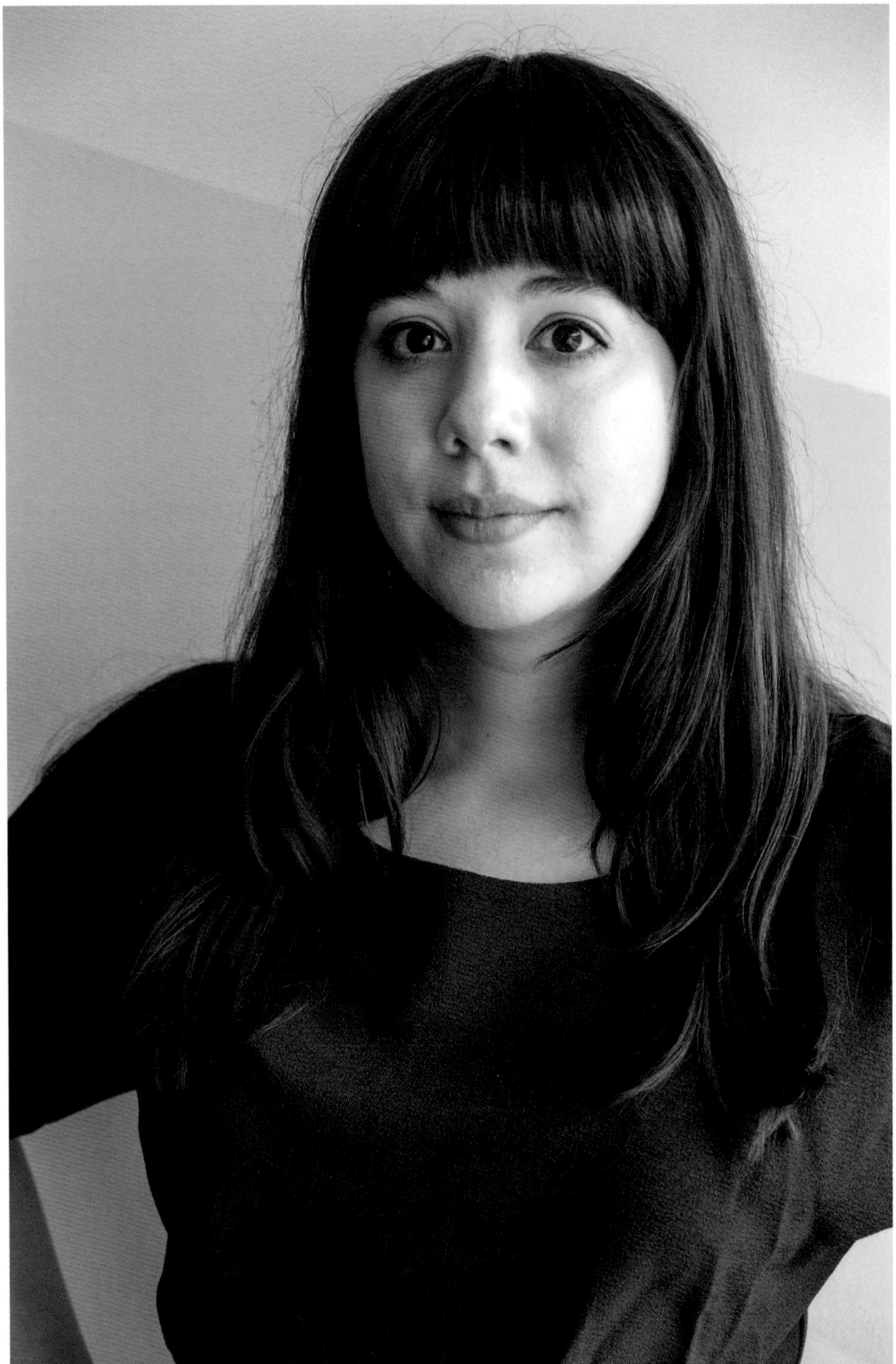

SAMANTHA GLADU

From age 15 to 17, I was officially living with my grandma, but I stayed with my boyfriend most of the time. He was six years older than me. When I was with him, I kind of felt like I was on my own and had independence. There were so many people in my family household that it was really easy for me to slip through everybody's attention.

I found out I was pregnant three months before my 18th birthday. I had my first-ever job, at a party store, and I felt really sick at work. I was puking. On a sleepover with some of my friends I took a pregnancy test. I found out I was pregnant while Kanye West's hit song *Gold Digger* was blasting.

It felt like an exciting moment because no one in my friend circle had dealt with a pregnancy. We weren't sure what the next step was. At first, because of my lack of understanding about my options, I was like, "Oh, I'm having a kid." But my mom had been 19 when she had me and it was not my goal to be a young mom.

I tried to tell my partner about it and that is how I realized that he was cheating on me. I decided to tell my mom. Both my mother and my boyfriend made it really clear to me how challenging it would be to have the baby. One thing that my mom said to me that really hit home was, "If you do this, your boyfriend is always going to be part of your life. Do you really want that?" And I did not. That part terrified me and made me want to cut ties and to be able to do so cleanly.

I went with my soon-to-be ex-boyfriend to Planned Parenthood in a neighboring suburb to get a pregnancy test. They explained to me my options: have an abortion, have the kid and put it up for adoption, or have the kid and be a parent. I knew what I wanted to do, and I scheduled an abortion probably within three weeks of finding out that I was pregnant. When it happened I was just under eight weeks pregnant. The issue of money didn't necessarily come up because I think my boyfriend understood that this was a small price for him to pay to not have a kid.

When we got to the clinic for the procedure, I was really frustrated because they told me that before I could be seen they had to have a signature from my mom because I wasn't 18 . . . I was really mad. I am still mad about it, frankly.

When we got to the clinic for the procedure, I was really frustrated because they told me that before I could be seen they had to have a signature from my mom because I wasn't 18. This was just a couple of months away from my 18th birthday. . .I was really mad. I am still mad about it, frankly, and that has inspired me to get into politics and advocacy. My mom had to call out of her job at Home Depot to come sign for her daughter to have an abortion. It was so humiliating to have to get permission.

The days after my abortion I felt really lonely because nobody in my friend group had had that experience, so they didn't even know where to begin in terms of being supportive. Not only did I have an abortion, my boyfriend had been cheating on me. My mom wouldn't really talk to me about it and I didn't tell my grandma because I didn't think it was necessarily her business. I didn't go to school for a few weeks and I almost didn't graduate because I became so sad after everything that had happened. The breakup and the circumstances of the relationship were really hard on me. It was a rough time. My mom and I had big blowout fights.

After high school, I moved to Portland along with a lot of my friends. I started dating someone I had a big crush on and eleven years later we're still together. No kids, no desire to have kids. He had a vasectomy. He's helped me learn and grow a lot from some of the things I experienced when I was younger.

I think about how hard it was for my mom when she had me. I also reflect on what an awesome community leader my grandma was in her world. I wonder what it could have been like if the horizon was more open to her economically and socially.

I decided I wanted to work on abortion rights issues. I volunteered in a few different capacities with several organizations, including being a patient advocate. Now I'm on the board of two organizations.

In my day job I'm the executive director of Next Up, which is an eighteen-year-old nonprofit organization that engages young people in progressive systems change and politics. We seek to amplify the voice and leadership of young people ages 16 to 35, and connect youth with their political power. When I started running this organization and I was doing my first round of one-on-one meetings, I actually led with my abortion story. I share with people that I got into youth activism because I had barriers to abortion access, like my mom having to sign permission for my abortion because I was under 18.

Oregon has the most expansive reproductive health protection law in the country. It makes abortion coverage available regardless of the type of insurance you have, regardless of immigration status and gender. There's no time limit here in Oregon as to when you can have an abortion. We still find, however, that gestation, geography, incarceration, misinformation from fake clinics, and federal health plans limit access to abortion. There is always more work to be done.

I've come to include abortion in every part of my life. I've become such a fan of the organizations that advocate for abortion rights. I also recognize how important it was for me to be able to have an abortion.

I even include my abortion story in my art and my music. Both of my punk bands have songs about abortion. One is called *Papa Don't Preach, Part 2,* about having an abortion rather than keeping the baby. Another is called *Abortion Fund,* from the male perspective of calling an abortion fund for their partner. The message of both songs is that abortion is normal, abortion is fine. When my bands play, people come up afterward and share their stories and say thanks. I also have a few dresses that say "abortion" and one that says "Abortion is a Human Right." I wear them sometimes when I perform.

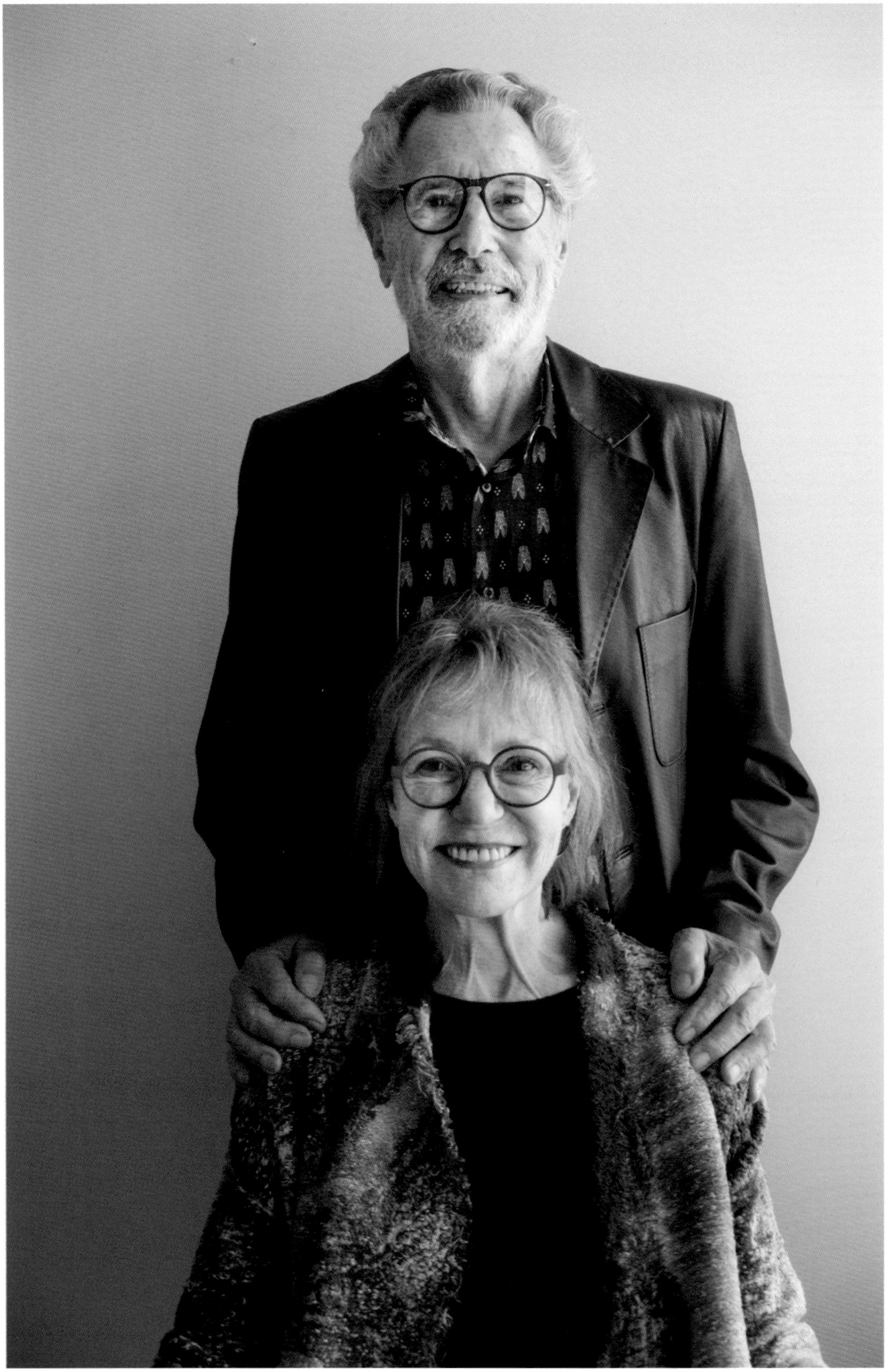

GLENNA HALVORSON BOYD AND
CURTIS BOYD

Glenna Halvorson Boyd and Curtis Boyd

Glenna: Everything I know about abortion counseling I have learned from patients. This all started in Dallas, Texas. I had married my college sweetheart and was in the midst of divorcing him. A friend worked for this doctor who was opening the first freestanding legal abortion facility in Texas. I was hired to train the first batch of legal abortion counselors in the state of Texas.

One day, this peculiar man showed up back in the clinic's surgery area. He was not authorized to be back there, and was making the patient I was with very uncomfortable. I tried to throw him out. That's how Curtis and I met.

Curtis: I was recruited to do abortions by the Clergy Consultation of Problem Pregnancies, a multi-denominational group. I saw patients only referred by them. That's where I was recruited to do abortions.

The model was developed by Harold Moody, a Methodist minister in New York City. He thought we would be some kind of a protocol to guide young women to abortion services when it was still illegal in the '60s. They set up guidelines for conversations with the women: What is your story? How long do you think you've been pregnant? They also checked out the places and people they would be referring the women to.

So, I thought, whatever counseling they're doing is making a big difference. I wanted to carry that forward, but I didn't know how to do good counseling. There were a lot of feminist women coming out of the woodwork then. I thought we could train them to do counseling, but I didn't know how to train them. That's where Glenna came in.

Glenna: In many ways, I'm a very predictable product of a feminist father and a feminist mother. My father was a Norwegian immigrant, and he was a devout atheist since the age of 5, because the Lutheran God of hell, fire, or damnation scared him. My mother was an agnostic. In fact, they were anti-religious.

I was expected to achieve great things. I majored in five or six different things as an undergraduate and got my bachelor's degree in English literature. I later got my doctorate in psychology. In my 50s, I went to nursing school and got my RN.

Curtis: I grew up in a provincial community in central East Texas, Henderson County. My family was part of a foot-washing Baptist church. There were a lot of them in the South, still are some. They were part of the great Pentecostal movement that occurred in the South. I became involved in church early.

But I was more interested in why things were, what life was all about. No one was very good at answering these questions. I had this incredible memory and people thought I was extremely intelligent. If you have a good enough memory, people are going to think you have an extremely high IQ. I also had this unusual sort of fierceness of the Old Testament prophets, to defend the faith. So, even in junior high, I would take on anyone in a religious debate to defend the faith of our Father, of the elders. I was very good at that.

My father wanted me to go West Point or Texas A&M. Well, I didn't want to be a career military officer. But, I could not say no to my father. I honored my father, I was respectful of him.

Eventually the church elders called me to the pulpit. I did preach for a while, but I realized it was not really what I wanted to do. In fact, I had a much more eclectic religious view, a broader one, about this thing called God. One day this sister from the church came up after I had preached. She knew that I had been thinking about going to medical school, and she told me God had called me to a greater purpose. She said, "You can't fulfill that role, and be a doctor too." Well, I knew right then, I'm going to medical school. That was my out! If I go to medical school, then I can't continue this preaching career.

Glenna: I'm an atheist but my beliefs are not what matter in the counseling session. So we explore what the woman's religious beliefs are since they will play into her decision as to whether or not she will have an abortion and how she's likely to feel about it.

What I've come to appreciate is that the majority of our patients do hold religious beliefs. This may in part be because we practice in New Mexico, which is Hispanic, and Catholic largely, and in Texas, which is part of the Bible Belt. If you ask, "Have you talked with your God about this?" many have. Others will say, "I was afraid to." If you give patients an opportunity to talk with their God, to reflect, to talk with you about their beliefs, there's a shift in feeling, in tone that's very powerful.

WHAT I'VE COME TO APPRECIATE IS THAT THE MAJORITY OF OUR PATIENTS DO HOLD RELIGIOUS BELIEFS. . . . IF YOU GIVE PATIENTS AN OPPORTUNITY TO TALK WITH THEIR GOD, TO REFLECT, TO TALK WITH YOU ABOUT THEIR BELIEFS, THERE'S A SHIFT IN FEELING, IN TONE THAT'S VERY POWERFUL.

Curtis: A lot of the women come feeling that abortion is wrong, and women who do have abortions are bad. Liberating them from some of that feeling comes from asking, "What kind of God do you believe in, a loving God, a forgiving God? Do you think you're a bad person? If you do, let's talk about that." You talk about their feelings and the meaning it has for them. You've got to just listen, to let them talk it out. They decide either one way or the other.

Glenna: We do individual counseling. The essential part of it is giving the woman space and time that is hers, where she has your full attention to talk about how she feels about the pregnancy, about ending the pregnancy, and what that means to her, and to the most important relationships in her life. That may be the man by whom she's pregnant, or her parents, or the children she already has.

Back in the '60s, the women went to the ministers at Clergy Consultation for practical information: where to go for a safe abortion and how to get there—which is not counseling. But in listening to the woman's story, the ministers sent an invaluable message: Your life matters. Your plans and hopes and dreams count . . . in my eyes and in God's.

The secret is for the counselors to close their mouths, allow silence, and listen to what the patient has to say. For some of our patients it's the first time that anybody has listened to what's going on inside of them as they navigate this important life decision. For some, it's the first time that anybody has truly listened to them about much of *anything* in their lives.

Curtis: The medical model has traditionally been prescriptive, advice giving. Doctors typically don't make the best therapists or counselors. They talk, they don't listen. Therapists listen, they don't talk.

Abortion is not the problem. The problem is the consequences of the unwanted pregnancy. If a woman can feel that she is looking to what is best for her, the children she has, the children she wishes to have in the future, her extended family, society even, then she is going through a moral decision-making process.

OUR WORK IS NOT PRIMARILY ABOUT ABORTION—AS IMPORTANT AS THAT IS, AND AS SIGNIFICANT IT IS IN OUR LIVES. WE DO IT IN AN EFFORT TO ACHIEVE WOMEN'S RIGHTFUL PLACE IN SOCIETY AS ONE OF RESPECT AND EQUALITY, WHERE A WOMAN HAS AUTONOMY OVER HER OWN BODY.

Women who come to us are behaving as ethical, moral beings. They think seriously about what they're doing. They value the fetus. I value the fetus . . . I can value the fetus, and I can value the needs of the pregnant woman, both at the same time.

We've seen a 13-year-old girl want an abortion. You ask her what she's been thinking about as she's come to her decision and she says, "Well, I'm a child myself. I can't be a good mother." So, you ask her what it means to be a good mother? She replies, "to raise a child that has some opportunity. I want my family to be proud of my child." A 13-year-old can go quickly beyond self. She's going through a moral decision-making process, and she doesn't get credit for it. She mostly gets that she is using abortion as birth control. Well, of course, abortion is birth control, of course she is.

It's unfortunate that women feel such gratitude toward me when I do their abortion. It's an ordinary medical service. You can be grateful for kindness, if you were shown kindness, and had good care, and service. When they say, "Thank you, doctor, you were very kind." And, I say, "You're welcome." That's enough. I'm working for the time that they don't need to feel so grateful for what should be a simply done, readily available medical service.

The issue really is religion, and Glenna's talked about this. This is a religious war on women and on their right to have an abortion. The anti-abortion forces, while they are actually a minority, through their successful political action, have corrupted the political system, legislators, judges, medical community. They are doing everything they can to prevent women from having abortions.

My grandmother was a midwife, and she did abortions. My mother told me long after my grandmother died. My grandmother never knew, in the 1960s, that I was doing them either. If she were still alive, I think we'd have a lot to talk about. I would like very much to talk with her.

Glenna: Over the past few years, we've had to deal with more legal harassment by protestors and by legitimate bodies of the state that have been corrupted by the antis. Those things are really wearing and demoralizing. In terms of the protesters, and the death threats, I learned when I had cancer that I'm basically a fatalist. I can make myself miserable, and worry, and put a lot of energy into that, and let it ruin my life. Or, I cannot. It's a question of where I place my time and energy and attention.

Curtis: This is the life we have chosen. We continue today for the same reasons we've always been doing the work, because it's important, and we can make a contribution.

Glenna: It's all about the place of women.

Curtis: For all of history we've had patriarchy. Now, we're talking about moving toward egalitarianism.

Our work is not primarily about abortion—as important as that is, and as significant as it is in our lives. We do it in an effort to achieve women's rightful place in society as one of respect and equality, where a woman has autonomy over her own body.

Glenna: She has rights, and those rights do not disappear because she's pregnant.

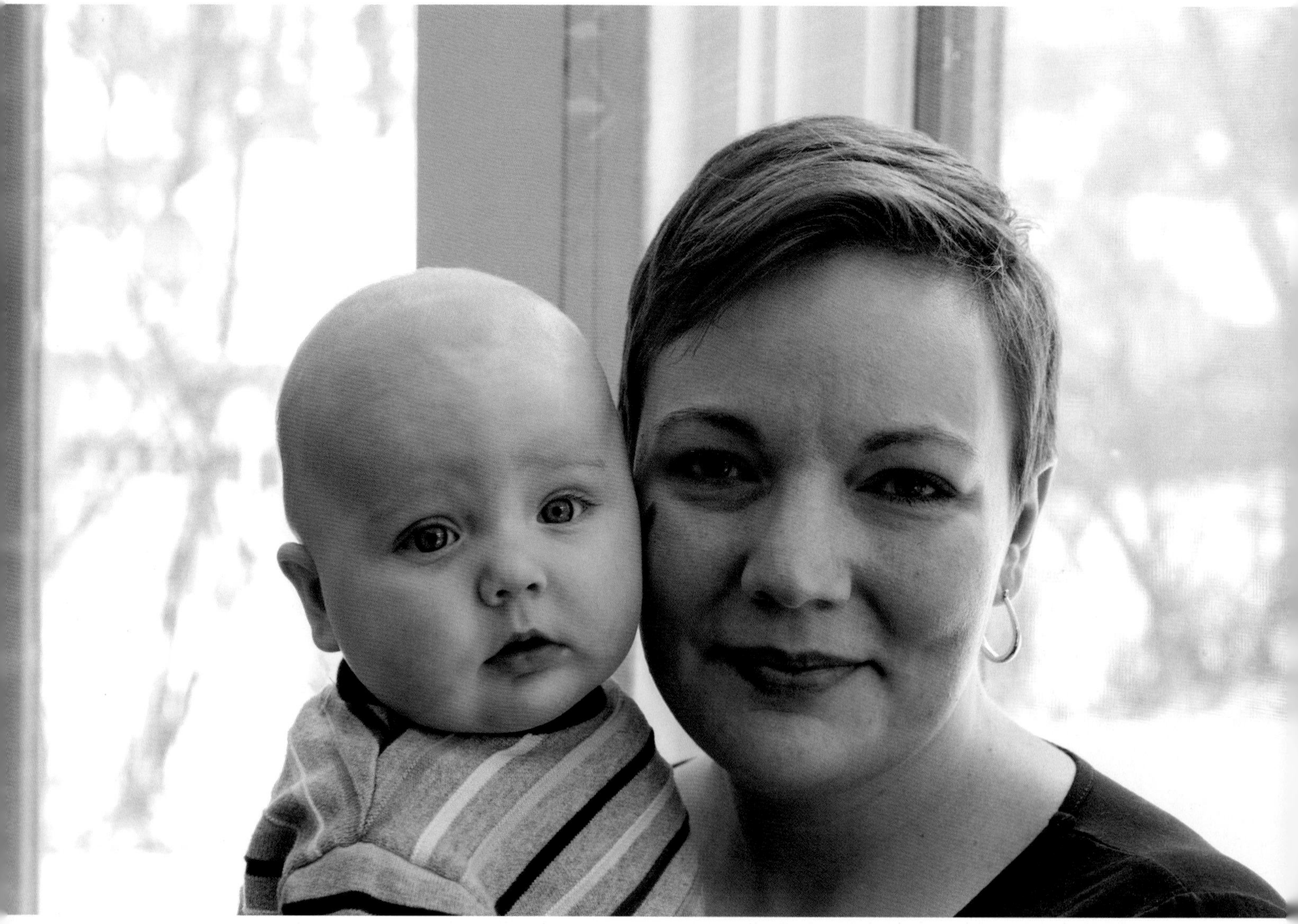

MALLORY McMASTER

Mallory McMaster

MY ABORTION STORY started five years ago, the week before my first wedding. I was crash dieting, like a lot of brides do. I felt so tired and bloated. The day of my wedding, I couldn't zip up my wedding dress because my boobs were too big, and I've never had boobs! I knew something was up, but I assumed it was just stress.

Going into the marriage, I had a lot of doubts. It was an abusive relationship. I wasn't financially secure. I didn't see a way out of it. I went through with it because that seemed like my only option. About a week after my wedding, I was still feeling sick and bloated. I was nauseous. I thought I'd eaten bad Christmas ham, but it turns out I was pregnant. I'd been using hormonal birth control.

I was surprised and disappointed to find myself pregnant. After all, I was a reproductive rights advocate and champion at that point. I remember asking, "How did this happen?"

When I found out I was pregnant, I started thinking about daycare costs. I was working a standard hospital shift, 7:00 a.m.to 3:30 p.m. There were no daycares open early enough for me to drop a baby off. We made too much money for public assistance, but barely enough with our incomes combined to cover rent and student loan payments. Really, though, there was never any doubt in my mind that I would have an abortion. It was the only possible thing for me to do. My husband was supportive of that decision. He was a terrible person; he recognized that and didn't want a child at that time either.

I was really lucky, because I live in Cleveland, where we have one of the best abortion providers in the country. I knew what to do. I didn't have to Google how to get an abortion. I had people I could talk to about it, and I had health insurance that covered abortion, which is something not a lot of people in the country have. I was able to get everything squared away. I chose to have Valium, which was $75. The cost of the abortion would have been $535. I was able to use my flexible spending account to pay for the $75 for Valium. All in all, I didn't have to spend anything out of pocket and that was really nice.

I went to the clinic for the abortion, a surgical D & C. My husband came with me. It was a comfortable, safe experience for both of us. I was nine weeks pregnant when I finally had the abortion. The protesters recognized my car and didn't even bother to yell at me that day. They knew me because I had been working at the clinic escorting patients from their cars to the entrance of the clinic and the NARAL Pro-Choice Ohio office is in the clinic, so I spent a lot of time there.

Although I breezed through it, every time I saw a barrier that would normally trip someone up, I was very aware of the fact that I had so much privilege and I was so unbelievably lucky in my situation not to have those barriers. After the abortion, I hugged the people at the clinic. I went home. For the first time in several weeks I wasn't nauseous. I hate being pregnant. As soon as the abortion was over, my hormone level started to drop and I felt hungry for the first time.

Afterwards I went on with my life. My marriage fell apart. It continued to be abusive, violent, and completely unhealthy. About a year later, we were able to get divorced. I didn't think about my abortion that much. I was grateful for it, obviously. I knew what a monumental decision that was to protect my future.

I started dating my current husband and things just kept getting better from there. I went back to school for my degree in nonprofit administration, and I love my work. We bought this great house and have a wonderful child. I knew every step of the way that it wouldn't have been possible if I hadn't had that abortion. I was grateful and appreciative of the decision I'd made at the time, but I had no idea how it would continue to affect me throughout my life.

My husband and I are from the same small village of three hundred in rural southern Ohio. It's considered Appalachia and it's so impoverished, underfunded, and in crisis that when I went to Ohio State University, I got a special minority tutor, because of where I lived. But a lot of the values my husband and I grew up with, like taking care of the people in your community, led us to work as activists and compassionate citizens today. Now I write about abortion and do consultant work in a bunch of different areas. One of my projects is working with our local county Board of Health on their teen sex-ed program. I write content, help with the website, do their social media about sexual health.

I'm aware that abortion is a very deeply personal and inflammatory issue for a lot of people. I also welcome that and seek out opportunities to challenge people's convictions on abortion, because I feel if they realize their neighbor has had an abortion they're not going to listen to what the politicians are saying. They are going to think about their neighbor, the actual people involved.

I really appreciate it when I can help people think about abortion in a different perspective. My own mother, for example, wasn't very comfortable with abortion when I started doing this work. When she learned about my abortion story, she asked how far along I had been. I told her I had been nine weeks along and it wasn't really a big deal and how much it changed my life. She was very supportive that I'd made that decision, because she could see what it did for me.

I firmly believe that I'm never going to change people's opinion if they are anti-abortion, but there are still people in that gray area where they're uncomfortable with abortion because they don't know a lot about it. But they're willing to think about the people. That's when you can change their hearts and their minds.

Had I not had an abortion, I would never have been able to finish school and get a job. I never would have been able to completely remove myself from my abusive marriage, because we would have had a child together.

When I think about my abortion, I realize it let me build my life the way I wanted it: Supported by a partner who I wanted to spend the rest of my life with and wanted to have a child with. My son is 5½ months now, still not sleeping for more than two or three hours at a time. Wonderful child in every other regard, but it's frustrating at 3:00 in the morning when I just put him down twenty minutes ago and I'm up again. Knowing that I wanted this and this is something I chose makes it a little easier to get through those really hard times.

I have enough money to pay for full-time daycare. We can buy any gadget or swing that might give us a twenty-minute break here and there. I have a supportive family and community, and a house where I can store all of the stuff. I'm realizing that had I not had an abortion, I would never have been able to finish school and get a job. I never would have been able to completely remove myself from my abusive marriage, because we would have had a child together. That would have continued to put me and any future children at risk. It would have damaged my career.

As an abortion storyteller, every time I share my story, someone shares theirs back with me. Wherever I am, in print or speaking at an event, someone pulls me aside to share their story. For a lot of them, it's the very first time they've done that. They're not all positive like mine. Some people regret their abortion or the circumstances of their abortion. Some people feel deep shame and stigma. But they all need to talk to someone about it, to feel connected.

I think the statistic is that one in four women will have had an abortion by age 45. That means one in four women are not talking about their abortion, because stigma keeps them quiet. Whatever their story, we need to give people a space to talk about their experiences so we can bust through the stigma.

Shalitha Mitchell

I'M A REALLY fertile type person. I know my body, so I knew I was pregnant. But I went to the doctor for the urine and blood test just to be sure. At first, I was kind of excited about having another baby. I have three children—a 10-year-old daughter, an 8-year-old son, and a 20-year-old daughter who is out on her own now. I had said when I had my son that I wouldn't have any more children; that I was done. But, I got the feeling I maybe wanted another.

When I got pregnant this time, it wasn't the right time to have a baby. I was stretched out, on an emotional roller coaster. I didn't have my own place. They sold the building where I was living and I can't find another place right now. For now, my mom has the kids staying with her. My mom and dad aren't together, but my dad, he's around and he helps out. It's hard to have my kids somewhere else even though I see them daily.

You know your body has to be right to have a baby. You can't be stressed out. I felt there were too many obstacles that I have to jump through right now.

I wouldn't want to bring a baby into this stressful situation. You know your body has to be right to have a baby. You can't be stressed out. I felt there were too many obstacles that I have to jump through right now.

I have five sisters and two brothers. They're all here in San Francisco, except one in Texas. I try to get together with them every time I can. I'm very family oriented. I love to be with my family. There's nothing else that's so important to me.

I didn't talk to my mom about being pregnant because she doesn't really believe in abortions. She wouldn't disown me or anything like that, but still. I talked to my sister and

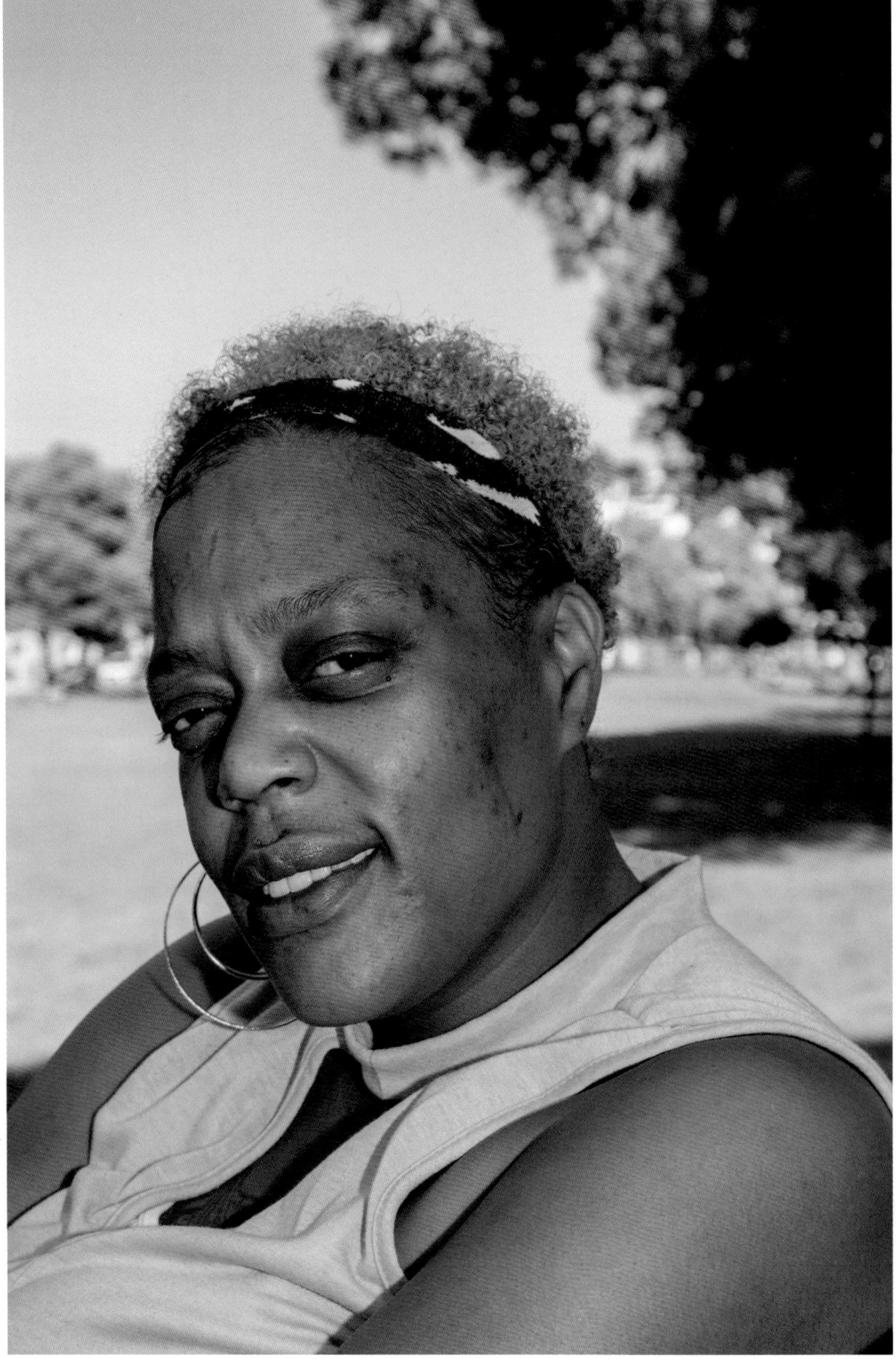

SHALITHA MITCHELL

my cousin and a friend. Those three people were supportive. They've been through that and they know it's a horrible feeling sometimes. There's an emotional attachment. So you just get over it.

I had other abortions when I was younger. When I was young I had more of an I-don't-care attitude. I didn't have any attachment to the pregnancies, it was just "oh well."

This last time, because I thought I wanted to have the baby, it was a hard decision. But it just wasn't the right time to bring a baby into the equation. The father involved said he was ready for either one—the abortion or the baby. I knew what I needed to do. I made the decision to have an abortion.

MOST WOMEN FEEL SHAME HAVING AN ABORTION. THEY THINK THEY ARE GOING TO JUDGED. I'D LIKE TO SAY THAT WE, AS WOMEN, ARE THE STRONGEST BEINGS ON EARTH. YOU KNOW, WE ENDURE A LOT. IT'S REALLY HARD.

It was really early on. If it had been four or five months, well, I don't mean to judge anyone, but that would have been harder. It would feel more like a baby, not a fetus.

Once, a long time ago, I was five months pregnant. The baby was kicking and everything. The baby died inside me. I had to push it out. That was really hard. It was worse than an abortion. The emotions and hormones go up and down.

Once I decided to have this last abortion, I knew where to go for the procedure. At the clinic they don't automatically give you an abortion but tell you all your options, including adoption. I didn't want to talk about them. I knew what they were. I had been there a couple of times before. I just wanted to get it over. The doctor told me what was going to happen even though I already knew. It was a suction abortion. I was awake. I was so drained. I hadn't slept in a couple of days. I worried about my kids.

Most women feel shame having an abortion. They think they are going to be judged. I'd like to say that we, as women, are the strongest beings on earth. You know, we endure a lot. It's really hard. Like they say, "Oh, you had an abortion." It doesn't happen like that. You have so many emotions. I was pregnant at 17. Do I have the baby or not? I did and was a mother at 17. When you have to make a tough decision about your own life, you're not any less for it. If you can't have a child at that moment, it's OK.

As women we have the right to choose, to make that decision for ourselves. One thing I don't do is judge anyone. Like I said, the women who get terminations later on in their pregnancy, I don't judge them.

I used to work in a shelter for women who were pregnant, a safe haven. The men didn't care at all. It was sad to see how the women were disrespected, like they were nothing. It's unfortunate.

I wish that we women could be more appreciated because we do a lot. We make the world go around. We do so much and most of the time we are not recognized for it.

Shiloh Modisett

IN COLLEGE I dated a guy off and on for about a year and a half. About three weeks after we broke up for the last time, I found out that I was pregnant. By the time I knew that I was pregnant, I had turned 21. I was in the midst of summer school and trying to finish my classes so I could graduate the next year.

I knew that if I stayed pregnant, I wouldn't graduate from college on time, or maybe ever. I think a lot of that was fear, based on shame. I thought if I had a baby, my life was over. I know now that wouldn't have been the case, but my life would have been much different. I wasn't emotionally mature enough, I think, to make the decision to have a baby.

At first, the only person I talked to about my situation was a good friend. I didn't want anyone else to know. After I decided to have an abortion, I called the guy involved to let him know. He really didn't fight me. He just said, "I wish you would do something different." I think he would have liked to have the child. He was a nice enough guy, a smart enough guy, but not for me. He had shown me in a lot of different ways that we were not supposed to be together. Probably he offered to help, but I really don't remember the specifics of our conversations, mostly because I didn't want there to be much of a conversation. I knew what I needed to do. I had to be really confident with that.

That was in 2004, so I was on my desktop computer, making sure to erase my browser history. I didn't want anyone to know I was researching where to have an abortion. I felt I needed to control the information. I was looking for a Planned Parenthood office because of their reputation, but the nearest office only did exams. I found three or four crisis

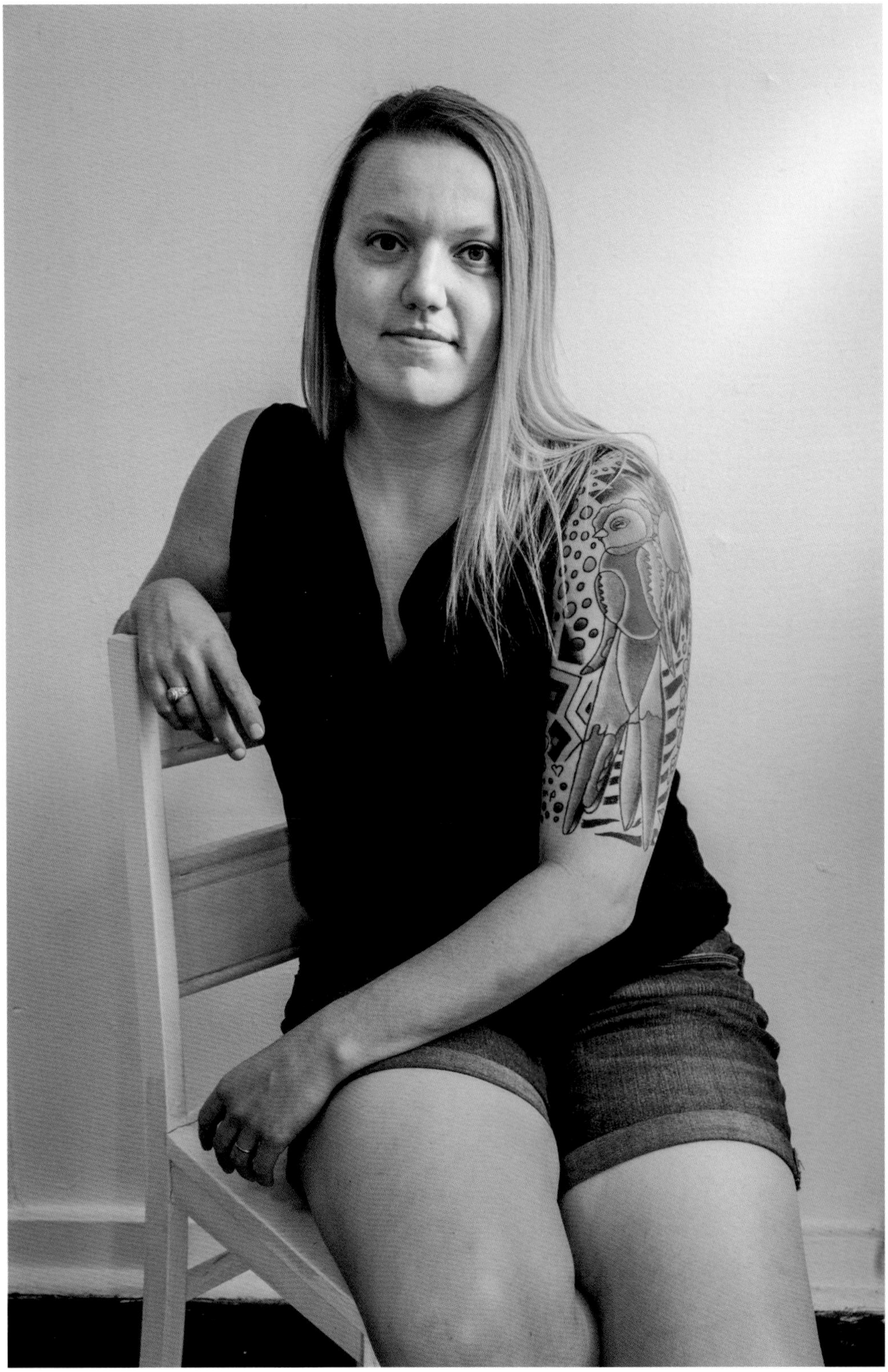

SHILOH MODISETT

pregnancy centers. Luckily, I was astute enough to figure out that their aim was to talk people out of having an abortion. Finally, I found a clinic and came to Houston for the abortion.

I didn't have the $400 to pay for it. When I arrived and the clinic told me they didn't have a payment plan and needed to be paid in full in advance, I almost had a meltdown in the counselor's office. I was able to pay $100 that day and my ex-boyfriend promised to pay the rest. He didn't. One lesson that my mom made sure I knew was that you have to protect your credit score. You pay your bills on time. You do not let things go to collections. By the time I found out my ex hadn't paid, the $300 owed to the clinic had gone to collection. I was devastated and felt shame times ten. I borrowed the money from a friend and paid her back over time.

Before my abortion I hadn't heard of anyone who had ever had an abortion except for my mom. When I had the conversation with her about getting birth control, she told me about her abortion. Basically, she said, "Please, just don't get pregnant." I think she must have been 21 or 22 when she had her own abortion because it was pre- Roe v. Wade.

Even though my mother had had an abortion, I didn't talk to her when I got pregnant. Between the ages of 14 and 24, my mom and I didn't have a great relationship, mostly because we're so much alike. We're both very stubborn and very competent in ourselves. As an older adult, I regret not having had that conversation with her. I think we could have related.

Actually, I had two coming-out stories to tell my mother: coming out about being queer, which I had previously shared with my mom without a problem, and coming out about having an abortion, which was scary. I just felt more able to talk about being gay.

The biggest thing that made me want to share my abortion story was seeing how women are being treated now. It's not just the challenge of access to abortion, but health care in general, the attacks on Planned Parenthood. That's the first reason. I think the second is, as an adult, as someone who is supporting myself, it was easier to talk about my abortion. There's less risk in telling the story. And I'm not worried about my reputation now. I was worried about it then.

In 2017, I was asked to be part of a theatrical production, Oral Fixation. I would be one of six or seven storytellers talking on stage about our abortions. I realized that before I could get up on stage and tell the story, I had to talk to my mom. I had to. She couldn't find out on Facebook that I had an abortion. Also, I also needed to ask her permission to say that she had had an abortion. That was risky because my mom was pretty private. When I told her, she was fine. She wasn't disappointed. She was curious. She wanted to know if I was OK, and then she wanted to know why in the world I would get on a stage and talk about it. She also asked if there would be a video of the show because she wanted to share it with her friends!

After I told my mother about my abortion, I felt like I was released from years' worth of pressure to be a certain way or maintain a certain set of expectations. I had always felt that the worst thing I could do was to get pregnant and have an abortion. Once we had spoken, I felt like, "Well, I'm good for the rest of my life."

Since I told my story the first time and have started talking more about having an abortion, a lot of folks have come to me and said, "Me too." I don't know if my mother had the same thing. Unfortunately, I didn't get to follow up with her. My mom passed away almost a year ago, suddenly, from a heart attack at age 67. Our abortion conversation happened ten months before she died. I'm so glad that we had that conversation. I would've had a whole lot more regrets and a whole lot more questions about our relationship if I wasn't able to share that with her before she died.

Actually, I had two coming-out stories to tell my mother: coming out about being queer, which I had previously shared with my mom without a problem, and coming out about having an abortion, which was scary. I just felt more able to talk about being gay. She asked me if I was ready to deal with all of the stigma that came with it, looking queer or whatever. When she asked me what I would do if a future employer didn't like that I was gay, I told her that I wouldn't want to work for an employer who felt that way. It took her a while to get used to me being OK with turning down a job if I couldn't be out. But she got it. She and Shelby, my partner, really loved each other. That was huge for me.

I wanted to be a parent my whole life. I don't think I've been ready until Shelby and I got together. Now, Shelby and I are married and we want to have kids. For us, it's interesting because we have to make a very conscious decision. There are lots of steps involved, to adopt or try to get pregnant, or whatever.

I think that the only way we relate to each other is by sharing our stories and being honest and vulnerable when we can. It's taking the risk of putting yourself out there. It's literally just saying, "I've had this experience." There can be so much judgment as a result of telling your abortion story. To me, it feels very, very similar to coming out about sexuality or gender identity. You run a risk when you say this is my reality, and you may or may not accept that. If you do, wonderful. If you don't, I then have a grieving process to go through. Even though stigma exists, I feel much less confined by it.

Reflecting on this last year and a half, I wish I would have given my mom the opportunity to love me at the time of my abortion. She would have. When I find myself talking with friends, I want them to know it's worth the risk of sharing as opposed to holding in all of the pain and fear.

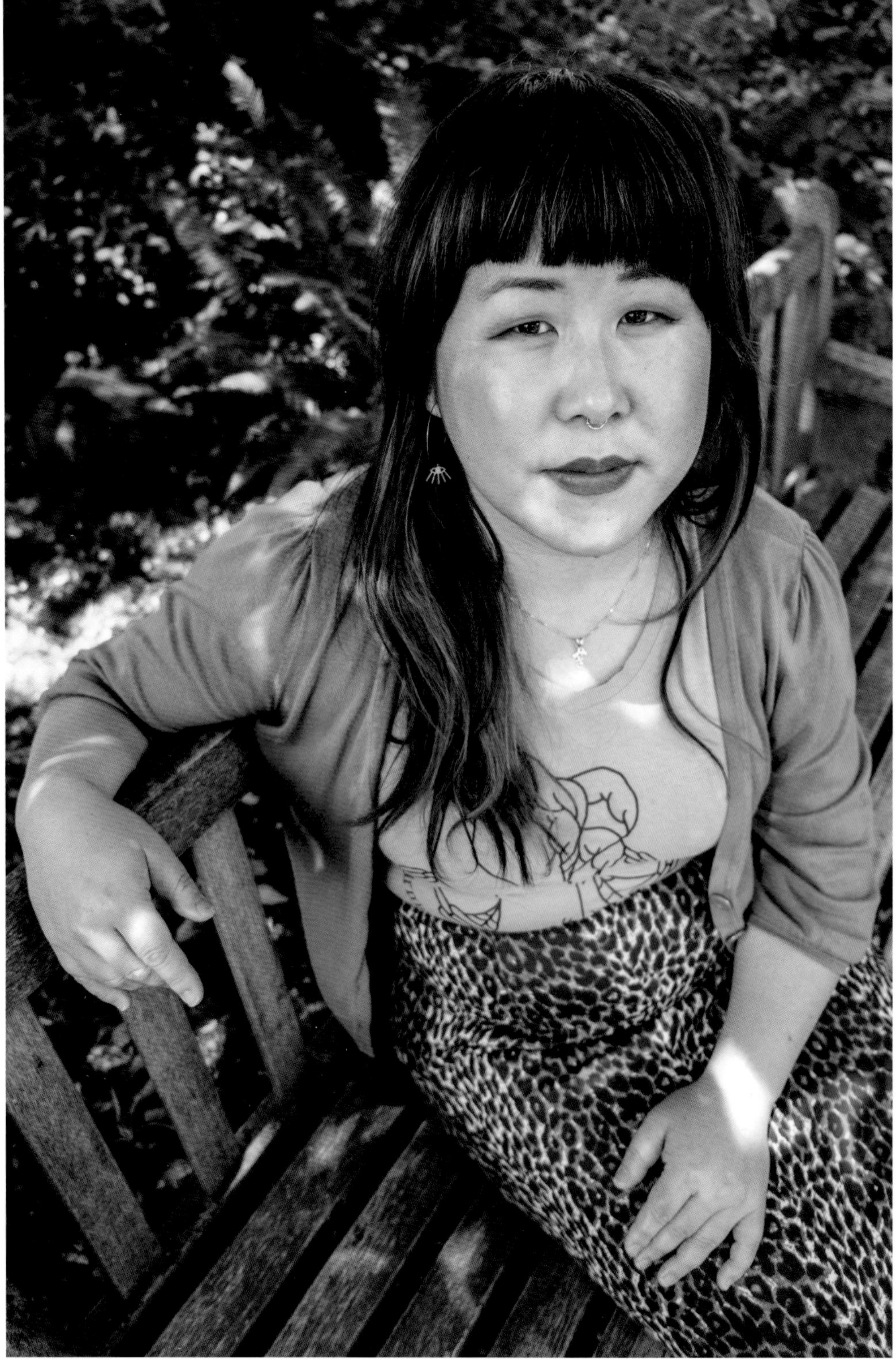

A’MISA CHIU

A'misa Chiu

I AM A mother, but it's taken a long journey to be at ease with becoming one. I'm a *Yonsei Nikkei,* a fourth generation Japanese-American. My four family names are Matsushima, Nakaoka, Takaki, Kaneko. We find significance in naming the generations to track how many generations deep we are into our immigration story.

When I was pregnant with my daughter five years ago, I had this conversation with a chaplain who studied family dynamics. He told me that in terms of children, you have to count your abortions and miscarriages as well, and sometimes people name them. I never thought about my first pregnancy as a child, but I liked the idea of naming the experience. I chose the term "ashless death" because there's no grave, there's no ashes. There's only a memory. I named my aborted pregnancy Pearl. Someday I'll tell my firstborn daughter about Pearl. Naming it gives it value. I'm not trying to erase it or make it disappear. I will own it and name it.

I never thought about my first pregnancy as a child, but I liked the idea of naming the experience. I chose the term "ashless death" because there's no grave, there's no ashes. There's only a memory.

My abortion was at the end of my junior year of college. I had just turned 21. I was in a non-committed, tumultuous relationship with somebody I worked with. I was a barista at a coffee shop on campus and we had an on-again-off-again relationship that lasted for a couple of years. He was the first partner that I had sex with. It was like a big deal. I was a young person and he was slightly older than me, a philosopher-writer-chain-smoker-alcoholic type. I lived in a community of experimental writers. We hosted a lot of readings and those readings became house parties. That was the lifestyle that I was living in college.

Suddenly I hated working as a barista. I couldn't stand the smell of coffee. I was getting nauseous all the time. I ignored it for weeks. One day, my partner and I were sitting and smoking cigarettes and I said, "You know, I just don't like the smell of coffee anymore. It's so weird, it makes me sick nowadays." He looked at me funny and suddenly it dawned on us both. I was really scared. At the drug store we used the self-checkout line because I was really embarrassed to buy a pregnancy test. We bought a really expensive one, because I had to be sure. This was not a drill.

I stood in my bathroom alone. I had no idea what I was doing, except that I needed to pee on a stick. I waited for what felt like an infinite amount of time. Time slowed down. When those two lines appeared on the test, it felt like my world was imploding on itself. I started to take in large gulps of air. I held onto the towel rack in front of me to steady myself. My head started spinning, everything turned blurry, my whole world felt like it stopped. All I could imagine was the faces of my community mocking me and judging me. The weight of failing to make something of myself came crashing down on me. How could I have failed everyone, especially myself? I felt a deep amount of shame. I was supposed to be the one with a lot of potential.

One of the values I grew up with was one must fit into the community you live in. I felt pressured to not shame the community and not stick out too much. The ironic part is that my own parents taught me not to be a trend follower, to be a free thinker and an independent woman. There's a saying in Japanese American, "The nail that sticks up will be hammered down." That phrase is key in understanding how my community operates. Anyone who speaks up or chooses an alternative lifestyle must face the reality that the community may try to suppress them into conforming. As a budding artist or as a free-thinking person, you don't want to conform and just be status quo, but at the same time if you stand out, you will be hammered down. That was the conflict in how I was raised.

My partner and I had a lot of conversations in the next coming weeks about what we were going to do. At one point, we were sitting in front of the computer looking at the developmental stages of babies. He pointed to a picture of a fetus and said, 'This is the baby and how big it is." He wanted to get married and have the baby, but I didn't believe that for a second. I made it clear that I had decided to terminate the pregnancy. When I called the clinic, I thought it was going to be like a one-day wait. Instead I had to wait four weeks for an appointment. I had an abortion when I was ten weeks along.

A friend from high school had told me that she had an abortion a couple of weeks before, and I ended up at her doorstep the night I found out I was pregnant. I told my brother a year later, the night before I graduated. It took a couple more years for me to tell my mom. My mother was supportive, surprisingly sad that I went through it alone. She was a practicing reproductive health-care nurse and pro-choice, so I knew on some level that she was going to be OK with it. It took me more than five years to tell my dad. My dad and I never talked about these kinds of issues, it just felt so personal. I was embarrassed, I just never knew how to bring it up.

I began talking about my abortion publicly when I participated in a documentary that Vanessa Yee, my friend from college, was making. *The Laundromat* is about airing your dirty laundry and exploring how and why Asian-American families are steeped in silence and secrets. The interesting part is how the documentary interview process seeped into my real life in a way I didn't expect. It challenged me to confront my silence with my own family.

The Laundromat was made about four or five years after my abortion. The director and Vanessa said they would be showing this documentary in shared spaces that we occupied in terms of Asian-American community. She told me she wanted me to very, very sure that I wanted my story in the film. That is when I finally told my dad, the day before the film crew was going to film at my parents' house

I think for my mom and my dad, it was very personal because they were in the film too. In fact, my dad spoke a lot in the documentary about his feelings about not knowing about my abortion. Because of the documentary process, I was finally able to process my emotions around the abortion. Before, there had been moments in my life where if someone said the words like pregnant or baby, I would just shut down. I would have to leave the room for fear of a panic attack. And yet it wasn't about my decision to have an abortion. I never doubted my decision.

What I didn't realize is there are consequences to deciding to have an abortion. You get pregnant and you don't want to have a baby and you decide to have an abortion to get rid of that problem. But my new problem then became having the stigma of having the abortion and all of the mental spiraling down that I experienced.

After I had my abortion, my life went to shambles, I spiraled down to a dark place. I couldn't live with people. I could barely go to school. I could barely get to work. I suffered a deep depression and crippling isolation. I cried every night for many years.

My spouse was there for me when I was in my deep depression and the beginning of our relationship was him helping me heal, talking to me, walking me through some of those dark times. We've been together about fifteen years now. We have two children, a 5-year-old and a 1-year-old. I eventually got therapy. I started creating artwork and writing around my abortion. I became stronger as I became comfortable with my own story. It was the process of becoming public with my story and owning it, that really helped me overcome the hurdle of shame and depression.

It took me many years to be able to be OK becoming a mother. I thought that I would never have other children, because it would be too hard emotionally. But as time passed, so did these feelings. When I got pregnant with my eldest child, I was scared. How would this pregnancy affect me? Would it send me into depression again? Are my demons going to come back to haunt me? Fortunately, they didn't.

In 2015 I created the *Hidden Motherhood* zine. That was a big moment for me because I was passing this out to strangers, to my family, to my friends. It was the first time I documented my story in an artistic way. My daughter had just been born and so I dedicated the zine to her as well.

I started creating artwork and writing around my abortion. I became stronger as I became comfortable with my own story. The process of becoming public with my story and owning it really helped me overcome the hurdle of shame and depression.

Poem by A'misa Chiu

I took back the night I lost my virginity,
I took back the night we laid in a drunken puddle,
I took back the night I got pregnant four days after my 21st birthday
(at least that night was quiet, comfortable),
I took back the night of the abortion.

Not a regret but a reclaiming.
I still had a sadness within me that was unfamiliar.
What saved me was I found a community of people who sole purpose was to serve others.
They fought for justice, they advocated on behalf of others.
In my heart, I joined the cause, the fight, the movement, the revolution.
I was so tired, I forgot to feel sad. I grew tired of being a pity party.
I met other women who had, had abortions,
more than one,
several,
many over the years,
mostly hidden moments, not shameful, just hidden.
The things unspoken,
the date marked on your calendar for no other reason except
a silent acknowledgement.
We mark our bodies with tattoo memorials
for the babies of abortions have no place of rest,
No gravestones,
no ash remains,
we walk like queens,
3, 4, 5 abortions,
we are fertile ground.
Our bodies transformed to hold life,
our minds continue to hold what our bodies stopped holding onto.
We do not forget.
It is all just whispered,
talked about in hush tones.

from "Hidden Motherhood," by A'misa Chiu [zine ©A'misa Chiu, 2019 All Rights Reserved]

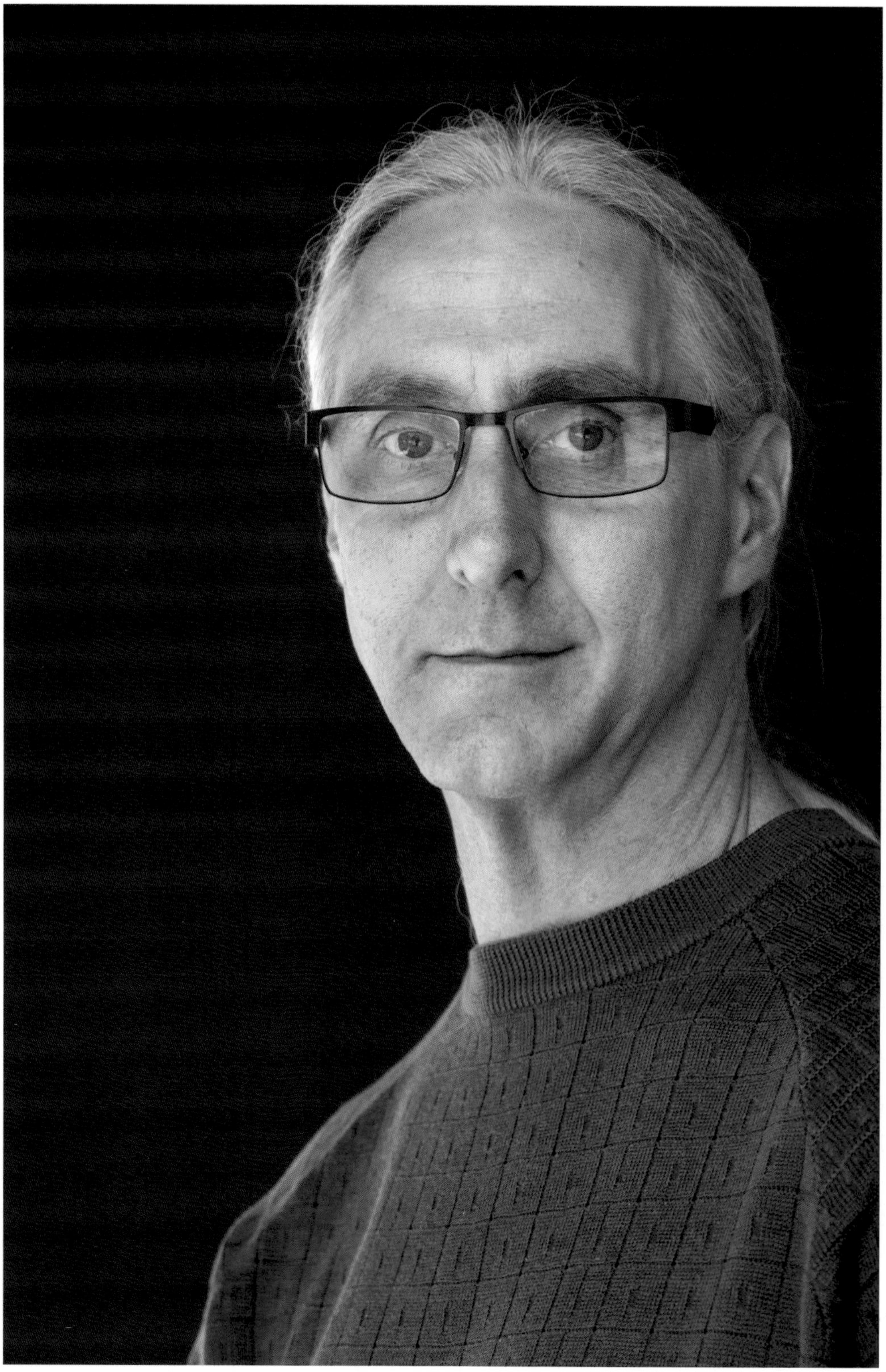

MONTE JONES

Monte Jones

OUR FIRST CHILD was conceived and died at 20 weeks old. We named her Faith. That was twenty-two years ago. My wife and I had been married almost three years when we got pregnant. But the pregnancy from the beginning was very difficult.

At our eighteen-week ultrasound, we were hoping to learn the baby's gender, but we could tell things were not going well. The baby was very small, and there wasn't very much amniotic fluid. That prompted more rounds of tests. Ultimately, an ultrasound on the baby's heart showed a very severe cardiac defect, and the amniotic fluid continued to drop. Without amniotic fluid, babies can't develop healthy lungs. There was no way for her to get enough lung function to survive, on top of the other organs that didn't work.

AT OUR EIGHTEEN-WEEK ULTRASOUND, WE WERE HOPING TO LEARN THE BABY'S GENDER, BUT WE COULD TELL THINGS WERE NOT GOING WELL.

I was at medical school at the time, so I spent the day at the medical school library researching this issue. I found out there were zero case reports of any child surviving this kind of situation. Our choices were to continue carrying the child to term or near term, and then deliver her and watch her suffocate, or to end the pregnancy early and try to help her suffer less. My wife, of course, couldn't bear to hold on anymore, and we knew we had to let our daughter go.

My wife worked for a hospital that is run by the Baptist church. She was insured through them, and we were in the process of scheduling the abortion there. However, a hospital committee met and decided that this was just an elective termination of pregnancy. They didn't get into the details of the fact that the pregnancy was hopeless. They just thought, the baby's got a heart defect, and that my wife and I didn't want to deal with that. This was far from the case.

We weren't allowed to have the abortion at her hospital, where she worked as a nurse, where she was insured, and where all her friends and support were. We were forced to drive an hour to Fort Worth to have the abortion in a different hospital. There, the doctor induced delivery and our daughter was stillborn at 20 weeks. She never took a breath.

When we were back at home, just trying to heal, to recuperate, my wife's hospital called. At the time the hospital was self-insured, so they just paid out of pocket for all their employees' medical care, as long as it was at one of their own facilities. They told me since we had the abortion at an outside facility, we were expected to pay for it. That just set me off.

Long story short, an attorney advised me we had a good case. He gave me great advice about dealing with the hospital, and if the hospital wouldn't give me what I wanted, to call him back. He didn't even try to take on the case; he was just supportive. I'm not sure he'll ever know how much it meant to have that one sympathetic ear that we had from no other quarter in our life. Eventually, I had to put on my white lab coat and stomp into the hospital CEO's office and kick up a fuss. I had to threaten to sue before they convened the ethics committee, and the chairman of the committee, wisely, apologized in person. They paid for everything.

People were loosely supportive. Everybody seemed to really shy away from the tragedy. When it comes to facing death and dying, a lot of people just can't do it. And through the twenty years I've been an oncologist, I've learned that a lot of times what people need when there is a death is just to not feel alone.

THROUGH THE TWENTY YEARS I'VE BEEN AN ONCOLOGIST, I'VE LEARNED THAT A LOT OF TIMES WHAT PEOPLE NEED WHEN THERE IS A DEATH IS JUST TO NOT FEEL ALONE.

That one good thing about the whole nightmare was it was kind of a bonding time for my wife and me. That was the time we became "us." We were all we had.

We now have three boys, ages, 17, 19, and 21. They're wonderful young men. I'm very proud of all of them. I love them deeply. But I still think of Faith fairly often. I always wanted a daughter, and she was the only one I had. So, when I see a bride being walked down the aisle, I'm reminded that I'll never get to do that for her.

My wife is very supportive of my telling our story. I think it's therapeutic for her too.

Just to put it out there that abortion happens in all kinds of different circumstances, to married couples with planned pregnancies like ours. You just can't rush in and judge people based on what makes you uncomfortable. You owe it to your fellow humans to understand where they're coming from, understand the agony they're in. Honestly, I think we have more in common between pro-choice and pro-life than we have differences. Nobody wants there to be more abortions. We just disagree on how to get there.

Shortly after we lost our daughter, I was looking for some support for us, and then for myself, frankly, because you know, fathers don't get a lot of attention when there's a miscarriage or a failed pregnancy. I went by the Planned Parenthood Clinic in Dallas to see if they had any support groups for parents that have lost a pregnancy. As I was walking up to the door, there was a lone protestor across the parking lot who shouted at me and called me "daddy." I wasn't in a very good place at the time, and I sort of lost it. I ran over and screamed in his face that he should probably carry a weapon if he's going to talk to me like that. He was rather taken aback. I could tell he didn't have a weapon, because he was afraid. I didn't touch him, but I certainly was not willing to sit there and let somebody call me "daddy."

You know what would be nice? To open up people's minds on both sides, because I really think we could have conversations that we're not having. We don't have to agree with each other to have a conversation. I appreciate where pro-life people are coming from. I don't think they're coming from a bad place. I just think they're going about it wrong, and going about it with a lack of empathy.

I'd like to think I could try to have a conversation with the demonstrator who called me "daddy" outside of Planned Parenthood. I would probably have to meditate for a good sixteen minutes beforehand, to really just get myself slowed down enough to where I wouldn't go off on my tangents. I would hope I could at least stay on my side of the street and say, "Look. I want to hear your side of things, but you've got to know, I'm not necessarily going to agree with them." I would love to sit down with him and say, "You know, my daughter was already dead before we had the abortion. She was not going to survive, and you made it worse. Is that really what your goal was? You didn't bother to find out why I was there. You didn't bother to find out what I was looking for. You didn't even find out that my daughter was dead already. You sure didn't say, I'm sorry you had to go through that."

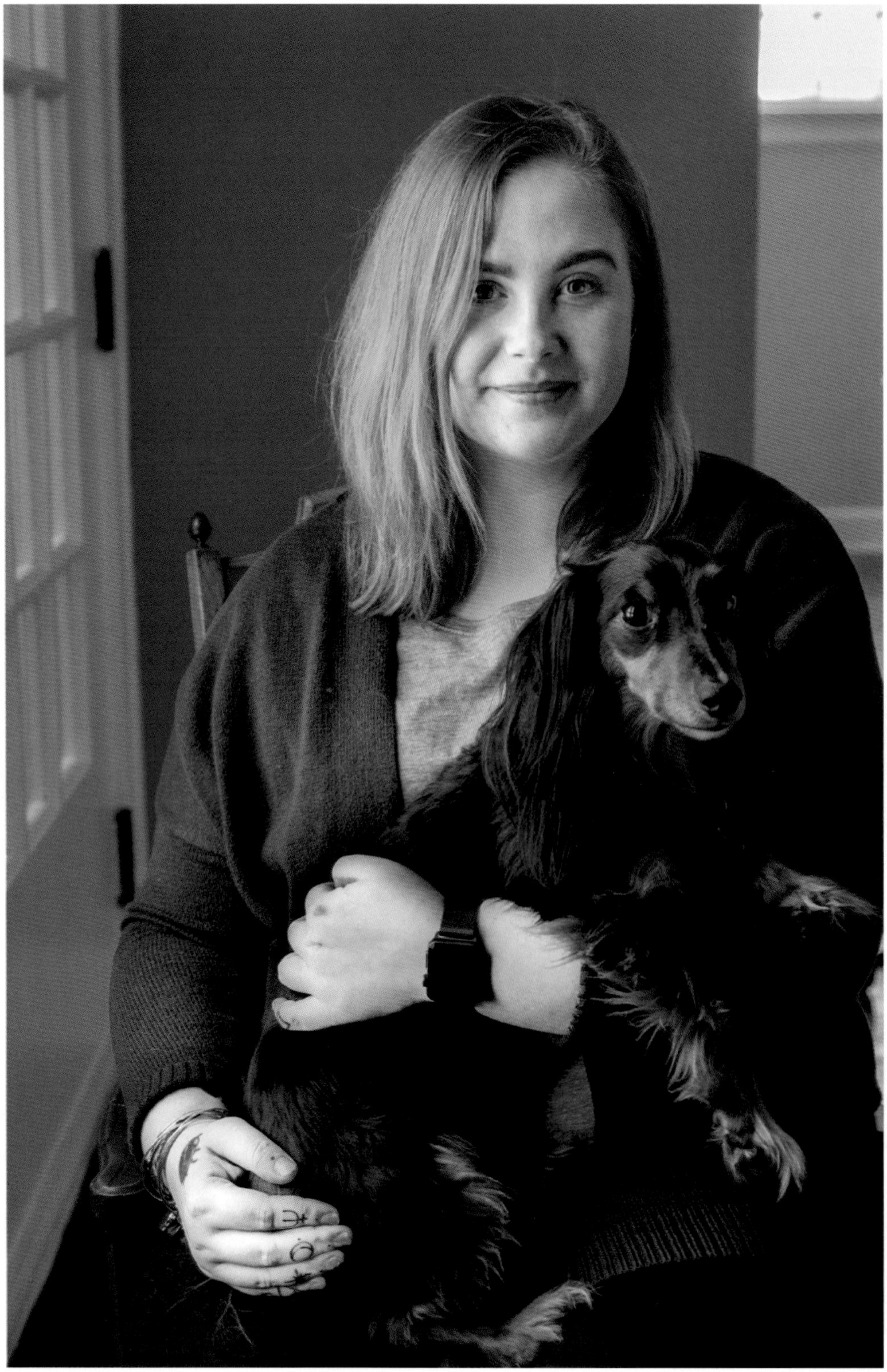

HOLLY BLAND

Holly Bland

WHEN I GOT pregnant at age 19, I freaked out. I knew the second that I peed on the pregnancy test that I was pregnant. It didn't give me any time to, like, recoup and think about what was happening. It was like a movie, me sliding down my bathroom door crying my eyes out. I just remember this meltdown.

There are no abortion clinics within an hour of Ashtabula, Ohio, where I lived. It's a very small, conservative town, northeast of Cleveland. The internet was flooded with "crisis pregnancy centers." These are the fake clinics that just try to trap a woman. A lot of the websites even say "abortion" on them to reel you in. But then abortion is like the only part they don't give you any more information about.

When I called those places, they all wanted me to come in to talk about "your situation." I'm like, "I want to schedule an appointment for abortion. Is that what you do?" I think four different clinics were like that.

I had my abortion at a clinic in Akron. I was five weeks pregnant when I found out and seven weeks when I was able to have my procedure because of Ohio's twenty-four-hour waiting period, and my schedule. I was working two part-time jobs at Giant Eagle and Dairy Queen, averaging at least fifty-five hours a week. The abortion cost $600. I didn't have any savings, just a little bit of a cushion for extra bills. I used that and maxed-out a credit card. My partner contributed a little bit as well. I mean, it was a large chunk of money.

The only person I involved was my partner at the time. He was in the military. We were unsure about his future in the military: Would he be gone for a while, or was he coming back to go to school? But even if he was going to be home, I still would've had an abortion because I was just not ready.

I felt like my partner was emotionally supportive, but now looking back on it, I think that he was also pretty sad about it. I'm pretty sure on the day of my abortion, he cried. But I was just so happy. The second I was done, I was like, "Can I have a Big Mac now, please?" I couldn't eat the morning of the abortion, so afterwards I was starving.

I DEAL WITH BIPOLAR DISORDER. THAT MAKES IT HARD TO EVEN CARE FOR MYSELF, WHICH IS ONE OF THE BIGGEST REASONS WHY I KNEW IMMEDIATELY I WANTED AN ABORTION.

I am great right now. Today, five years later, I feel confident about my decision still. I don't ever have a day where I think, "Damn, I wish I would've brought that pregnancy to term." But I do get angry because in those five years, bans and restrictions have just gotten worse in Ohio and clinics have closed.

Everybody has a different reaction to her experience and that's completely valid. I'm one of those cases where I just wanted it gone. I didn't want to be pregnant. And even thinking about a future with children now, I don't think I want kids.

I deal with bipolar disorder. That makes it hard to even care for myself, which is one of the biggest reasons why I knew immediately I wanted an abortion. It's why I feel I'll never have the capacity to care for children. My mother was the same way. I'm not saying she was a bad mom, but she definitely struggled being bipolar herself. Now that I'm an adult dealing with all of these things, it makes sense.

I don't deal with large life changes well either. There is often a very large tipping point for my mental illness, and I just don't feel it would've been good to carry a pregnancy to term with all of these things going on— work, school, home.

A lot of people feel shame or stigma over their abortions. If people would just sit down and listen for a minute, they would see that people who have abortions aren't awful humans. There's awful humans everywhere. So there might be a couple of awful people who have had abortions. But just because they had an abortion doesn't make them awful.

I didn't tell my mother until two years ago that I had my abortion. I could talk to her about anything, but I felt that she would want to impede my decision because she always wants to try to do what's best for me. I told her because I was going out to LA to do a photo shoot for *Cosmopolitan* for a story about abortion, including mine. I couldn't just go to LA without telling her why I was going. She just started crying, not because she was upset with me, not because she didn't believe in abortion access or anything like that. She was just upset that I didn't tell her that I had an abortion. She was like, "Honey, why would you go through that by yourself? I wish you would've told me." Then she told me about an abortion she had after she had me. That was a nice conversation. It felt good to have that moment with her.

Right now I'm the administrative assistant for an abortion clinic. I work there full time and I'm going to college with a journalism major. I'm not sure my path will be in journalism, but I'm hoping that it coincides with abortion and reproductive justice.

I feel like people have the capacity to change. One reason I feel like that is because my dad and I have had multiple conversations about my abortion and my work with reproductive justice and abortion access. He's not overwhelmingly like, "Oh my God. I can't believe you're doing this amazing work." But he's definitely not upset about it anymore, which I feel is an improvement, and it shows that people can change their minds if they really think about it.

My grandfather is still really upset about it. He doesn't talk to me about it. He just pretends that I don't work at an abortion clinic. He calls it the health clinic. He will not respond to anything that I say about abortion.

I would really just like to see people be more compassionate about why people need abortions. The people who support all of these restrictive laws and legislation and bans don't know the first thing about what it means to need an abortion.

I won't say that I haven't been hostile toward people arguing with me about this subject, because I have. But I've learned and I've grown up a little bit, so I try to approach people who are anti-choice in a respectful manner. Obviously, nothing will get done if we're yelling at each other, right? I try to give the same compassion that I received when I had my abortion.

So many things affect a person's decision to have an abortion. Mental health does play a role, and that's a part of the conversation that's been left unsaid.

People should know there's no one way to feel about your abortion experience. I never felt any regret or remorse about my own abortion.

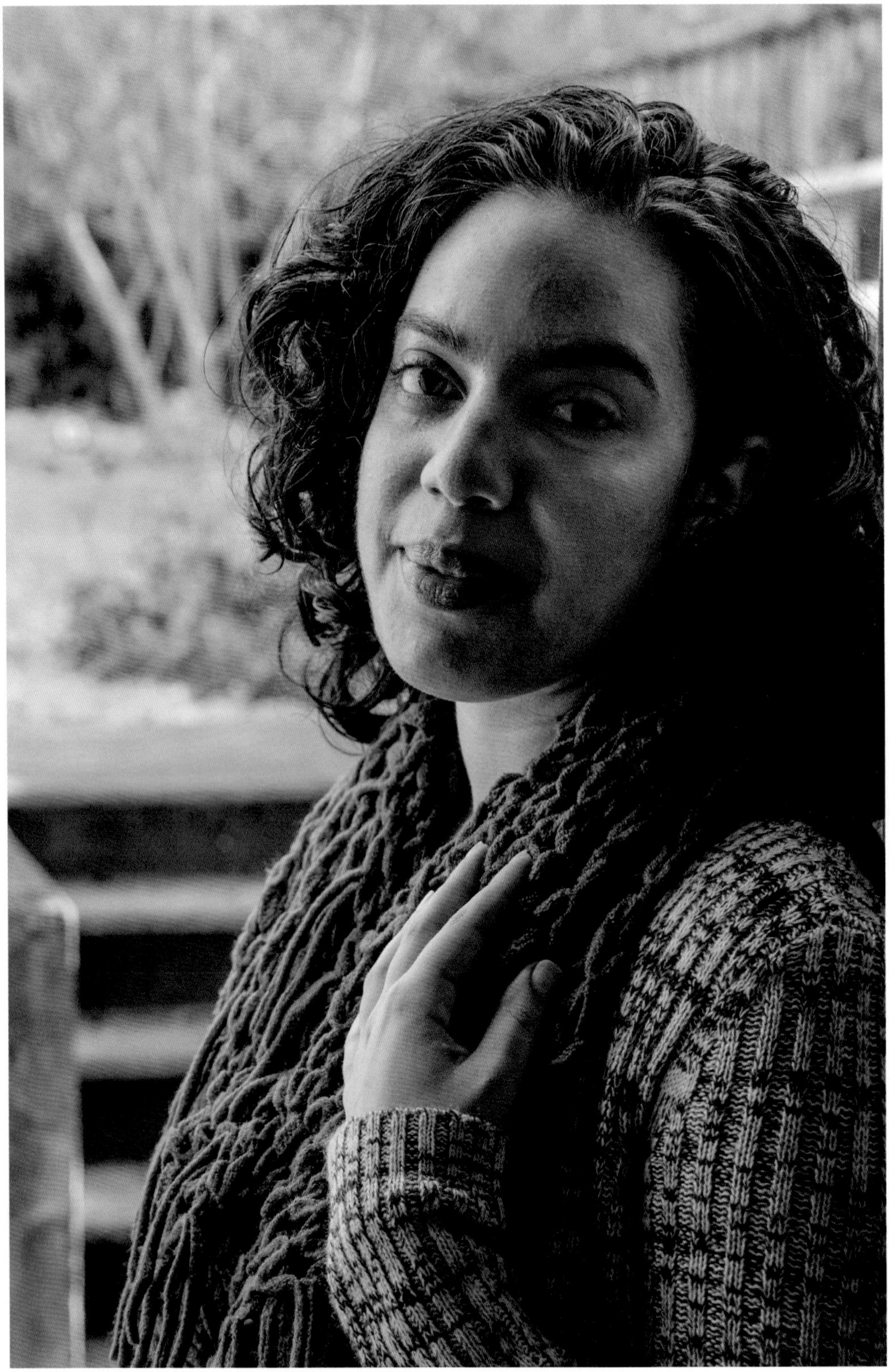

SARINA IRIZARRY

Sarina Irizarry

THREE YEARS AGO my life took a turn with health issues. So I started working out, eating healthy. And then, within six months, I was diagnosed with an autoimmune condition, and that totally changed my life. At that point I made a career switch.

I'm in my second year of a Master's program studying Integrative and Functional Nutrition. It has been a life-changing journey, really, from how I talk to other people to how I take care of myself, relationships with friends. I would say in the last six to eight months I have really worked on putting myself first.

You know sometimes life just doesn't work for you anymore, how you used to do things.

My first abortion happened in the spring of 2008. I pretty much knew right away that I would have an abortion because I was in school, planning to have a future, and having a baby was not something I was wanting and willing to do. To have that responsibility, I was just not ready for it. My partner at the time felt the exact same way. He was supportive and went to the appointment with me.

The clinic didn't feel comforting. It felt very cold and sterile. First, I had to make an appointment to make sure I was pregnant, then a "consultation," then the procedure. So all together it was three appointments over three weeks. It was very early at the time of my abortion.

But I do remember the second appointment. You go into a room and you quickly speak with a practitioner who says, "Well, here's a video on making a choice." I sat in a room by myself and watched the video. It was a really small room, with a TV, really old school. The film just talked about making a decision. It was pretty neutrally weighted. To be honest, I was not happy that I had to sit through that. After I left that appointment, I knew that I would come back for the procedure.

When I returned for the procedure, it was sort of a lineup. I could see all of the other women, before and after the procedure in the recovery room. It was hard because it felt like there wasn't privacy. There were a lot of women in the room who experienced different emotions. You were actually in a hospital bed with your gown. It just felt like a factory. My partner was in the waiting room.

I got over this abortion pretty fast. I'm a writer. I write poems. That was my therapy. I wrote about it. I'm a thinker. I thought about it. I talk out loud to myself a lot. So I never reached outside of myself for therapy or help. At the time it just felt like an experience I had and it was something that I owned. It was just something that happened. I'm thankful I was able to have the procedure and get it done in time.

The abortion experience that stays in my mind happened years later, in 2014. That was three months after I was diagnosed with my autoimmune condition. Again, I knew automatically that I was pregnant. So it was like, "Oh gosh, this is bad timing." I'm still young. I still had school. I was working full time and trying to figure out what to do next.

I went through a lot of shame and guilt and judgment for myself. Why did I let this happen again? I was frustrated because we had used a condom. I was protected, and I'm not sure of what exactly happened.

My partner was definitely supportive of my decision to have an abortion. So we had lots of talks about it. And that was therapeutic for him and me. But he was leaning more toward, "Oh, maybe we should take a stab at this and try to raise a child." And I said, "Are you crazy?" I decided to have an abortion.

There were a lot of sad moments in the months following the abortion. A year later my partner kind of brought it up. It took him some time to process it, to be honest with himself and to me, and say, "Yeah, I was sad about it. It hurt me and I still think about it from time to time."

My mother wasn't against abortion whatsoever. Growing up, she definitely talked about it, saying she had friends that had abortions, that she's had one herself, but she didn't really expand on it. It happened to her when she was younger, before she got married. So I didn't tell my mother about my second abortion until much later. I felt there's a kind of stigma that it should only happen when you are young, and after that you should know better.

A few years ago, when I started volunteering for a talkline for women who have had abortions, I told my mother about it. We are very close, my mom and my sisters and me. She thought I was volunteering because I had guilt. I wasn't doing that out of guilt. But I thought it was so interesting that she thought that. That's pretty much the last time we ever talked about my abortions.

During trainings for the talkline, I heard several women on a panel share their abortion stories. That was the first time I ever heard stories to my face. It was very comfortable, a very safe space, very informal. We gathered around the table. I just thought how brave and courageous these women were.

After my first year at the talkline, one of the support staff came and asked me if I would like to be on the panel and tell my story. I felt very embarrassed and ashamed because I had had more than one abortion. But they are very trusting women. I said that I would tell my story. So I was on a panel with two other wonderful, amazing talkline volunteers. I cried and cried and I could barely get through my story. I didn't expect that. I was trying to keep my composure. I needed some help to calm me down.

I felt amazing after I told my story. I felt that I wasn't judged at that point. I felt that I did the right thing, for myself and for others. I mainly focused on the last abortion because it affected me so much and it was so recent. And that validated so much for me. If I hadn't told the story of my last abortion, it would be such a missing piece to my truth of who I am. Yes, I was raised by my mom to not be afraid of who you are, to always be yourself. As long as I can remember I was always encouraged to speak my truth and what I stand for.

So now I feel more secure with myself to admit and tell my story and not be ashamed of it. Now my fear of judgment is just an outside noise. I can completely accept myself.

I realize that your story is part of who you are and always will be in whatever capacity you want it to be. You don't have to feel like you conquered it or you are over it. It's your story and it's part of your journey. And so whatever way it pops up in your life, it can pop up ten years later and you can finally talk about it, it's still OK. For a long time I just judged myself too much. So now I feel more secure with myself to admit and tell my story and not be ashamed of it. Now my fear of judgment is just an outside noise. I can completely accept myself.

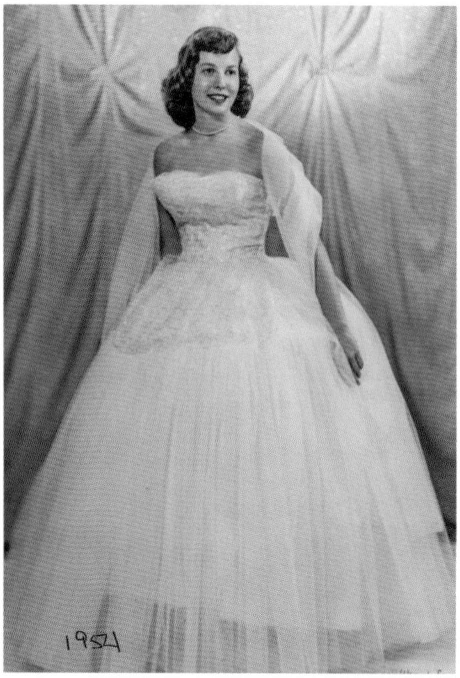

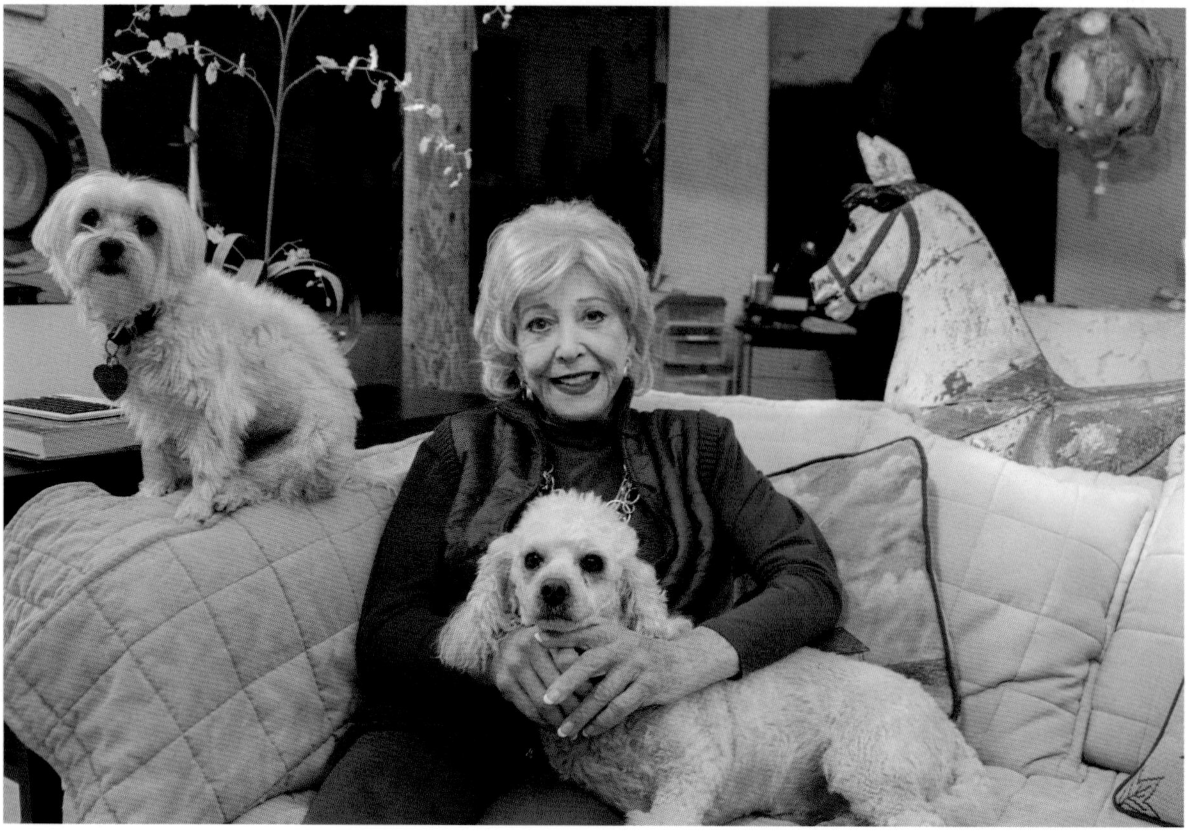

LANI MEIN

Lani Mein

AT THE TIME of my abortion I was freshly out of college in Virginia. I met a man who I could almost say was the love of my life, and I got pregnant. He would have married me. That was not the problem.

I realized I was too young to have a baby. I had been in school all my life. I was just about to step out in the world and be a real person instead of a child. I wasn't in a situation to become a mother, with or without the child's father. I just knew that I was not fit to be a mother at that time. Period. It would have ruined my life and probably the child's life. And I've never regretted the decision.

My abortion was in 1954, almost twenty years before Roe v. Wade. I never talked to anybody about it. My biggest concern was that my parents—my father really—would never know about it. My mother had taken off when I was young and married somebody else. She wasn't a particularly good mother. My father never knew about my abortion, ever, ever, ever, even when I was grown up and older.

I HAD A BACK-ALLEY ABORTION IN NORTH CAROLINA. IN THOSE DAYS, SOMEONE, NOT NECESSARILY A DOCTOR, STARTED THE ABORTION WITH A COAT HANGER.

My boyfriend, who lived in Norfolk, Virginia, had inquired to find out how to get an abortion. I had a back-alley abortion in North Carolina. In those days, someone, not necessarily a doctor, started the abortion with a coat hanger. You bled all over the place and you ended up in the hospital. The hospital seemed to be vaguely aware of what was happening. There was no criticism or government intervention or anything like that. That's how people did it then.

Thank God, I had the man I was in love with. He came with me to the abortion. I really wasn't alone. I think when you are really alone you may question your beliefs or your decision. I didn't question my beliefs. I knew without question that having the baby would be a huge mistake for two human lives. Period. That may have been selfish but we do have to take care of ourselves, don't we?

Was I afraid when I had my abortion? There's always a little fear when you are in extreme pain and bleeding. But it got the job done. Afterwards I used to worry a bit, wondering if I could have children when I was ready to have children. But you can't wallow in self-pity or worry about what-ifs. As things turned out, I did have children when I was ready to be a mother.

My life has turned out quite well. I was sent to boarding schools, one of them being the National Cathedral School. I probably spent as much time on my knees in church and in Sunday School as anybody you know. I went on to take drama in college and tried to be an actress. I did not have the fortitude to make it in the big city. I was more comfortable riding a horse in the country. Eventually I went to interior design school, and that became my profession. I ended up in San Francisco, where I met my late husband. We had two children and now I have two nice grandchildren.

I may have shared my abortion story with some best friends over the years. I don't remember the need or urge to do so. It was totally in the past and I moved forward.

When NARAL (National Abortion and Reproductive Rights Action League) became active in San Francisco, I wanted to jump on that bandwagon, to make my abortion a positive thing. It was a bit like coming out of the closet. Abortion has been around forever. It's time we open the closet door.

Decades after my abortion I got hold of some little gold hangers. A jeweler had them left over from the gay rights movement, when they signified gays coming out of the closet. I gave them out at a luncheon. They are a reminder of the many abortions, including mine, that happened with hangers in back alleys, before Roe v. Wade.

My advice to a woman contemplating an abortion is to be confident in yourself. Don't let yourself be all uptight and confused.

I believe that having a baby is a big a step to take if you don't know what you're doing. We should have to get a license to reproduce, like getting a driver's license.

Some people want to have a child more than anything in the whole world. They want to be a mother even if the father will not be around. That's fine. Some people believe in Jesus Christ, that's fine. I don't happen to, but I believe there is a spirit somewhere out there.

As far as I'm concerned, the climate for reproductive rights is now in the dark ages. It hasn't moved one bit from where it was in the '70s. Recently it has moved backwards. The religious right has moved into the Republican Party and has changed everything that has happened in the last twenty years. And I used to be a Republican.

We do live in a puritanical country. People have just had too much religion shoved down their throats. And that's so ingrained. How do you tell somebody to look away from their religion? We have men making decisions about women's bodies. Politics have entered our bedrooms.

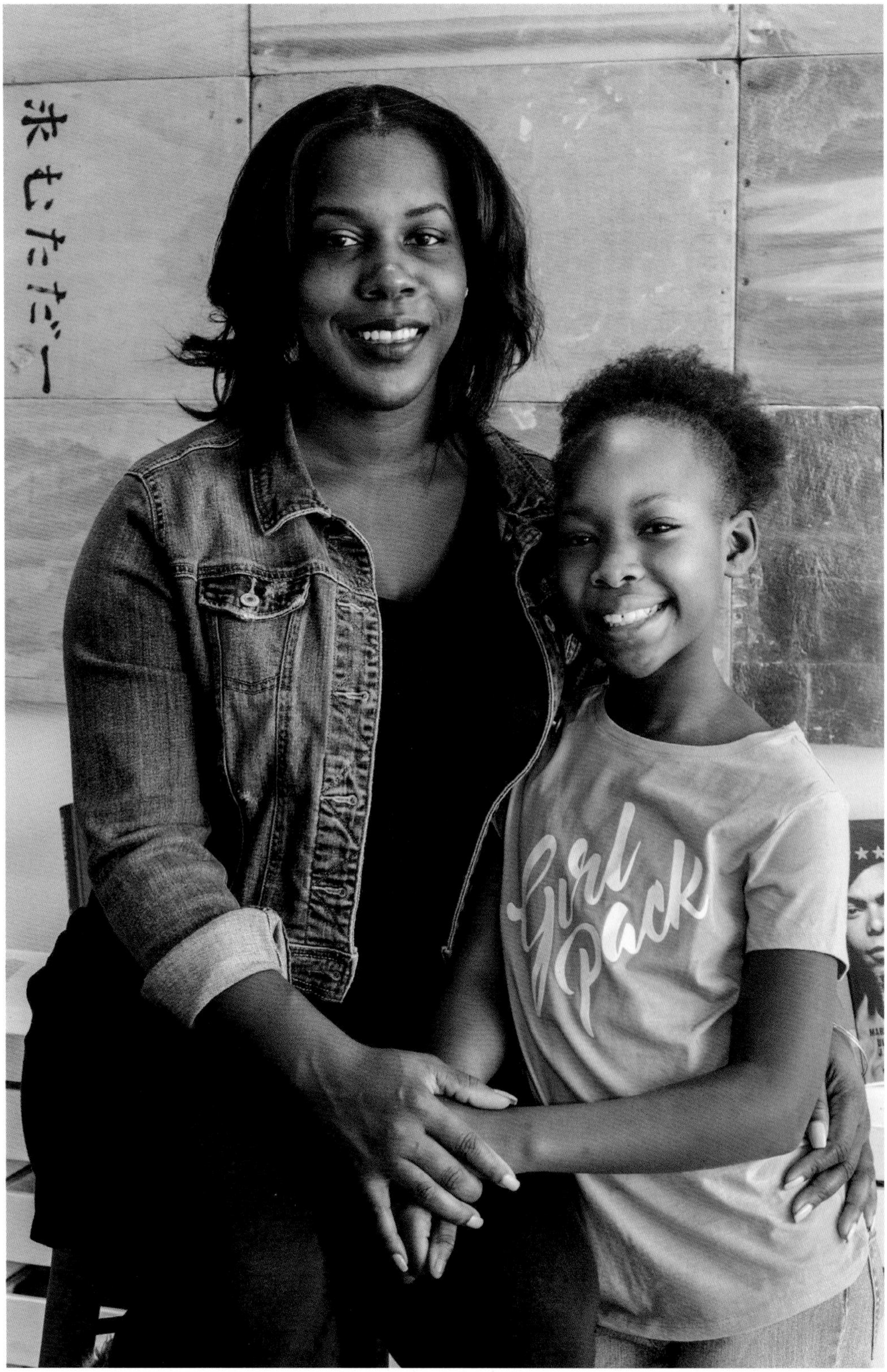

BRITTANY MOSTILLER

Brittany Mostiller

WHEN I BECAME pregnant in 2007, I had three small children: a newborn, a four-year-old, and my oldest was six. My family and my niece and sister were all sharing a two-bedroom apartment in Chicago. I was working part-time at Jewel, a local grocery store. I knew that I just could not afford to have another child financially, mentally, or emotionally. I couldn't.

I called the abortion clinic to schedule an appointment. At the time an abortion cost about $600 or $700. I was enrolled in Medicaid but I didn't know that Medicaid didn't cover abortions at the time. So, I chose to go to the County Hospital, which would have cost $50. But when I got there, I found that I was fourteen weeks along, and their limit was twelve weeks.

I was distraught. I was scared not to have the procedure. My mind was made up on it. That was the easy part for me. Accessing it and actually having the funds to pay for the abortion was the hardest part. I struggled to figure out how to come up with the money. If I had to wait for two more paychecks, I would then be about fifteen or sixteen weeks along and my procedure would cost about $900. I ended up borrowing money from my sister, from my great-grandmother, and receiving about a third of the cost from the Chicago Abortion Fund.

I went to a small, local clinic that performs first- and second-trimester abortions. The clinic was on the far North Side of Chicago. I'm from the South Side, I didn't have a car, didn't have a license, so I had to take public transportation. Plus, I wasn't familiar with the

North Side. It was almost a two-hour trip. I had to miss work. It was not easy trying to navigate that as a 23-year-old young woman. Definitely outside my comfort zone, but I knew it needed to be done.

I wasn't frightened by the procedure. When I'm dead set on something, I'm just determined to do it. It was just a part of the journey and what I needed to do in order to not carry this pregnancy to term and to live the life that I wanted. It was just another hurdle, I will say that.

Right before my abortion in 2007, I remember telling one of my best friends at the time, while I was walking to Jewel to work, that I wanted so much more out of life. I had no idea how I was going to get there, but I wanted my own space, my own car. I told her I wanted to finish school. I had all these dreams, not really a roadmap, just a destination.

I have four daughters, ages 16, 13, 11, and 5. They fuel my passion to do this work.

When I received a grant from the Chicago Abortion Fund, I just knew that I had found my political home and my purpose. The fund is a thirty-two-year-old organization that helps women who can't afford their abortion procedures. The communities we support are mostly low-income communities of color. I started volunteering and joined the staff in 2013 as deputy director. I am currently the program director. I get to focus on what continues to make me smile and feed my soul: advocacy and community organizing. I love being on the ground, in the communities, talking to community members about reproductive justice.

I have four daughters, ages 16, 13, 11, and 5. They fuel my passion to do this work. I'm raising young women, and everything we're fighting for now will impact them at some point.

Volunteering with the Fund for those years, I saw and experienced things I never would have imagined. Traveling for the first time on a plane, speaking on panels, and just becoming this leader in my own right within this movement really changed me as a person. It changed me as a parent. So when I got pregnant with my fourth daughter, I wanted to carry that pregnancy to term. I had grown as a mother, and I wanted to experience that with my youngest. It was quite a different experience being pregnant and having a baby at 28 instead of 17. I just felt like I knew how to go after things I wanted, to find the resources I needed, or fight like hell if they weren't available to me. I was just a different person.

I want my daughters to be seen as full human beings. I want them to live in a world where anti-blackness is non-existent. I know that's a big dream. I want them to know that just because they are Black girls and will be Black women, that they can still do anything, even though they have fight to be seen and heard. Yes, there are many barriers, but you can still kick ass and do it. I also want them to seek the love and care and nurturing they deserve. I try my best to give them that.

Being a part of the reproductive justice movement, I have found some amazing people, some amazing Black women. They have held me, and I am here partly because of them. Even on my worst days when I don't know how I'm going to continue, especially as someone who's struggled with depression and anxiety most of my adult life, I turn to them. And I get love from them and I give love back to them when I'm able to.

I WANT MY DAUGHTERS TO BE SEEN AS FULL HUMAN BEINGS. I WANT THEM TO LIVE IN A WORLD WHERE ANTI-BLACKNESS IS NON-EXISTENT.

My mother and aunt shared our apartment for most of my young life. So besides my two siblings, I also had my cousins. I watched my mom work sixteen-hour days sometimes. She's a certified nursing assistant. When she came up here, she left everything in Alabama, including the car. We took a Greyhound bus up here. I watched her put herself through school to get her nursing certificate with three small children. We wore clothes from thrift stores. We were poor, but we never went without. She loved us.

As I begin to raise teenagers, I realize that my mother taught me perseverance. She taught me to be fearless. And I know now that leaving Alabama the way she did took a lot of self-determination.

Before I became a parent, I was a whole person and I never want to lose that. I talk to my kids about that. I tell them I'm your mommy, but I'm still a person with dreams and aspirations and a life.

My children definitely know about my work. They've been to protests with me. They've been to community outreach. They are a part of this world too. My 11-year-old has already told me, "I don't think I would have an abortion, but I support other peoples' decision to have one."

Folks have been fighting for reproductive freedom for decades and centuries and a lifetime. It takes more than complacency. Sometimes it takes gathering your people and talking to them, as simple as that. My family's views on abortion, I wouldn't say that they're changed. However, the conversation is different. What folks say about queer folk, or abortion access, in my presence is different. They think about things differently now. I don't want folks to not be who they are. I just think it takes some conversations, and we can start there.

This is not just my work. This is my life. Our reproductive decisions and our reproductive health are always going to be a part of who we are.

Patricia Defechereux

MY MOTHER IS Irish, born in Dublin, and my father is Belgian. I was born in Belgium and spent most of my life there.

I acquired US citizenship in 2016, but in my heart, I feel Irish and Belgian. The subconscious part of me is probably from all that I swam in when I was a kid, what I was immersed in when I was growing up. I feel like I'm sitting between two chairs.

I'm a scientist. I did research on chicken pox. When I gave birth to my daughter in Belgium, right before we came to San Francisco, I got chicken pox. It wasn't related to my research! It was such a traumatic experience because I thought I was dying. And then I got postpartum depression pretty soon after the birth of my daughter, but it was totally undiagnosed.

After I completed my PhD in Belgium, I moved to the States with my husband and 8-month-old daughter to do postdoctoral AIDS research. We landed in San Francisco at the peak of the dot-com boom.

It was a very competitive, very intense period that put an enormous strain on my marriage. We were over here in a different culture with an infant. We arrived, no support, a lot of financial strains. My husband started studying to be a marriage and family therapist. It was extremely challenging emotionally, the whole bit.

I didn't realize how much the chicken pox and the depression had affected me. I think that's why my abortion happened. When my daughter was about a year and a half, I got pregnant again.

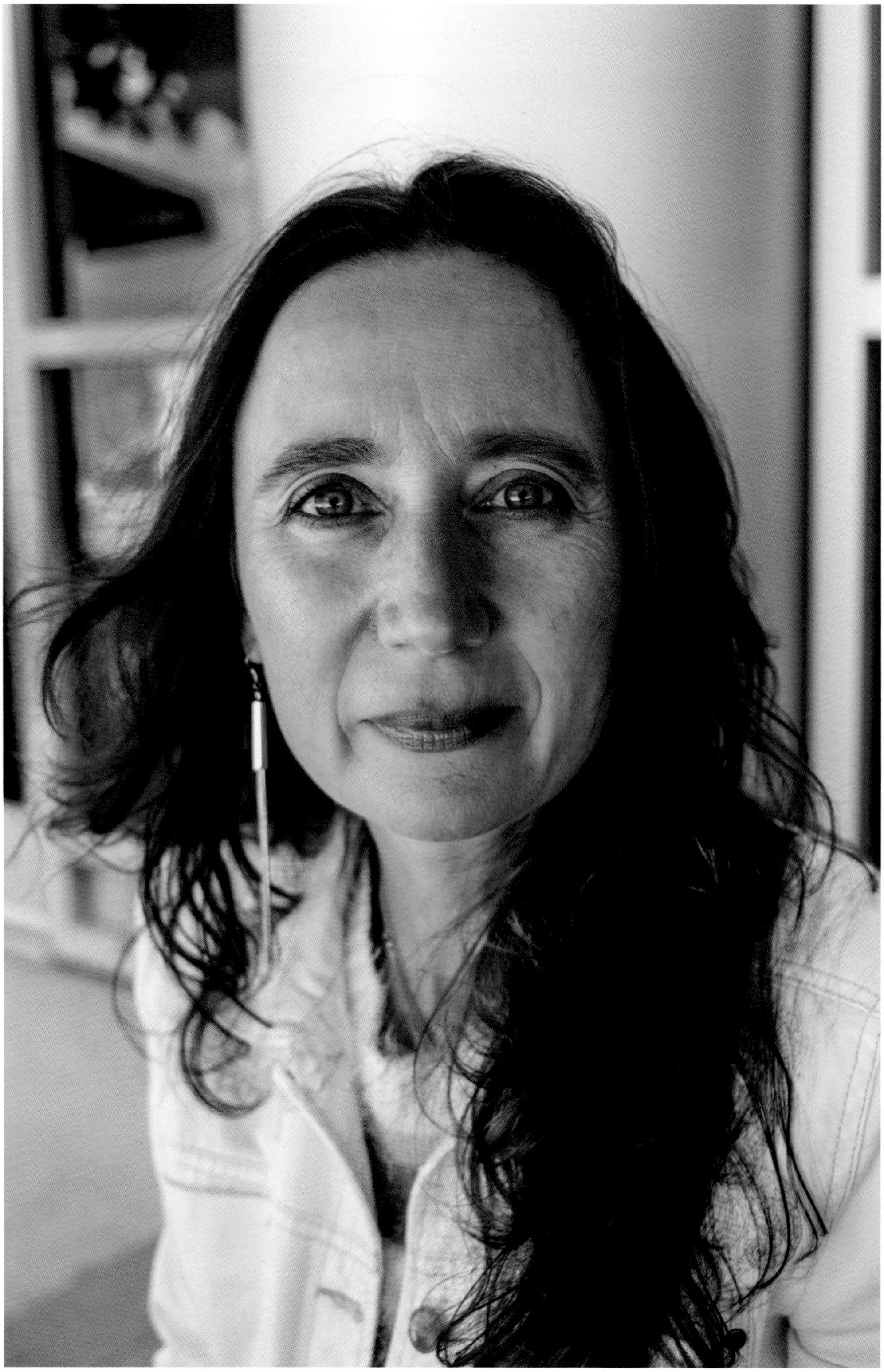

PATRICIA DEFECHEREUX

I wanted to have a second child but we couldn't have afforded to live here and have a second child without family support. And I was ill. I had depression. If we had gone ahead with the pregnancy, it would have meant going back to Europe. My husband was not really ready to do that. I wanted to go back to Europe. I would come home from the lab, I'd be crying. All I wanted to do was sleep. I wasn't really suicidal but I had dark thoughts and my relationship with my husband was unraveling. It was just such a chaotic time in our life.

At first, I wanted to keep the pregnancy, but the timing was wrong. Postpartum depression is really this evil demon that steals away years of people's lives. This was my first experience dealing with it and I think the decisions I made around that time were fraught with this extra layer of challenge. There's no doubt in my mind that if I had been supported by my network of family and friends in Europe, that we would have kept the baby. It was hard. It was hell.

I WANTED TO KEEP THE PREGNANCY, BUT THE TIMING WAS WRONG. POSTPARTUM DEPRESSION IS REALLY THIS EVIL DEMON THAT STEALS AWAY YEARS OF PEOPLE'S LIVES . . . THERE'S NO DOUBT IN MY MIND THAT IF I HAD BEEN SUPPORTED BY MY NETWORK OF FAMILY AND FRIENDS IN EUROPE, THAT WE WOULD HAVE KEPT THE BABY. IT WAS HARD. IT WAS HELL.

Having nobody to turn, to help me figure out what do, I remember calling my OBGYN in Belgium. Finally, a doctor who was working with me in the lab here helped me. I didn't know her very well, but I must have just gone up to her and asked her for help. She was very warm and caring. She helped me get an abortion at San Francisco General Hospital. The pregnancy was early on, early first trimester. I think I had a D & C, a dilation and curettage.

I remember the day I made the decision to go ahead with the abortion. I remember the day of the abortion. I remember the door going to the clinic. I remember being in the room. I remember the smell in that room. I remember waiting beforehand, almost passing out because my blood sugar dropped. It's such a powerful event.

My husband came with me. He held my hand throughout the procedure. It's funny, because we never much talked about it afterwards and I'm sure it contributed to the challenges we've had in our relationship afterwards.

The one person who was my support was my best friend with whom I was doing my postdoc at that time. Both of us were from Belgium. I shared all my struggles with her, including this unexpected pregnancy. I don't think I told my mom about the abortion.

I must have felt that she would be more judgmental. Also, I didn't want her to worry. She was so far away and she was already so worried about me.

Those years were extremely lonely and difficult. I still feel a sense of isolation, not having my family and my community close by; my old friends are not around. I think people work so hard here in the United States. It's all about work, work, work. It's not this way in Ireland and Belgium. There, it's more about family. People don't go to school so far from their parents and they don't set roots so far away. The parents, children, grandchildren are in the same town or in the next town up.

Afterwards my husband and I just drifted apart. We did one session of counseling. The therapist asked us if we wanted to split up. We both said yes, and to this day I wish we had done more work to make the marriage work. Maybe, had we done that, we'd still be together, but at the same time, we separated very peacefully.

What was terrible and still aches to this day is that my daughter really was devastated about the divorce. She was 2. She was angry about it for years and years and years. She talks about how hard it was.

I didn't tell my daughter about the abortion until a couple of years ago when she was 17 or 18. Her response was, "Why did you never tell me? I always wanted to have a sibling from you and papa that was the same blood." She has half siblings from her father's second marriage. She was really upset with me. She stormed out and the conversation ended there.

I think for her it brought back the pain of us splitting up, when she could have had a brother, a family life with us all together. Her reaction was not so much about killing a life. And, of course, that made me extremely sad because it's not the life I wanted for my daughter. That wasn't my intent.

I met my current husband in 2006. We have a son together who is now 8. I am convinced to this day that my son is the spirit of the pregnancy I aborted. I'm a scientist but I still am deeply spiritual. I have these beliefs in karmic connections. After the birth of my son, I had a second postpartum depression. I was very ill that time, I mean to the point of suicidal.

I just feel like nobody ought to ever judge you for doing what you choose to do because we try to make the best decision we can make at the time. I don't like to use the word "should," but we should not be punished for it. In this culture, people are being punished, not just an emotional punishment, but in really very tangible and dangerous ways.

In the United States, it becomes this crazy pro-life, pro-choice battle where people take guns and shoot people at abortion clinics. It's fucking ridiculous. Excuse my language, but it is already such a difficult decision for a woman. At least it was for me. It's an intense, emotional moment. On top of that, to have to deal with the judgment of society or your friends or your family, and then with being physically at risk because some fucking nut job thinks that you're killing lives and would shoot you or your doctor, it's ridiculous. It really is.

I'm a spiritual person and I really believe in preserving life. For heaven's sake, I've dedicated my entire life to saving lives and to fighting stigma, fighting HIV, which is also extremely stigmatized.

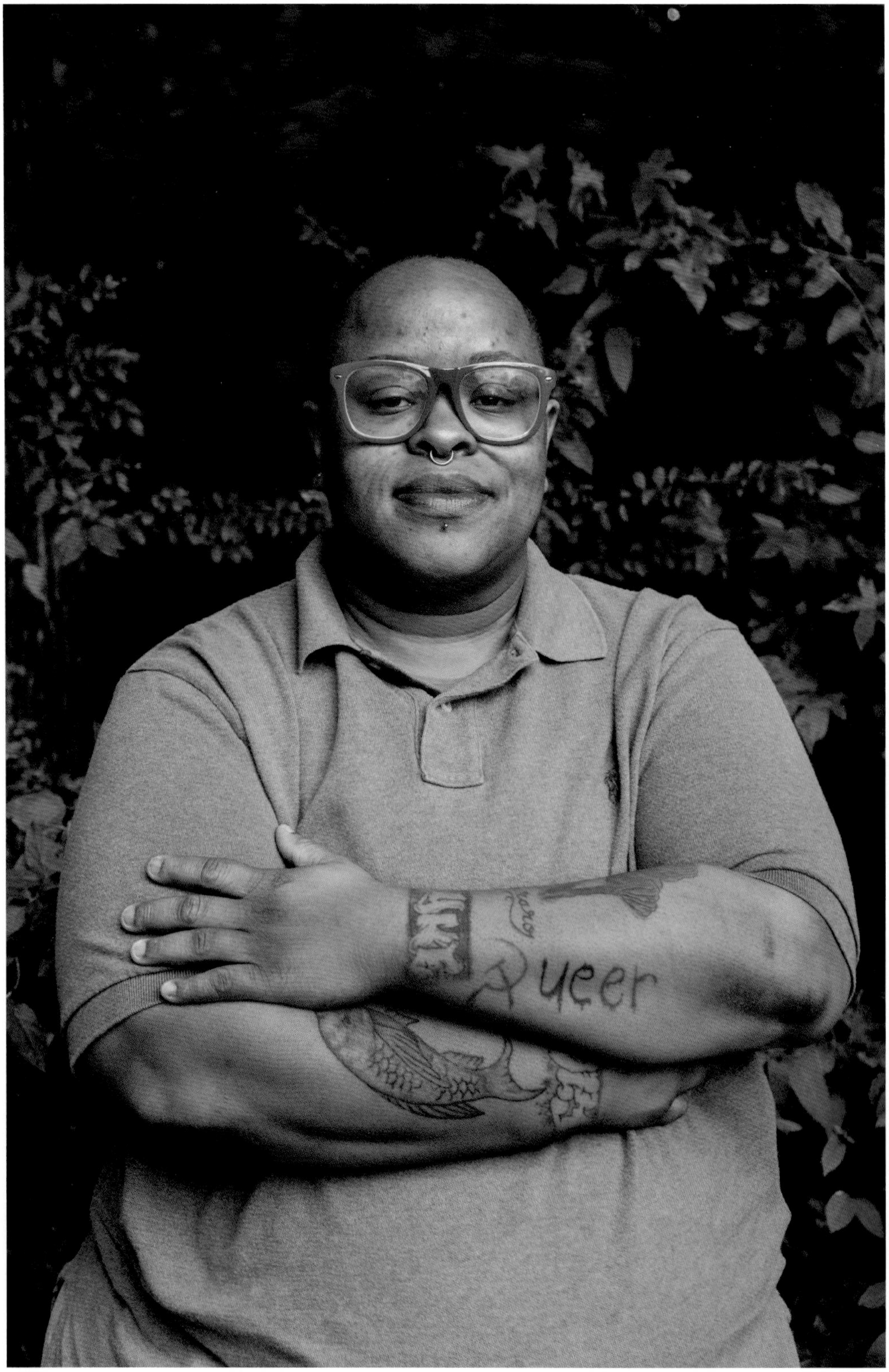

CAZEMBE JACKSON

Cazembe Jackson

I GREW UP in a family that was very proud to be a Black, very Baptist missionary. My mom was in leadership of the church the whole time I was growing up. My dad didn't really play that much of a role in our life growing up. He was around, but my mom was definitely the dominant parent.

I came out as a queer person when I was 12. Nobody took me seriously. My mom took me to my pastor's house. He basically said, "If you live this life, you will go to hell and hell is the worst place to go."

I think she has gotten used to me being queer, even me being trans, me being a social justice organizer. I talk about my abortion as it relates to reproductive justice and reproductive health, but I'm also an organizer who fights police brutality, who talks about race. I live my life in a way that says it's OK to be queer. It's OK to be trans. It's OK to be a Christian and have all of those things be together.

My abortion story is a story of so many things. I was a junior in college, and queer, mostly masculine presenting. During the week before finals, like everyone else, I was studying. I stayed late at the library; it might have been midnight or one in the morning. Normally, we would walk home with another person, but I stayed later than everybody that lived in my dorm and I walked home by myself. Four men in a truck approached me. I won't go into the details of what happened, mostly for my own sanity, but I was gang-raped by the four of them. They told me over and over it was because I was dressed like a boy. They knew that I was gay and that God wanted me to live a different life. Those were the things they said to me, as they raped me.

All four of them were Black, which just makes it so much more complicated. They beat me up and left me in a grassy space between the museum and the dorm. They all went to jail for six months apiece. The reason that they didn't get longer sentences—besides the obvious reason that the criminal justice system is a sham—is because I had asked them to wear a condom. Their lawyer argued that was consent, which the judge didn't buy, but also gave them shorter sentences because of it. About a month after that I found out I was pregnant. I also got an STD.

I called my mom to tell her that I was pregnant and try to figure out what I was supposed to do. Basically, she told me the reason this bad stuff had happened to me was because I was gay, which just made it worse because that's what the men said while they were raping me. But, she said she would come and pick me up, and I could come home. Of course, I had to say I would stop being gay. If I did that, she would help me get an abortion. So I said it and she took me to get the abortion.

I'm a non-binary trans person who uses he pronouns, who is actively trying to conceive a baby, and who's had an abortion.

There was a Planned Parenthood right around the corner, so access was easy. But it was hard to pay for. I got a payday loan for the $300 it was supposed to cost, but it ended up being more like $1,000. At the clinic, I took the pills and then, it was like, horrible. The worst diarrhea feeling I ever have felt and just pain. I wasn't prepared for that. My abortion wasn't a great experience, but what I appreciate still to this day is that I didn't have to worry about anyone pushing a whole bunch of Bible verses about me being gay. And, they had my mom wait in the lobby, so I got to talk to people by myself. The nurse even called a rape crisis center for me.

I'm a non-binary trans person who uses he pronouns, who is actively trying to conceive a baby, and who's had an abortion.

In 2017, I went to a retreat for abortion storytellers that Renee Bracey Sherman created. There was another Black trans person, and I was like, yes, I don't have to do this by myself! There's another trans person who already understands what I'm going through and what I'm talking about, about doctors, about the abortion, about all of the things.

Talking about reproductive justice is an uncomfortable topic for a lot of people on both sides. Non-trans people really don't understand how to shift their language to include people who have had abortions who are not women or even to talk about reproductive health in that way. I don't necessarily think that you have to replace "women" with "people" because I think it's very important that we talk about women having control over their bodies. I don't think that excludes trans people.

When I talk about women, I'm talking about women of all kinds, including trans women. I just think it's important to say, "Women, trans, and non-binary people," because that includes everyone. It took so long for me to be able to see myself as a part of reproductive justice because nobody was saying that trans people are a part of this. Nobody was saying that it's more than just women.

I'M A MEMBER OF BASICALLY AN ALL-BLACK QUEER CHURCH IN ATLANTA, AND I'M THERE EVERY SUNDAY THAT I CAN. THE GOD THAT'S IN MY LIFE DOES LOVE ME UNCONDITIONALLY AND LOVES EVERYBODY.

I used to say I was married to the movement because I didn't care about being in a relationship. I didn't care about going out and having fun. I cared about reading books and being in the street with people who were resisting oppression.

But now I'm in a relationship and me and my partner are actively trying to conceive. We're waiting for our appointment with the fertility specialist because we've been trying for months with just a third-party donor and I'm not getting pregnant. My doctor told me they're going to call this a geriatric pregnancy because I'm 38, and that I probably need some assistance with the fertility part at this point.

I'm going to carry. I got off of testosterone a year ago, so that I could start having my cycle again, so that I could get pregnant. I postponed my top surgery because I want to be able to breastfeed.

What I want to do is create a life in my body, give birth to it and then love it, and feed it, and take care of it as long and as best as I can with my partner. I feel secure enough that I could have a kid and that my kid will have a family that will love it and take care of it like a family.

Audre Lorde said, "We don't live single-issue lives, so we can't build single-issue movements." So I have to put as much energy into talking about my abortion story as I do into fighting for low wage workers, into fighting against police brutality, and against state violence toward Black people and poor white people and brown people.

I'm a member of basically an all-Black queer church here in Atlanta, and I'm there every Sunday that I can. The God that's in my life does love me unconditionally and loves everybody.

This is what I tell my mom. My God is big enough for me that it doesn't matter to me if your God is not accepting, because my God is enough already. Yeah, so I'm cool with it. It's fine and she gets to have her God.

The world I would like to bring babies into is one where they're able to just be a kid for as long as they can. I want them to not have to worry about if they'll be able to make a living wage or take care of themselves. I don't want them to have to worry about getting shot by a police officer. If they do happen to have ovaries, I want them to be able by law to have control of them, and whatever it is that they want to do with their body. I'd like that world for all of the babies that are not born. Yeah.

It took so long for me to be able to see myself as a part of reproductive justice because nobody was saying that trans people are a part of this. Nobody was saying that it's more than just women.

Margret Cawley

ONE OF MY first memories about abortion was seeing a bumper sticker on the car of a woman we went to church with. It was the heartbeat sticker, like "Abortion stops a heartbeat." I had no idea what the word abortion meant. I was maybe 7 years old. I went inside and told my mom that abortion was bad, and she said, "Well, wait a minute. That's not always true. Women need to be able to have them. When you're older you'll find out what it is."

I grew up not far from here, on the east side of Cleveland. My parents were liberal Catholics. I went to public schools through ninth grade and transferred to a Catholic high school where we even had sex education! I started college at St. John's University in Queens, New York, but realized I was really Midwestern and needed to come home, so I transferred to Case Western here in Cleveland. That was a rough transition and then some life events took shape and I've been out of school since then.

I'm 28 years old now and I have a 2-year old daughter. Eight weeks after my daughter was born, I got pregnant again. It was a very tumultuous time in my life. My daughter's father is a recovering drug addict. I just knew that I had to provide for my daughter. I decided that it would be impossible for me to carry the second pregnancy to term.

I was about eight or nine weeks pregnant when I called an abortion clinic in Cleveland. Well, I feel very fortunate that I live in this liberal bubble oasis within Ohio, Cuyahoga County. The next available appointment was about a week and a half away. If I had lived

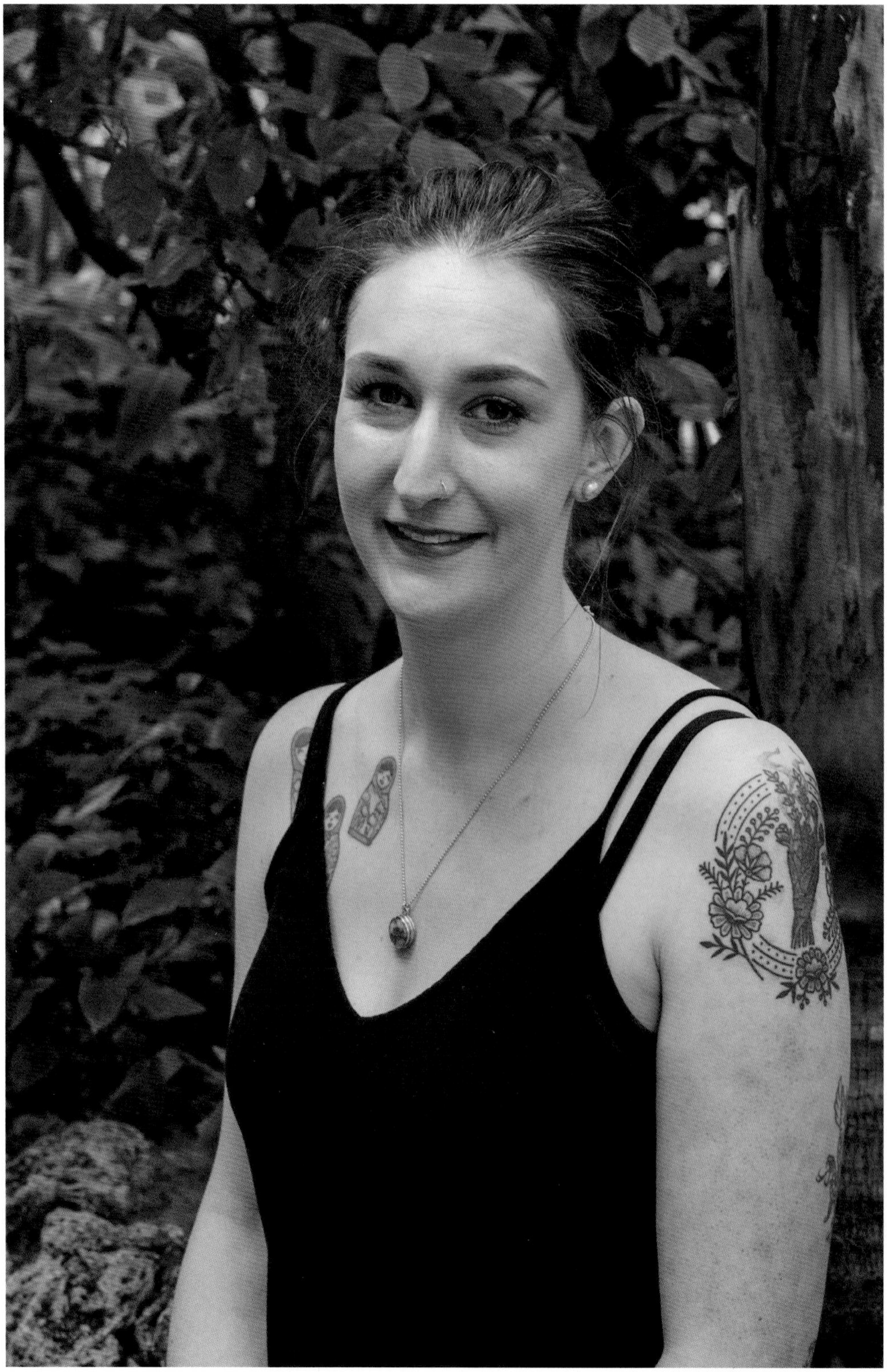

MARGRET CAWLEY

in Dayton or Cincinnati or Toledo it would have been way more challenging. Those cities are really struggling right now to keep their clinics open.

The first time I went to the clinic I went by myself. When I had my abortion, I was still on maternity leave. I had just gotten my tax refund, so I had the money and the time. It cost about $495. My boyfriend came when I had the procedure.

I had the abortion without anesthesia. At my stage in the pregnancy you were allowed to choose, so I just did it without anything. I don't like feeling loopy, especially not just twelve weeks after having gone through natural birth.

It was a pretty simple surgical procedure, the vacuum suction. It took about two and a half minutes. It felt like getting a Pap smear, which is uncomfortable, but pretty routine as a woman. The doctor was very professional and straightforward, but also very kind. Afterwards, they wheeled me into the recovery room. I sat in a recliner. They gave me ginger ale, checked on me, and asked if I was OK. They sent me home maybe a half hour after. I drove myself home, picked up my daughter, and carried on.

It sounds really weird to say, but I loved my abortion. That is not most people's experience in Ohio. If you're coming from down south, chances are you have a very conservative family and you're coming by yourself or with a female friend or an aunt. It's not normal yet to tell your employer that you need two days off during a three-week span of time to have an abortion. I could tell my bosses that.

The law in Ohio mandates a twenty-four-hour waiting period. You go to the clinic on the first day to have an ultrasound to confirm your pregnancy, see how far along you are, assess what procedure you'll need. That's when they make you pay the first part of the bill. You also meet with the patient advocate for a state-mandated session, where they basically tell you all your options. They have to give you a list of possible medical complications that could happen—like you could hemorrhage or die, all sorts of things. They tell you this in a way that is deceptive because they don't tell you statistics or rates of these things happening. They ask you how you feel about things, read you all this literature, offer you the opportunity to see the ultrasound and tell you if a heartbeat was detected.

Governor Kasich wrote a real nice little statement that the advocates have to read aloud. I just remember my advocate read me this whole thing and exhaled, "This is what I'm telling you. You can see the ultrasound." I just looked at her and said, "That's some state literature, isn't it?" She was surprised and agreed that's exactly what it is.

Most of the advocates are really passionate people, but they only have about fifteen minutes to talk to you after they get through all of the state jargon. Their job after the session is to actually file a report on why you're having the abortion. And you still have to schedule the second appointment to have the procedure. That can take three days to two weeks depending on how busy the clinic is.

On the second visit, you have to meet with the physician. They basically explain everything to you again. You have to sign a whole bunch of paperwork. It's a lot of sitting and waiting around.

Ohio has a twenty-week ban. One of the girls I know passed over from the first trimester to the second trimester, and she couldn't get an abortion anymore in Ohio because of that twenty-four-hour waiting period. An abortion in the second trimester is a more invasive procedure and it would've cost $400 or $500 more. She wasn't going be able to get that much money before she reached the twenty weeks. So she carried the pregnancy. She had a miscarriage and was really devastated by it. She went from not being ready for the pregnancy to fully embracing it, which is a roller coaster of emotions to go through in one pregnancy. It was really heartbreaking.

> **I FELT LIKE MY ABORTION WAS A SOUL-SEARCHING EXPERIENCE FOR ME AS A NEW MOTHER. MY ABORTION WAS MY FIRST MAJOR PARENTING DECISION. I FEEL LIKE I GAVE MY DAUGHTER A GIFT IN HAVING IT.**

When I was at the clinic doing the paperwork for my abortion, there was this little half-sheet of crumpled paper that said, "Do you want to participate in a fellowship? There's a stipend." So I filled out the form. This turned out to be the most amazing thing that I've ever done.

The fellowship is education and training for women to become pro-choice advocates in the community in their own ways. We did a lot of group exercises with writing, public speaking, podcasts, lobbying, and panel discussions. In some ways it was almost therapy. It's a very tight-knit group of women who are ready to go, "Yeah!" This fellowship and the friendships I've made are the coolest things that ever happened to me.

I'm in the second year of the fellowship now, doing an independent project researching the kinds of practical support offered by local and regional nonprofits. I'm compiling data to help nonprofits create strategies and programs for women accessing abortions from the different areas our major clinics serve.

My abortion gave me so much peace of mind. I felt like I was in good hands the whole way. I didn't feel much stigma. I felt like my abortion was a soul-searching experience for me as a new mother. My abortion was my first major parenting decision. I feel like I gave my daughter a gift in having it. It also gave me an opportunity to navigate a really tumultuous situation in my personal life, and I'm grateful for it.

More than anything I feel gratitude. When I look at all the ways that I really get to experience my daughter developing because I have the time and the energy to commit to really being with her, I sometimes pause and think that I wouldn't be able to do this if I had had to go through another pregnancy and raise another child.

I'm also pleased that my boyfriend is a happy part of our lives these days. He has more confidence and is working hard every day to be a positive force in our lives.

My daughter is the brightest spot in my life. Almost on a daily basis I am just grateful that I was able to have the procedure. I want my daughter to feel comfortable in her own skin, in her own body. If she needs a simple medical procedure like an abortion, I want her to be able to choose to talk to me or not. In my dream world, she presents her insurance card and the procedure is covered. She goes in and can have a same-day procedure; she doesn't have to read state literature that uses the word "baby."

I would like people to know from my story that it can be a positive experience, that you can make this decision in spite of the stigma, you can make this decision in spite of laws and restrictive legislation, and that it's OK to be confident in your decision.

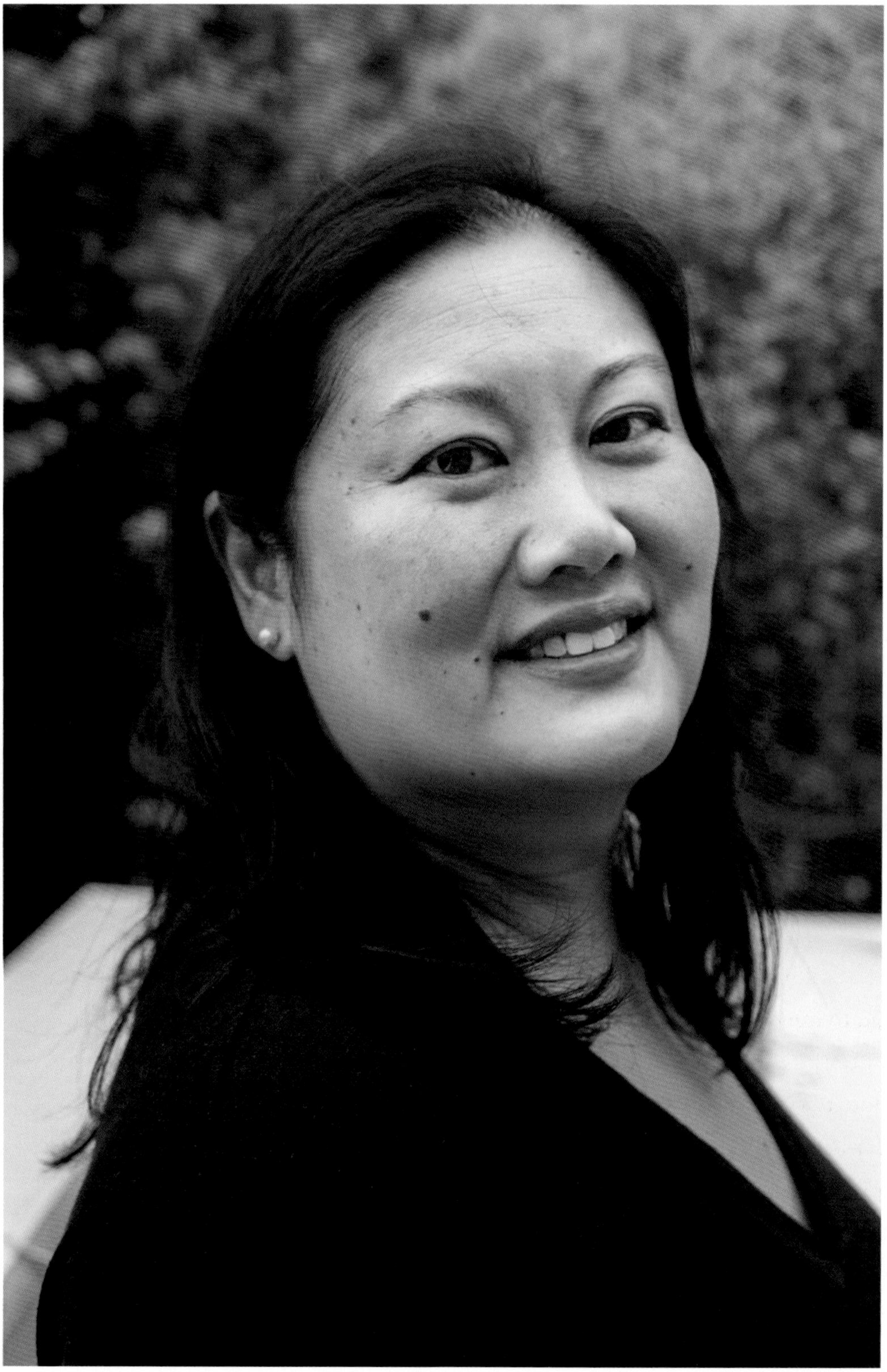

KARBO TAM

Karbo Tam

MY MOM ALWAYS told me it was my job to concentrate on my studies because that would be the gateway to everything else. My mom and dad emigrated from Taiwan and Hong Kong, respectively, in the '70s. They were really hard working. We lived in San Francisco's Tenderloin district and they owned a laundromat.

It was so intense as an immigrant family just keeping our heads above water. My mom's very practical and she drove the dynamic in our family, where everything was goal-oriented. Whenever I joined things like volleyball in school or when I sang in a choir, I explained them to my mom as things that would look good on my college applications. Enjoying volleyball or music wasn't a reason to participate. I was the first person in our family to go to college.

I felt a responsibility to my mom and dad who had given up so much so that my sister and I could go to the best schools, and have the things that we needed. Sometimes I almost felt like two people. At home, it was all focused on being a student. At school, I could be a little bit more free and enjoy some of the things that were developing in me. I kept the two worlds fairly separate.

So many things were not talked about in my family, including sex, relationships, and feelings. I haven't actually talked about my abortion very much. I'm crying now because the abortion was when those two parts of my life came together in a very real way.

I was in high school when I had my abortion. We had finished our final exams and I had missed my period. I bought a pregnancy test at the grocery store. It was positive. I was super scared. My boyfriend certainly wasn't prepared to be a father. He had already moved away to college. I knew I couldn't have a baby or be a mother.

I felt very much that telling my family I was pregnant would be a disaster. This was the exact opposite of everything they had hoped for me. And, of course, they didn't know that I was sexually active. In the Chinese community, like it's almost assumed that you're asexual and then you find a husband and then you get married and have a baby.

Luckily, I had close and resourceful friends to talk to. We found Planned Parenthood's phone number in the Yellow Pages. We called, and Planned Parenthood helped me figure out how to pay for the abortion using Medi-Cal. I went to the office and applied for Medi-Cal, and then we set a date for the procedure. I had only one friend with a car, but we got the dates mixed up and arrived on the wrong day.

When we talked about rescheduling, the counselor was really kind. She said Planned Parenthood wasn't required to tell my mom or my parents at all. That was my decision. But it planted a seed, and so I told my mom. It was a little bit out of necessity because I couldn't ask my friend to drive me again to the next date to have the procedure. The first thing that I told my mom was please don't kick me out of the house. She was very disappointed in me. She just started crying and crying. Nonetheless, it felt OK to have told her and she accompanied me to the procedure. She was in the waiting room the entire time, sobbing. I think it was painful for her too.

I had a surgical abortion. It was my first pelvic exam. It was my first anything with the physician down with my genitals. I'd been seeing a pediatrician still at that point. It was pretty uncomfortable.

There was a woman, maybe a medical assistant or a nurse, who accompanied me through the different steps of the day. I felt so grateful to have the support that I kind of wanted from my mom. I still remember what she looked like—she wore purple-rimmed glasses—and how she made me feel. After the procedure, I went back in to hug her and thank her. I remember feeling like, "Wow, she made such a big difference for me. I hope that someday I can return the favor."

Anyway, we took the bus home. My mom and I never talked about it again.

I'm so grateful that I had a safe choice, a protected choice. Even though I ended up telling my parents, the law protected me from having to do that or get their permission, which I am so grateful for.

I went to medical school thinking I might not do anything related to women's health, but I kept coming back to it. I wanted to contribute in an individual way where people could trust me and I could help them. Even though providing abortions is a pretty small part of my practice today, it's probably the most rewarding part.

When I went to medical school in Philadelphia I met a much more politically diverse group of people. It blew my mind that there are people who are anti-choice. A large group of colleagues didn't even agree with providing contraception and safer sex education to the women's shelter where we volunteered. Conversations with them weren't very productive, but they propelled me into being more political about abortion. I realized that I was very lucky, that not everybody in the country had the choices that I had, that our laws here in California are actually so great compared to other places. I joined Medical Students for Choice, which gave me some tools to evaluate what I really believed in and to talk to people on the other side about how we can work together.

Those tools helped a lot in trying to bring termination services to our hospital. We were challenged by nursing staff who were primarily Catholic, Filipino women and men who didn't want to participate. In partnership with our ethics director, we had meetings where we talked about what it means to be a medical provider, what brought us all into medicine. Everyone, similar to me, wanted to help people.

We talked about whether you can make the comparison to a person who comes in because of a drug overdose or alcoholism issues that resulted in massive liver failure, or somebody who's brought in with gunshot wounds because they were participating in street violence. You may not agree with that person's lifestyle or the habits that have led to the medical problem, but your calling in being a nurse or a physician is to help the people who come to you for health care.

YOU MAY NOT AGREE WITH THAT PERSON'S LIFESTYLE OR THE HABITS THAT HAVE LED TO THE MEDICAL PROBLEM, BUT YOUR CALLING IN BEING A NURSE OR A PHYSICIAN IS TO HELP THE PEOPLE WHO COME TO YOU FOR HEALTH CARE.

I want to think that my colleagues believe that I am providing termination services because I believe in it. It's part of medicine and part of my role as an obstetrician gynecologist. Others may have different beliefs, but they still trust me as a physician and as a person. It makes me feel really good that I can be open and do what I believe in, and still be a physician for all these people.

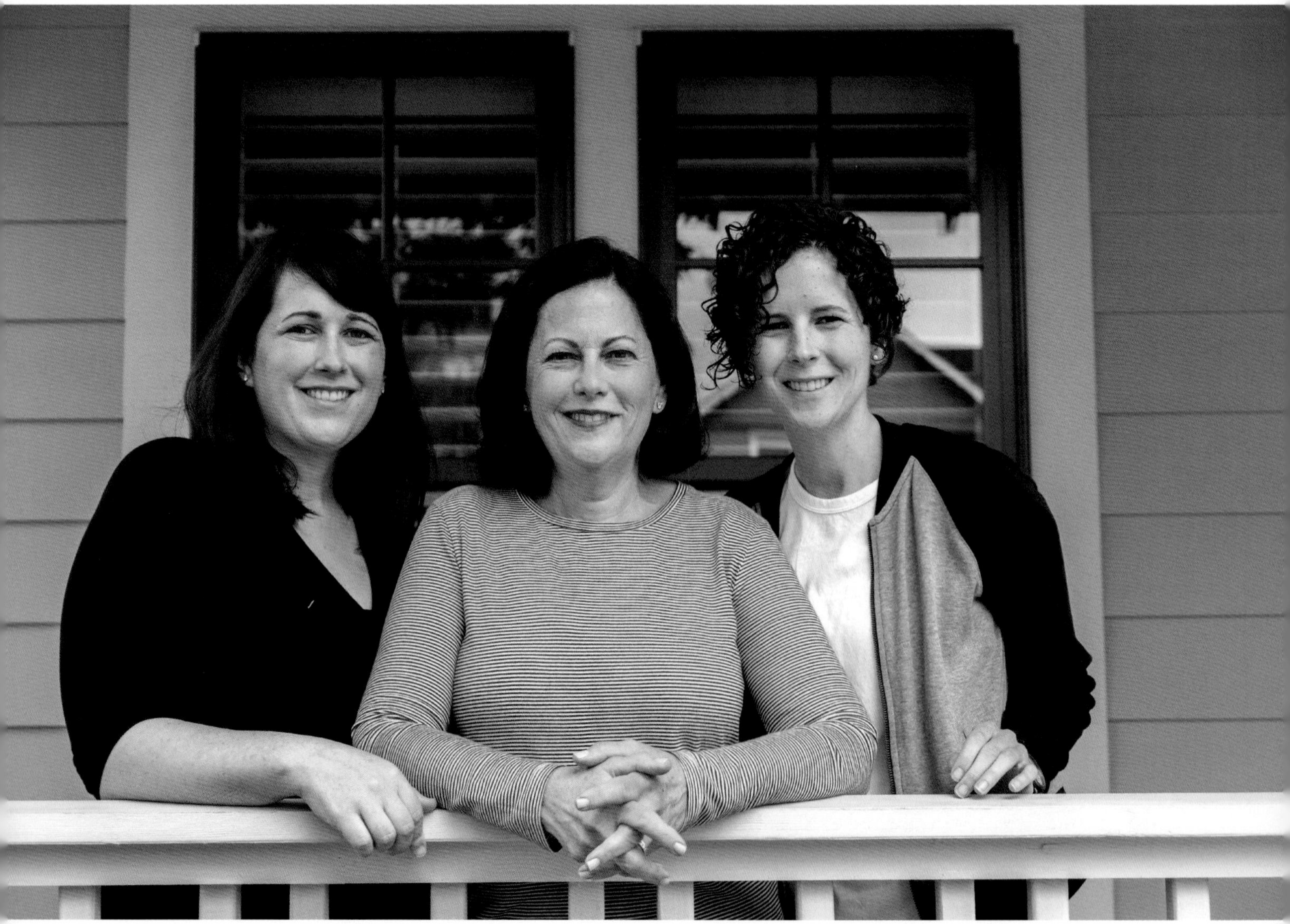

BETH, SHERRY, AND BRETT MERFISH

The Merfish Family—Sherry, Gerald, daughters Beth and Brett

Sherry: As we were growing up, the message was, "Do not get pregnant." When my mother told me about the birds and the bees, my first comment was, "I have a sister, there are just two of us. That's OK mom, you only did it twice." I got the message that sex was not a healthy activity or a normal part of living.

In the fall of 1972, I was a college senior at the University of Texas. The pill had just become available. But getting the pill would be acknowledging myself as a sexual being and that seemed dangerous. Nonetheless, I cautiously started to acknowledge myself as a sexual being. But I still held a lot of guilt about having sex outside of marriage.

A few months before Roe v. Wade, in '72, I got pregnant with Gerald, now my husband of forty-five years. When I thought I might be pregnant, we went to the student health center at the University of Texas. In those days, you needed a blood test to find out if you were pregnant. I can remember where I was, what I wore when I found out I was pregnant. I was stunned. But I had never shied away from tackling a problem.

Fortunately, our counselor told us about a clinic in New Mexico where I could get an abortion.

Gerald: I had a bit of money in a savings account. I withdrew some of that and we got a loan from the university emergency aid fund.

Sherry: Before our top-secret excursion to New Mexico, we went to San Antonio for the Jewish High Holidays. There I was on Yom Kippur, the Day of Atonement, sitting in a synagogue, knowing I was pregnant and had scheduled an abortion. I remember sitting in the temple and the sound of the chorus changed to the sound of crickets. I felt I had a black mark on me.

Gerald: It was tumultuous for me, but I was worried about you. You were burdened for both of us.

Sherry: I had no way of preparing for my abortion. I walked through those clinic doors feeling like I was entrusting my life and my future fertility to people I didn't know. I was about to be 21 years old.

At the first appointment, the doctor was distant. He didn't make any sort of human connection. When we returned the next morning, I still can feel myself putting one foot in front of the other, putting on a gown and sitting in a circle of eight women.

One woman was sobbing uncontrollably. I wanted to comfort her but it was very clear that you were supposed to stay in your seat. Also, I didn't want anybody to identify me. A nurse gave us pamphlets about contraception. With such self-assurance, she said she was sure we would all be repeat customers at the clinic. I remember thinking to myself, although birth control methods can fail, I will never be here again.

Gerald: I think what I was most scared about was our ability to conceive children later.

Sherry: Back on campus after the abortion, we focused on plans for our graduation and wedding. When I shopped for a wedding dress with my mother, I looked in the mirror and the white wedding dress appeared to be black!

Although I was a feminist before my abortion, afterwards my commitment to women's rights was strengthened. I was very aware of my privilege; that I had been at a big university with resources. That I was white. I couldn't help but think about women whose choices were so much more restricted and the desperation they faced.

As I continued my work for women's rights, I realized I was a part of a movement. My own mother, who died of breast cancer at age 47, was starting to understand why I was a feminist. I took her to hear Gloria Steinem. I saw a glimmer of her understanding that this wasn't a phase for me. Had my mother not died so young, I think eventually we could have had the conversation about my abortion.

ALTHOUGH I WAS A FEMINIST BEFORE MY ABORTION, AFTERWARDS MY COMMITMENT TO WOMEN'S RIGHTS WAS STRENGTHENED. I WAS VERY AWARE OF MY PRIVILEGE; THAT I HAD BEEN AT A BIG UNIVERSITY WITH RESOURCES. THAT I WAS WHITE. I COULDN'T HELP BUT THINK ABOUT WOMEN WHOSE CHOICES WERE SO MUCH MORE RESTRICTED AND THE DESPERATION THEY FACED.

I have advocated for women for more than four decades, including sixteen years working at Emily's List, a political action committee dedicated to electing Democratic, pro-choice women candidates. But I told no one of my abortion that entire time.

When my daughters Brett and Beth went off to college, I was determined they would not leave without knowing my abortion story. Certainly, they knew where I stood on the issue. They had been at protests with me. They had put together birth control packets at Planned Parenthood for their bat mitzvahs. But hearing about my abortion revealed a new dimension about me. I think they were both shocked.

Brett: In 1999, I was a very young 18-year-old, still an adolescent really. I remember wondering, "Why are you telling me this now?" It seemed to be a much bigger deal for her to tell me than it was for me to hear it. I was surprised, but it was just an experience she had that she had kept secret. By 2013, I would occasionally ask her why she hadn't told other people. Her answer was, "It's private. That's my thing to tell and it's a secret." I didn't tell any of my friends because it wasn't my story.

Beth: Maybe I'm more judgmental than Brett, and that's why I remember having a different reaction. I remember every single moment when my parents dropped me off for college. We were in the hotel room and my dad said, "Well, I'm going to leave the hotel room now." Which felt like a very strange thing to do.

My mom set the emotional stage by prefacing her story with, "I never want you to think there's anything so bad that you can't come to us with it.'" She also told me never to share this story with anyone. Ever." At the end of it, she asked if I had any questions. I was dumbfounded, I could not think of any questions. Then my dad came back in the room and he said, "Do you have any questions for me?" And I was still dumbfounded.

Afterwards, it seemed like there had been a shift in how I knew her. Not that I judged her, but I felt like I needed to figure out how this information fit into the person I knew.

Brett had already known for two years, and she didn't tell me even though we talk about everything! I was fiercely pro-choice, but I had internalized the narrative that other women did this. Not my women, not my hero. It took a while, and I actually remember, like a year later, I brought it up to my mom. I said, "Are we ever going to talk about it again?" And she said, "We can talk about it again." It was never mentioned again. It wasn't a disclosure that turned into a dialogue. I felt like it was my mom's deep, dark secret.

I WAS FIERCELY PRO-CHOICE, BUT I HAD INTERNALIZED THE NARRATIVE THAT OTHER WOMEN DID THIS. NOT MY WOMEN, NOT MY HERO.

Sherry: I wish I could change that, but at the time I was still dealing with the stigma.

Beth: Going to an Emily's List conference with my mom a couple of years later helped me assimilate the information. Her colleagues there were incredible people. We were all sitting in a restaurant having root beer floats. As they talked, one woman said she'd had an abortion. One by one they all told their abortion stories and I heard my mom talk for the first time outside of the family about her abortion. I thought, *Oh, my mom has a peer group!*

Brett: I am a lawyer at a public interest law center in Austin, where I lobby at the Texas Legislature. My mother was visiting in 2013, when State Senator Wendy Davis was attempting to defeat by filibuster a bill that would further restrict abortion in Texas. Together, Mom and Beth and I went down to the Capitol, stopping to get orange T-shirts—the color adopted by supporters of the filibuster.

Sherry: I had not seen a sight like that since we protested the Vietnam War. It incredible to see such a commanding presence. Everybody was wearing orange.

I'll never forget when we walked up and I was so excited, Brett turned to me and said, "Mother, don't get arrested."

Beth: At ten to midnight, the Republican leadership shut off the Democratic senators' microphones and tried to call for a vote on the bill even though the commentary wasn't over. They claimed Wendy Davis had violated the filibuster by having some help getting a back brace put on. It was ludicrous.

Brett: So we just screamed and they couldn't get any business done.

Beth: We knew that screaming, no matter how powerful we felt, was not going to win the vote. And we did lose. In my bedraggled state I just turned to my mom and said, "I just feel like if women talked about their stories more . . . "

Sherry: When we got in the car, Beth said she wanted to write an op-ed drawing parallels about disclosure between the gay rights movements and the women's rights movement and, "I want to use your experience as an example."

Beth: By then, I had written the op-ed in my head. At home I sat on my bed and typed it up. I had been processing this story for twelve years. I emailed it to my mom and went into the other room as she read it.

Sherry: My reaction was, "Let's go."

"My Mother's Abortion" was published by the *New York Times*. I was shocked and remain shocked that, forty years after Roe V. Wade, the tale of somebody's extremely early abortion was still newsworthy.

WHEN I PICTURE MY 20-YEAR-OLD SCARED BUT DETERMINED SELF, COULD I EVER HAVE IMAGINED THAT LATER I WOULD GIVE BIRTH TO TWO DAUGHTERS, THAT I WOULD SHARE MY STORY WITH THEM, AND THAT THEY WOULD BE THE ONES WHO WOULD ENCOURAGE ME TO TELL IT SO PUBLICLY?

When I picture my 20-year-old scared but determined self, could I ever have imagined that later I would give birth to two daughters, that I would share my story with them, and that they would be the ones who would encourage me to tell it so publicly? Who could imagine that trajectory? I couldn't have done it without them.

I wanted my story to be a catalyst. It was always about getting women to be more authentic about their lives and be honest with whomever they chose to share their story.

Telling your story is powerful and I want more women to feel empowered, to feel that they don't have to justify their choices, because no one knows better than you what you're prepared to do. I want other women to feel good about their choices, and above all, not to feel alone. Because they're not alone.

Gerald: And to know that there's just no shame to it. Shame on us that we weren't brave enough to talk about it while our parents were alive.

Sherry: Some of my older relatives called me after the story appeared to ask if I had thought about my mother when I agreed to publish it. I told them: "I was thinking about your daughters, your granddaughters, your sisters. That's who I thought about."

Beth: Last summer I had a miscarriage after having some prenatal testing. Had we known the test results before I miscarried, we would've terminated the pregnancy. That is something my husband and I want to talk about openly with our 2½-year-old daughter and the daughter we are now expecting. For us, it won't be dramatic, the way my mom did it. It will just be part of the story of how our family came to be. I hope I'm as good at parenting as my parents are; that she and her sister have the kind of bond that my sister and I have.

I'M PROUD OF MY MOM FOR BEING BRAVE WHEN SHE WAS 20 AND BEING BRAVE WHEN SHE WAS 60.

Each experience I have as a mother, gives me more and more compassion for what my mom has experienced. I can't hear my mom talk about going into the abortion clinic when she was 20 without crying. I went for a D & C with a husband who could hold my hand the whole time and doctors who were totally compassionate. My D & C was because of a miscarriage, but if it had been because of a termination, the experience would've been the same. I also want my daughter to know this about her grandmother's abortion experience when she's old enough to understand it.

Sherry: We have to own our stories.

Brett: I'm proud of my mom for being brave when she was 20 and being brave when she was 60.

Oriaku Njoku

I'M A FIRST-GEN immigrant. My dad came to the States to do his Master's at Michigan State University and my mom moved shortly after. Then we moved to Bloomington, Indiana, so my dad could get his PhD. After that we moved to Bowling Green, Kentucky, where I think we were the only family from Nigeria.

Igbo people—one of the 250 ethnic groups in Nigeria—are people of service. We were always told to never forget where you came from. Always remember your family. Family is not just your cousins, your sister, your brother, but it's our community. That definitely has come through with me in everything I do.

Ours was a fun household where there was lots of music and different cultural opportunities and experiences. Growing up, I was kind of a nerd, and there were a lot of expectations being the first born. There was a lot of pressure to live up to this ideal and make my parents proud by becoming a success, a doctor or a lawyer.

I went to the University of Kentucky. That is where I came out as a lesbian. Coming out to my parents was such a tough moment. My mom started crying. My dad said, even though it was hard, they would do what they could to support me. We had a family prayer and then I went back to college. Two weeks later my parents drove up to Lexington to see me. My dad told me that my being a lesbian was not "settling right with spirits." They were begging me not to be gay. He even said, "If we had known, we would've sent you to a convent." That's when I kicked them out of my apartment. Five years later they realized

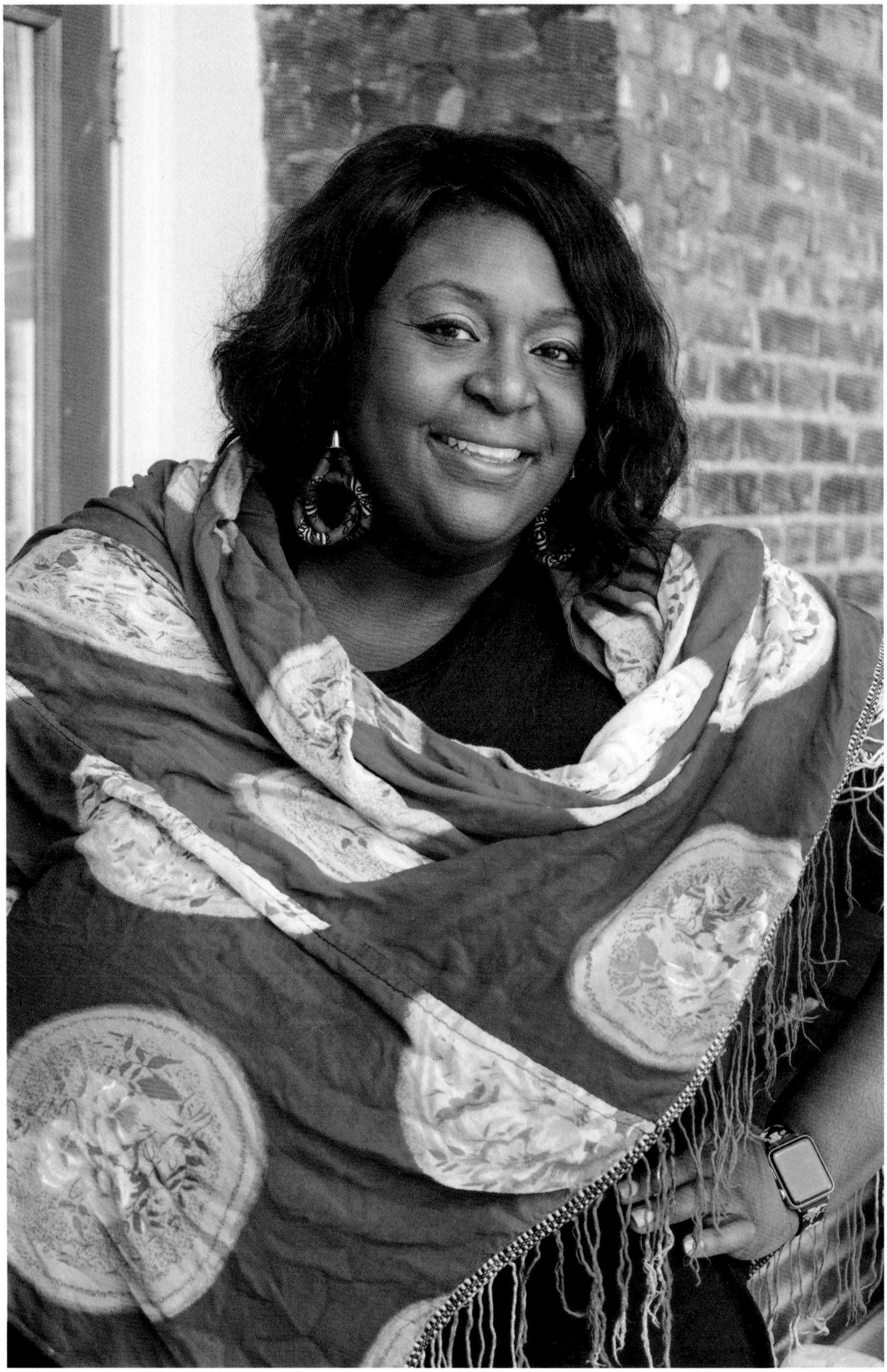

ORIAKU NJOKU

they wanted our family back. At that time, we really regained trust with each other. Now my mom is my best friend.

I do not have an abortion story; my sister Chi Chi does. Back in 2010, when she was maybe 20 years old, she was in some sort of relationship with a guy who was just really shitty. Basically, he raped her and she got pregnant. She phoned me: "Bubby, I am pregnant. I need to have an abortion. Can you help?"

I remember saying, "If you decide to keep it, I would help raise it, if that's what you want. I love you."

The closest abortion clinic was in Nashville, Tennessee. At the time I was barely making $300 a week working retail and could barely pay my rent. She called my brother, who came up with the funds to help pay for her abortion. A friend drove her to have her abortion—a medication abortion—at the Planned Parenthood Clinic in Nashville.

Since then, I have told my mom about the work I do in reproductive justice and about wanting to start an abortion support group. When she said she'd love to come to that, I asked her what she would say to the group. And she's like, "Well, a lot of people have this stigma and shame and feel like abortion is this bad thing. It's not the end of the world. Sometimes it's an opportunity for other things to happen." That was a great conversation.

I started out working on immigration when a friend introduced me to the idea of reproductive justice, which is so intersectional. It relates to immigration and gender justice, and race. All of these things come into play when people make decisions.

To start with, I went to work at a clinic where they did abortions. I saw folks from all over the South, but not one white person was in the waiting room. These women were having to travel from Tennessee, Alabama, and South Carolina to get their abortion. There I was on the phone, trying to find funding for their abortions: National Abortion Federation, the National Network of Abortion Funds. And I was like, "Y'all, we have to do something to show up for Southerners in a more meaningful way."

Technically, there was no fund that served the state of Georgia. In that moment, I realized that if we start a fund, it has to cross state lines. If someone is in Atlanta and they have to travel somewhere else because they've passed the gestational limit here, their funds would be able to transfer with them. For us, as long as you're a Southerner in the region we work in, we're going to support you as best as we can. Our fund is called Access

Reproductive Care–Southeast. It provides support for those in Alabama, Florida, Georgia, Mississippi, South Carolina, and Tennessee.

We balance the abortion funding piece with education and advocacy work in the community to de-stigmatize abortion. We launched a billboard campaign in Georgia. There are three versions that say: "Abortion is health care." "Reproductive justice is unconditional love." "Trust those who you love to make decisions about their bodies."

Ninety-six percent of people in the state of Georgia live in a county without an abortion provider. That means folks are traveling at least an hour and a half, two hours, or more to get to an abortion clinic. Our hope is that if you're coming into one of these major cities, you will see one of these billboards and at least feel some sort of affirmation or support for what you are doing. It's positive messaging that's counter to this negative anti-messaging that we see and hear every single day. There's also a digital pledge associated with the billboards to make a commitment to use your voice for reproductive justice, to speak out when you see something that's awful in the news and media. The other part of the pledge is to make a commitment to join our practical support volunteer network. Right now that is a group of about sixty people, who help people crossing state lines or people who need rides, lodging, or childcare.

I just firmly believe that we wouldn't be here without the amazing work that Black and brown women have done in the past. I'm able to do this work because there are people before me like Loretta Ross, and others who started reproductive justice, who have created this environment to do this work.

I just firmly believe that we wouldn't be here without the amazing work that Black and brown women have done in the past. I'm able to do this work because there are people before me like Loretta Ross, and others who started reproductive justice, who have created this environment to do this work.

The thing that makes me be positive in this particular moment is that I know we're doing the right thing. We're fighting for our basic human rights. And I know the warrior is in me. We're going to ultimately win this fight.

Yes, abortion is available, but is it fully accessible? I feel like this is our time, especially for the voices of Black women, LGBTQ folks in our community, and Southerners to really start speaking up and advocating for ourselves. We are committed to making sure our people continue to get safe, compassionate health care.

Jon O'Brien

I WAS BORN in 1965 in Dublin, Ireland, in a small suburb called Drimnagh. It's a particularly rough, working-class neighborhood. My family was Mom, Dad, and three brothers. Mother had worked in a printing shop. She stopped working to have children, as women traditionally did. My father was a skilled toolmaker and an incredibly hard worker.

I am a Catholic in good faith, believing in a woman's right to end a pregnancy.

The four of us were unruly brothers. My mother very often had us at the dinner table while my father was working late. The three things that she said you can't talk about at the table were politics, sex, and religion. I've built my whole life talking about all three of those things because, at the end of the day, they're very important for us from both a philosophical and a values-based point of view.

My mother really put it upon me: "Whatever you can do for women, you should do."

My parents are very religious people, not in that conservative way, but in that Jesus-was-a-radical way. They read the Bible every day and took us to church every week.

There are many things in Catholicism that are absolutely wonderful. It's not just about going to Mass on Sunday. It's not just about confession. It's not just about all the sacraments. It's about living a life that tries to put into practice the principles of equality and fairness and love.

The sadness, of course, is that if you listen to the bishops these days you'd think it was all about trying to get contraception out of the Affordable Care Act. They're so stuck in the pelvic zone. They're so focused on contraception, abortion. The Church hierarchy is so

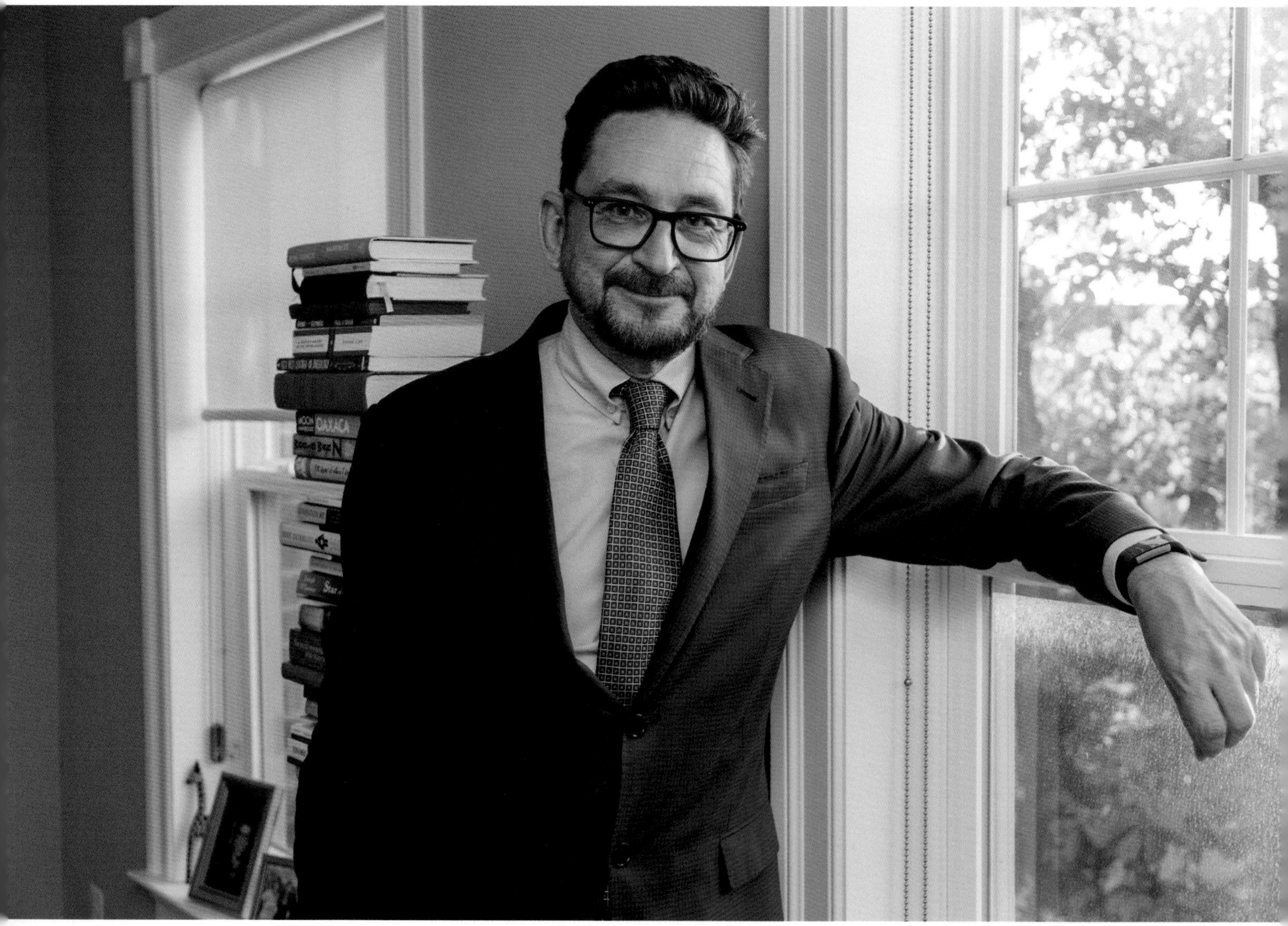

JON O'BRIEN

preoccupied with this myopic view of humans. It's a view that's built upon power and the ability to enact that power over others.

To give an example: In the 1920s, when Ireland gained its independence from Britain, there was a power vacuum. The Catholic Church had played a very important role, both practical and symbolic, in the Irish Revolution. But now you had all these laws on the statute books, including heavy censorship of magazines, newspapers, books, and films. This greatly limited your access to culture, thought, and change. From the bishops right down to the priests and nuns at a local level, the hierarchy wielded enormous control over Irish life.

There was a referendum in 1983 to amend the Irish Constitution to protect and defend the right to life of the unborn. The Catholic Church used the pulpit to really put the fear of God, literally, into people. It worked and the referendum passed.

In the 1980s many of us really wanted to change the world, and we wanted to change Ireland. Quite a lot of friends of mine had become teenage moms, which meant the cycle of poverty would go on, or even be worsened once you have one or two more kids—especially if the father is not around to help.

I also knew that some girls were forced to sneak away to England to have abortions, and I knew that wasn't a happy situation. Plus, there were so many cases of sexually transmitted diseases.

In the Republic of Ireland, I began working at the Family Planning Association, an independent group that set out to provide contraception. With them, I set up various services for young people, including contraceptive services and a hotline that people could telephone to get advice. I began writing advice columns in newspapers and magazines. At one point, I ended up being convicted for the illegal sale of a condom. Eventually, we were able to change the condom laws in Ireland, which I'm very proud of.

The Irish activist Ruth Riddick educated me about abortion and about how much the laws hurt poor women who can't exercise their autonomy because it costs money. Even here in the United States, if you're working two or three jobs, how can you take time off work? Not to mention the distances you might have to travel in order to find an abortion provider. I could really see how supporting abortion rights fit together with the same social justice message that my parents brought me up with.

I became critically aware that what I experienced in Ireland I was seeing played out again and again in places like Lithuania and Poland. I saw how hell bent the Catholic hierarchy was on holding back women's reproductive health. That's when I met up with Catholics for Choice.

The Catholic hierarchy doesn't get up in church anymore and preach that contraception is wrong. They lobby behind the scenes. They bully and flail politicians to acquiesce to their agenda, in order to pass laws on contraception that are either restrictive or completely forbid it, and to make abortion unavailable.

The Catholic hierarchy has always held that abortion is wrong, that it's sinful. But, its reasons for this have changed over the years. Originally, it had nothing, absolutely nothing to do with the idea that the life in the uterus was the equivalent of a born person. It was because, back in the eighteenth century, doctors of the Church were looking at fetuses through microscopes. They thought what they saw were fully formed. They were not.

Then, there's the "perversity view." Back in the day, if you were pregnant by someone other than your husband, then you must have done something wrong, illicit, sinful. So, it was really the sex that was the sin, not the abortion.

When a bishop or a priest gets up, and says something like "abortion is murder," I believe that they genuinely believe that. I think a lot of Catholics don't believe that even though we know it's a serious thing to end life in the uterus. Now, it doesn't mean that you don't have to take seriously what the Catholic hierarchy says, but this is maybe the most important part of what I'm going to say to you, and why I can tell you that I am a Catholic in good faith, believing in a woman's right to end a pregnancy.

St. Augustine and Thomas Aquinas, two of the most important fathers of the church, didn't believe that a fetus in the early stages of development had the same quality as a born person. That's very important.

We believe, just as St. Thomas Aquinas and St. Augustine, that the most important thing is to follow your own conscience. This doesn't mean you get up in the morning and just go off and do whatever you want. It means that you look carefully at what the Catholic hierarchy teaches. You look carefully at the implications of your decisions, especially their implications for others, and then you go ahead. The teachers in church have said that you must follow your conscience.

It would be wrong when you go through the Pearly Gates to say, "Well, I was just following orders." As Catholics, we can't say that. So, when a woman makes a decision to have an abortion, she's following her conscience, she's doing the most Catholic thing she can do. When a woman makes a decision not to have an abortion, she's also following her conscience. When we use contraception, when we're gay or lesbian, the most important thing to do as Catholics, is to follow our conscience. A properly formed conscience requires going through the process of discernment that I believe women do go through in making the decision to have an abortion.

When a woman makes a decision to have an abortion, she's following her conscience, she's doing the most Catholic thing she can do. When a woman makes a decision not to have an abortion, she's also following her conscience.

At Catholics for Choice, we give voice to those Catholics who think and believe and act differently than the hierarchy of our church. It gives them the backbone, if they're lacking it, or gives them the permission, understanding, and knowledge they need to stand up against a powerful hierarchy that wants to have its cake and eat it.

I met with some doctors who were struggling as to whether to provide abortions or not. One of them said, "Catholics for Choice, is that an oxymoron?" No, it's not, because Catholic women use birth control and they have abortions at the same rates as those of other faiths or no faith. Last time I looked, there's a hell of a lot of gay, lesbian, and transgender Catholics. Last time I looked, a lot of Catholics are divorced. So, don't tell me that our world view is not shared by the majority of Catholics in the world.

As Catholics, we don't believe the church is a building in Rome. It's not the cathedral here in Washington, D.C.. The church is *all* of the people, including nuns, priests, and bishops. But the hierarchy is the minority that fails to grasp the reality of what the majority's daily lives are about.

I'm a religious person. I'm Catholic. I don't want someone dictating to me that I can't practice my faith as I see fit.

At Catholics for Choice, we give voice to those Catholics who think and believe and act differently than the hierarchy of our church.

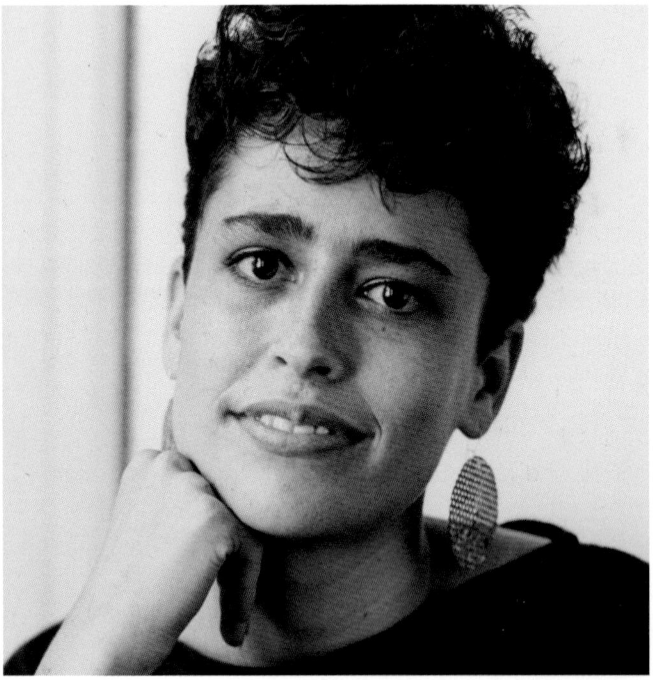

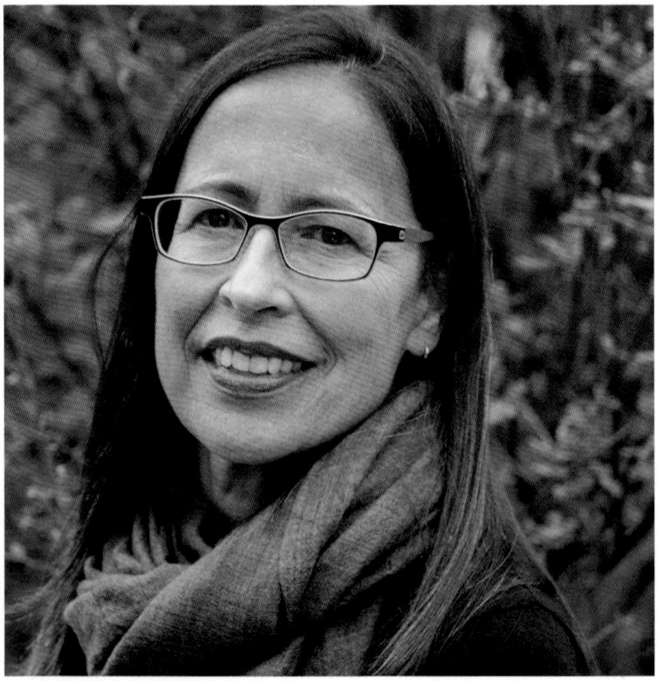

JULIE GEBHARDT

Julie Gebhardt

IT WAS 1983. I had finished with my schooling and was early in my hairdressing career. I had just ended a two-year relationship, and a month later found out I was pregnant. I wasn't with a partner then and it really didn't feel like the right time for a baby. I had not yet thought about whether I wanted to become a mother, I hadn't sorted out that decision at all. So when I realized I was pregnant it was pretty clear to me that I wasn't going to keep the baby. I was very independent and I was very oriented toward doing my own thing.

I had been going for my health care to a women's clinic—I think it mostly focused on health care for lesbians—but it was the place I went to. It felt good because it was a very small office and everybody was really warm and I was familiar and comfortable with the people there. I just felt that I wanted to have the procedure done there. So I lobbied them to help me.

They had never done an abortion on the premises of the clinic. But they had someone on staff who had done them somewhere else. She borrowed equipment to be able to do it for me there. So that's what happened.

I don't know why it didn't occur to me to go to Planned Parenthood but somehow I was attached to this clinic run by lesbians. I was very invested in the women's community and the lesbian feminist community. I had been a Women's Studies major in college.

I don't remember who paid for the abortion, but it must have been me. I was making pretty good money for my situation as a hairdresser and I didn't have a lot of expenses. Compared to my friends at the time who were working random jobs, I was making a good living.

A close friend came with me for the abortion and I went home the same day. I was not prepared for what it was like afterward. There were contractions, there was bleeding. When I went home it was a long, painful night, dramatic with all the bleeding. I was nervous. Was this normal? I was glad I still had my girlfriend with me. It wouldn't have been good to go through it by myself.

Afterwards I felt wiped out. I was very emotional about the whole thing. Although I wasn't torn about the decision, it felt upsetting, very heavy to me, sort of wrenching even though it was what I wanted to be doing. If it had been less dramatic and uncomfortable I might have felt more matter of fact about it. But it was so visceral. I thought, "Oh, that was a baby." And that was upsetting. I felt sad.

I actually ended up getting back together with my boyfriend, who was the father of the baby. I think I was so upset about the abortion that I went back into that relationship for another year, even though it wasn't right for me. The relationship was really over. And I think if I hadn't had the pregnancy and the abortion, I wouldn't have gone back to him. But it felt like a lot to handle on my own.

He had been away for three months, he had a summer job, and I told him about the abortion when he came back. He was torn up about it and upset that I hadn't made the decision together with him. I had just assumed it's my body and it's my decision. But it didn't feel that way to him, especially because he was a father already—he had two kids from his previous marriage—so it wasn't just a pregnancy for him, it was a baby. So it was complicated.

Having my abortion always felt like the right choice. I didn't ever have regrets. It was like going through something hard but still having confidence that I had made the right decision. I knew that everything was going to be OK but I just had to feel those feelings. And I think the hormonal element, the pregnancy hormones, make you so sensitive to your emotions.

After I had my abortion I did go back to feeling like an independent woman and didn't picture myself as a mother or even necessarily someone who would get married. Then I met Allen, the person I have been married to for thirty years. We were only married a year when I discovered I was pregnant. We hadn't even talked yet about whether having children was going to be part of our lives.

I normally used birth control but one night I didn't and I knew, even when we were making love, that we just made a baby. I just knew it. And then I didn't get my period and

I went to Planned Parenthood for my test, still with the attitude, "Uh oh, pregnancy." And then when the woman told me, "You tested positive, you're pregnant," I was shockingly flooded with happiness. And I had not anticipated that. I said to the woman, "I need to think about this because I feel really happy." And the woman said, "Oh, that's wonderful. We don't hear that that often." When I told Allen how happy I was, he agreed that we would start our family. I had my first son Victor when I was 28, and then six and a half years later I had my second son, Charlie. My boys are now 23 and 30.

When I was young, I wanted to be a teenager when I grew up. My sister had dolls and eventually did a lot of babysitting. But I was not maternal. I was not a person ever to like babysitting. But, ah, being a mother has definitely been the best part of my life. I feel it is the most profound thing I will do in my life and the most meaningful relationship. I did not anticipate that I would feel this way. It's my greatest joy.

Whatever was distressing about that abortion was not something I carried into the future with me. Because if I had gone ahead and had that baby, my life would have been really different . . . I might have stayed with that partner and that wouldn't have been good. I just didn't have the maturity yet to be a mother. It was much better that I had my children later, when I was more mature and ready.

I have shared my abortion story with both of my sons. I felt it was important to give them a complete picture of who I am, not just as their mom but as a person. And I parented that way anyway. I'm more than just a mom, I'm also an independent person. I wanted them to know who I was before I met their dad, to have my full story.

I HAVE SHARED MY ABORTION STORY WITH BOTH OF MY SONS. I FELT IT WAS IMPORTANT TO GIVE THEM A COMPLETE PICTURE OF WHO I AM, NOT JUST AS THEIR MOM BUT AS A PERSON . . . I WANTED THEM TO KNOW WHO I WAS BEFORE I MET THEIR DAD, TO HAVE MY FULL STORY.

I feel gratitude that I had the option to have an abortion, that it was a choice I could make for myself. I didn't do it lightly, and it wasn't without upset. It wasn't a cavalier decision. But it was definitely the right choice for me.

I'm immensely distressed at the direction things have taken in our country. I can't believe we are still discussing it and fighting over it. I feel, "Are you kidding me?" We won that right, and we're still fighting and it's being nibbled away at. I feel really incensed.

When I think about the 23-year-old who had an abortion, I can still find her in myself. I would say I am a more solid person, more grounded, a more grown-up person now. But I can locate that younger person within me.

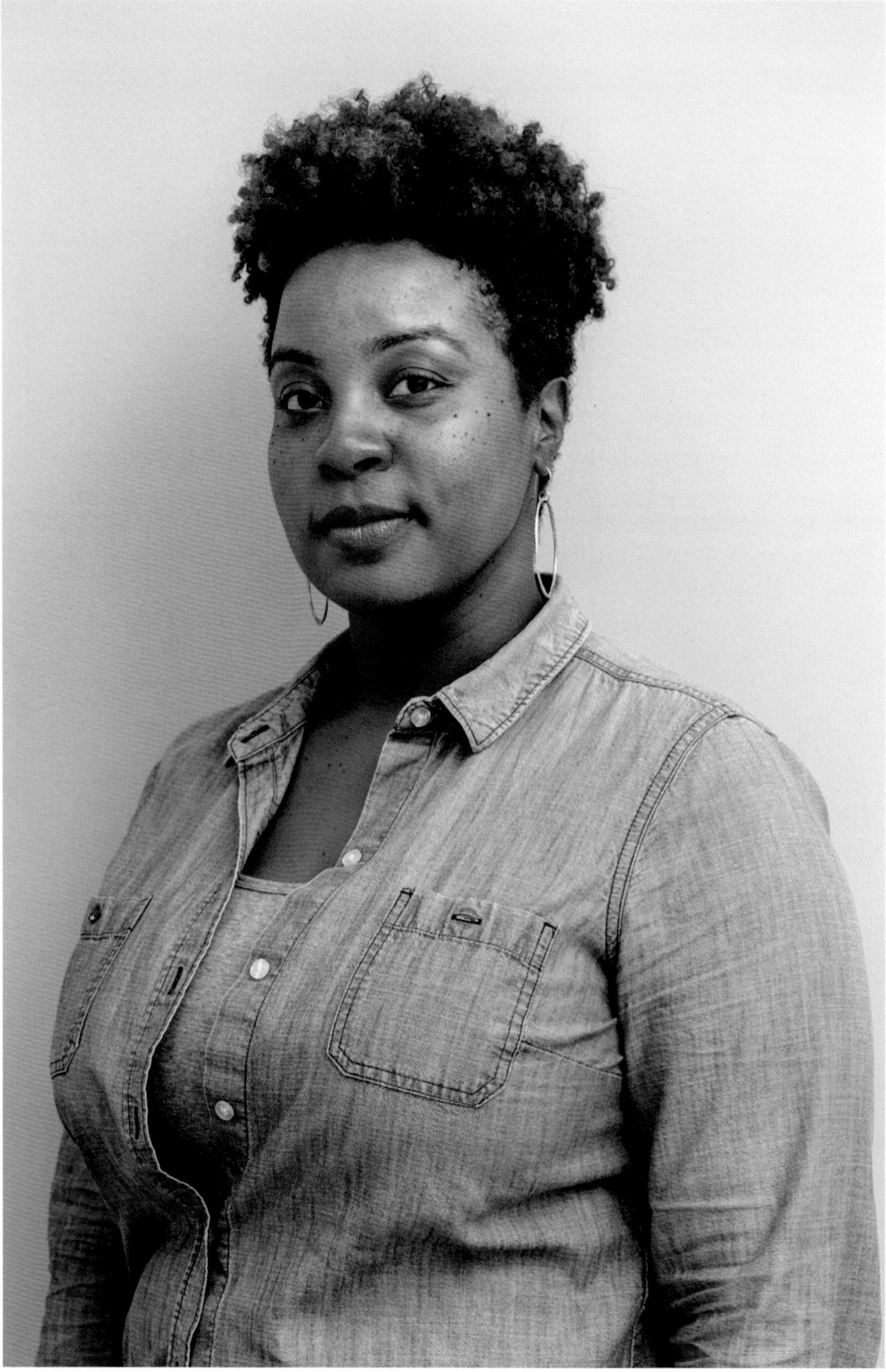

AZIZA JONES

Aziza Jones

I HAD AN abortion when I was 33. I was unemployed but working under the table at a restaurant in Chicago, doing odd jobs, making enough to pay my rent. At a friend's wedding in Washington, D.C., I met someone. There was this whirlwind romance, like you see in the movies. I was in Chicago, he in D.C.. We were just texting back and forth until I ended up going back to Maryland.

We used protection when we had sex but there was that one time. I was on the pill but I wasn't using a period app that would have said if I was ovulating or what was going on with my body. After we had unprotected sex, we talked about what we'd do if I got pregnant.

I came back to Chicago and kept going through life, trying to find a job and working when I could. I either missed my period or had some serious breast tenderness, so I thought maybe I should take a pregnancy test. I must have peed on fifty-five sticks. The tests kept coming back positive.

I didn't have health insurance, so I went to a clinic just up the street for a check-up and another pregnancy test. It came back positive. I remember walking home and sitting by a little tree. I called my mom in St. Croix. And she was like, "What's up, Baby." I'm like, "I'm pregnant." She's like, "Oh, Aziza. I support you in whatever decision you make. I'm 100 percent with you." I cried on the phone with her for a little while.

Then I called my boyfriend, the father of the pregnancy. He asked what I wanted to do and added that he would love to have another kid. He also said that he would have to make more money and that I'd have to move to Maryland. I was like, "Yay!" I'm 33. I'm a Black woman. Historically, Black women just bear the brunt of whatever they come up against—keep a kid, live paycheck to paycheck, go through the social services, go on welfare and food stamps—all that kind of thing. Just make it work. He admitted he didn't know if it was the right thing for us to bring a kid into the world. When I got off the phone with him I just sat around with my cat. I tried to put on my happy face around my friends while I was in turmoil trying to figure out what to do.

At Planned Parenthood, an abortion would cost $500. I didn't have a job, was barely able to pay my $800 rent. I ended up going to the Stroger Hospital at Cook County Hospital. An abortion there would cost only $75. I could definitely afford that! By this time I had decided to have the abortion. There was no way I was going to have a kid without having a job and being able to pay rent. Kids are expensive.

WHILE I WAS SITTING IN THE METAL CHAIR, I WONDERED HOW I GOT THERE. HERE I AM, 33 YEARS OLD, HAVING AN ABORTION, SITTING ON A METAL CHAIR . . . I STARTED SINGING SONGS IN MY HEAD SO I WOULDN'T HEAR THE PEOPLE AROUND ME. THE ONE SONG I HUMMED IN MY HEAD OVER AND OVER AND OVER WAS CHRISTINA AGUILERA'S "STRONGER."

I went to the hospital by myself. They make you come in first for a sonogram, then the procedure. You're in a waiting room with twenty to thirty women at various stages of pregnancy. After the sonogram they ask you if this is something you want to do. You sign the paperwork. Then they schedule your actual procedure.

It's a public hospital and they treat you kind of like cattle. You know when you see kindergartners and they hold hands following their teacher? It was kind of like that. We weren't holding hands, but we were walking single file through the nice, glistening parts of the hospital. We went down all these stairs to the bowels of the hospital. We ended up in a room with four or five rows of hard metal folding chairs, maybe five to six chairs in each row. Filled with women. They told us to go and take our clothes off.

After you sign more paperwork, you take this pill. Once you take this pill, you can't change your mind. I think there was one person who decided not to take the pill. The pill softened the cervix so they could go in and do the suction abortion.

While I was sitting in the metal chair, I wondered how I got there. Here I am, 33 years old, having an abortion, sitting on a metal chair. What decision-making skills was I not using? I had had many close brushes having unprotected sex. I thought maybe I couldn't get pregnant. Obviously, I could, because here I am sitting on this metal chair. I started singing songs in my head so I wouldn't hear the people around me. The one song I hummed in my head over and over and over was Christina Aguilera's "Stronger." I think there were two tears that ran down my eyes.

When it was my turn, they told me to get on the table, this won't be too hard. There were two or three people in the room. I don't think I had any anesthesia. I think they gave us some Tylenol after they gave us the pill.

After the procedure, they have you sit on a chair in a little room with this huge, ancient pad from like 1932 that goes from your belly button to the back of your spine. They make you eat a couple of crackers and drink something. You sit there for a little longer. Finally, you put your clothes on and talk to an outtake person. At this point they give you a brown paper bag with morning-after pills and two boxes of condoms. You sign more paperwork.

The outtake nurse said, "If anything happens you can always call us or come back in." I said, "You will never see me again." She said, "Yeah, I hear that a lot." I said, "No, you will never see me again."

I ended up moving to D.C. to be with the guy who was the father of the kid. We were together for four and a half years. We got engaged, but a few months before the wedding I realized this is not the right decision. I broke off my engagement and we parted ways. We're still friends.

I want people to be able to talk to friends and family. Don't sit in silence and think you have to take it all on yourself. Words are powerful.

I know the stigma is strong, especially in a family. I still haven't told some people in my family. My grandmother in Milwaukee knows that I work for an abortion fund, but I have never said I've had an abortion. She was born in 1927. I'm sure she knows women who tried to have abortions or tried to give themselves abortions and something ended up botched. It's just not a conversation that we have ever had.

I want people to be able to talk to friends and family. Don't sit in silence and think you have to take it all on yourself. Words are powerful. If you speak to people who may have resources, or know someone who has resources, you won't have to go to the bottom of a hospital and go through a procedure like I did. Use your words, talk to people who have an open mind and who won't deter you from doing something you have made up your mind to do. Talk to people who will help you find a solution to the issue you have at that time.

People from all walks of life have abortions. People who are rich and famous and people who are unemployed have abortions. Some people who are not making nearly enough money to scrape by and don't want to rely on public assistance have abortions.

If you want to have an abortion you should have one. But nobody should force you to have one.

Ava Torre-Bueno

MY MOTHER IS ultimately how I got into this field I am in. In 1962, I was 10 years old and my mother got pregnant. Our physician told her he could send her to a gynecologist who could do an abortion. It wouldn't be legal, but it would be safe. The gynecologist would charge $1,000 for taking a profound risk. That was a huge amount of money in 1962. My parents did not have any money. We lived in a housing project and we were broke.

Because there was not enough money to pay for a safe physician-induced illegal abortion, she had a self-induced abortion. She took a blunt plastic instrument and put it up her vagina through her cervix. Without an anesthetic.

She popped the amniotic sac. She labored and delivered into the toilet and flushed the toilet. Then she got very sick. She must have taken some bacteria from the vagina into the uterus. When she went to the hospital I thought she was dead because I wasn't allowed to visit her; I was too young. I remember our upstairs neighbor coming down to clean the bathroom. She told me we would get this all clean for when your mother comes home.

Afterwards, my mom got depressed. My dad got sad and overwhelmed. It was just a really tough time in our family.

In my late teens, my mom told me that my grandmother had had an abortion on the kitchen table, by the same doctor who later delivered me.

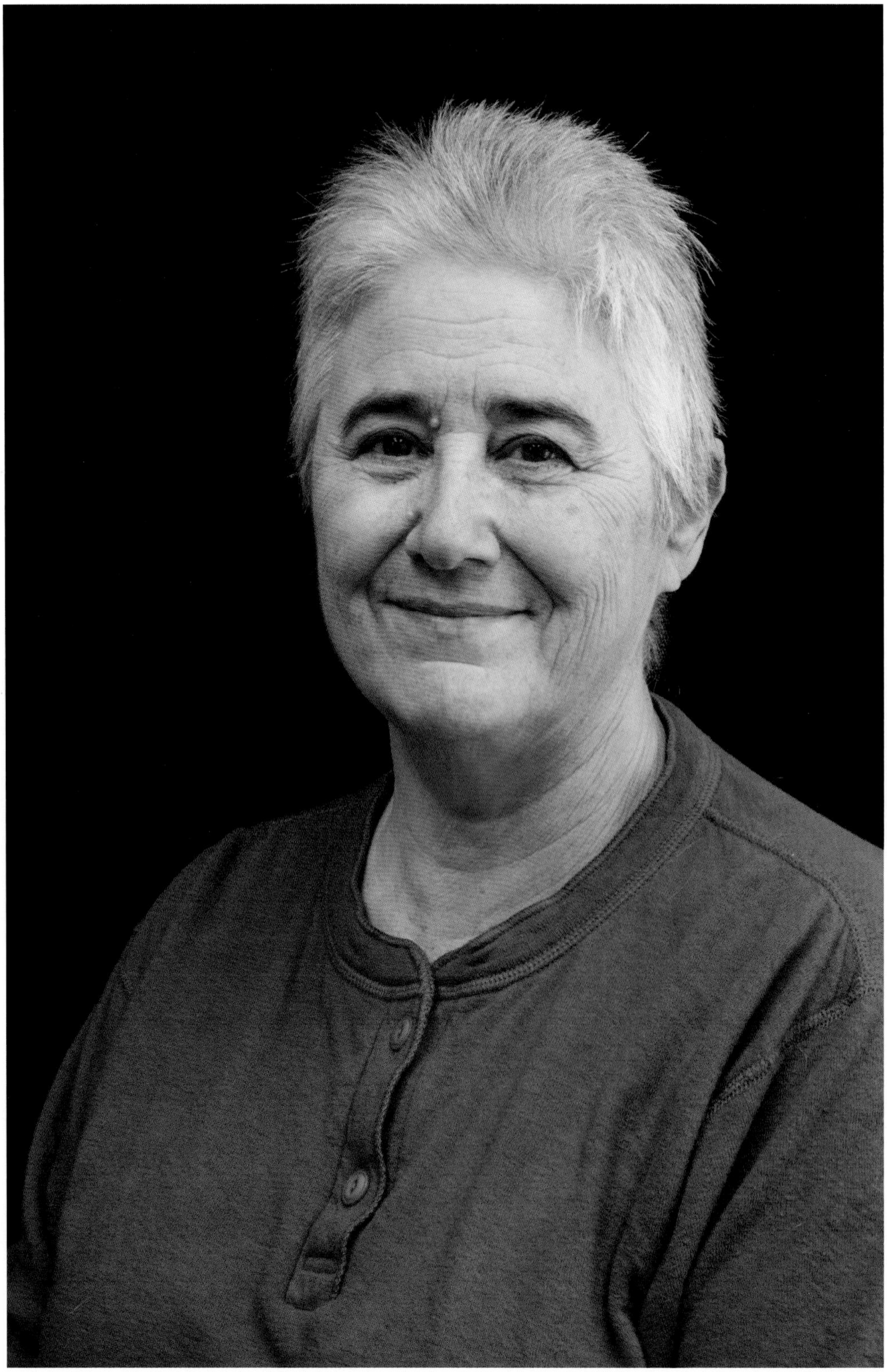

AVA TORRE-BUENO

When I was a kid we used to cross the 59th Street Bridge in New York City to donate old clothes and stuff to the Planned Parenthood thrift store. That's where my mother always took me and she explained the importance of birth control.

When I was still a student at San Diego State I went to work for Planned Parenthood. We did pregnancy counseling: doing pregnancy tests, giving the results, and talking to women about their choices. After ten years I went into private practice as an individual adult psychotherapist. My niche is post-abortion counseling. I'm the person to go to for pretty much all things reproductive.

Often people ask me how I could have spent my career working with such an intense subject as abortion. I tell them it's fabulous and it is such fun work.

I myself have never had an abortion. The first time I had sex I was 17. The man pulled out a condom and put it on, thankfully, because I was too stupid at that point and drunk, which is so normal. That's when I said to my parents, I think I should get some birth control. My mother took me to the clinic associated with an agency she worked for. The doctor popped an IUD in me and I had it for ten years.

In my practice, I see a self-selected population of people who are struggling after an abortion, which is only 10 to 15 percent of those who have abortions. The things that cause people to have trouble after an abortion, like guilt and shame, are the things I know about.

When I see men as clients, as part of taking their sexual history, I ask them if they've been involved in any pregnancies that they know of. That makes their eyes get big. Often, they've never thought about the concept of having been involved in any pregnancies. Sometimes they say, "Yes, I got a girl pregnant in college, and she had an abortion." I ask, "And how was that for you then? And how is it for you now?" And often it's fine. And sometimes it's like, "I've carried that around and felt guilty about how I treated that girl." Or, "I wish I could have been able to provide at the time but we both knew we couldn't do it."

In my practice, I see a self-selected population of people who are struggling after an abortion, which is only 10 to 15 percent of those who have abortions. The things that cause people to have trouble after an abortion, like guilt and shame, are the things I know about. Guilt is the dropping, sinking feeling in your stomach that you have done something wrong. Shame is this horrible feeling of wanting to sink into the earth and vanish. It is feeling that you are fundamentally flawed to the core. If you feel guilty about an experience, it activates your shame. If you weren't raised with shame, nothing gets activated. But a whole lot of people are raised with shame.

About a quarter of the people who struggle after an abortion are grieving a loss that was precipitated by becoming pregnant when they didn't mean to. The loss is almost never what the anti-choice people say it is. It is almost never, "I killed my baby." For the most part, the loss is other things. It can be the loss of innocence. There is the realization that sex is fun but sex has real consequences that I have to face now. That loss of simplicity is a profound loss.

A woman may have a really close relationship with her parents, and not be able to share this one thing with them, because she doesn't want to disappoint them. She doesn't want to see her dad cry. That gap between her and her parents can be a painful loss of connection. Another woman might have told a friend that she needed help and the friend turns out to be anti-choice. The friend accuses her of killing her baby. The friendship may be lost.

Mediocre partner relationships almost always end around an unplanned pregnancy. Another loss. Really good relationships generally get better around an unplanned pregnancy.

And then there's grief. About one-quarter of my clients haven't dealt with their grief. I help my clients grieve. They let me hold their hand figuratively and go all the way through grieving, and reassure them that they are going to be fine.

Many people who are having difficulty after an abortion, can't grieve that grief. Why not? Because we live in a culture where almost no one has any idea how to grieve. They're terrified of grief. They just need help starting down the path of grief, some encouragement and assurance that grief will not kill them. I tell clients that when you really let yourself grieve sometimes it feels like someone's taken their hand and grabbed the skin of your chest and gotten their fingernails under it, and they're pulling your chest off. It can feel like you're having a heart attack. But you need to know that grief has an endpoint and that there are gifts at the end of grief.

The other three-quarters of my clients are coping with the anxiety of finding out they were pregnant when they didn't mean to be. Whether you're 17, 27, or 37, becoming pregnant when you didn't mean to be takes all the oxygen out of the room. It's terrifying for many people—for men because it's out of their control, they totally freak out. Even very stable, grounded men get pretty whacked out.

Added to the anxiety is figuring out how to pay for it, the anxiety of going to a clinic, maybe crossing a picket line of people screaming at you that abortion is physically dangerous—which is completely untrue – the fear that you're going to die.

All this anxiety even though abortion is a completely safe procedure. It's brief, it's often pain free, although, yes, it can be painful. When it's done, you might feel total relief, or you might not. Afterwards some women are distressed. They are pro-choice, they wanted the abortion, they had it, yet they still feel a profound loss.

As a psycho-dynamically oriented therapist, I help people understand that what has happened in the past comes up and bites us in the present, even when we don't know that it's the past that's biting us.

We all carry boxes inside of us where old, unaddressed anxieties are locked tightly away. When these boxes are opened, it unleashes a flood of emotion, of visceral, body memories around a given event. Finding out you are pregnant when you don't want to be often brings up visceral memories that are disturbing and distressing. I want to help them understand and work through it. The memories may be childhood trauma; physical, verbal, emotional or sexual abuse or neglect. In our sessions, we get to what the real issue is in their life that they have been tripping and stumbling over.

People's capacity to heal is profound.

I can ask my patients: "What's another time in your hurt life that felt even remotely similar to how you're feeling now?" Sometimes just that question pulls the picture memory up. They remember, being 9 years old when their father had a heart attack, thinking he was dead and that it was their fault. Their visceral memory surfaced with one question. All the anxiety is their visceral memory.

I get lovely, lovely results. It's amazing how much people can heal if you're willing to take the risk of coming to therapy. People's capacity to heal is profound. People who are struggling after an abortion, women or men, need to know that this is all healable. You don't have to suffer your whole life with guilt or regret.

Ava Torre-Bueno is the author of Peace After Abortion, *Pimpernel Press, 1997.*

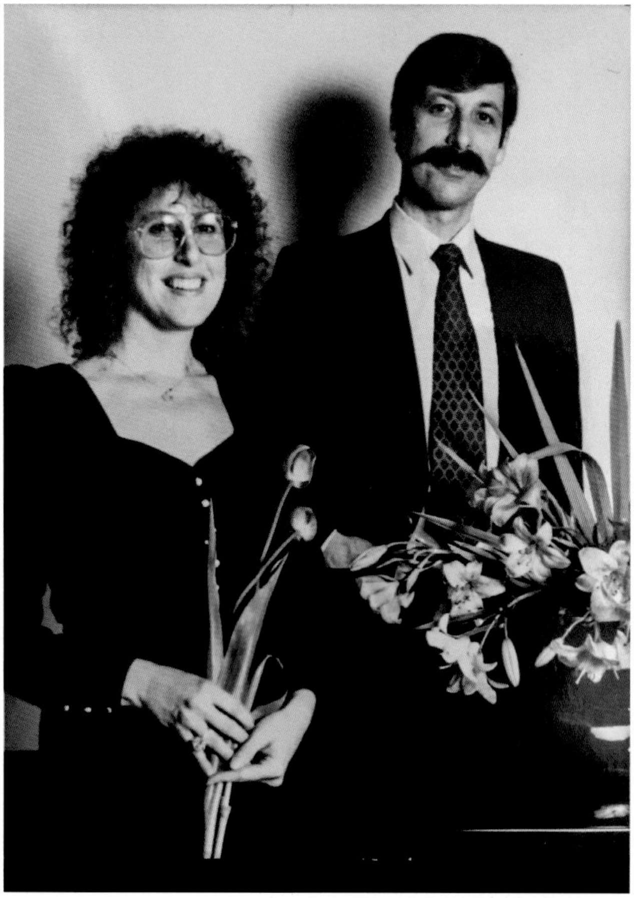

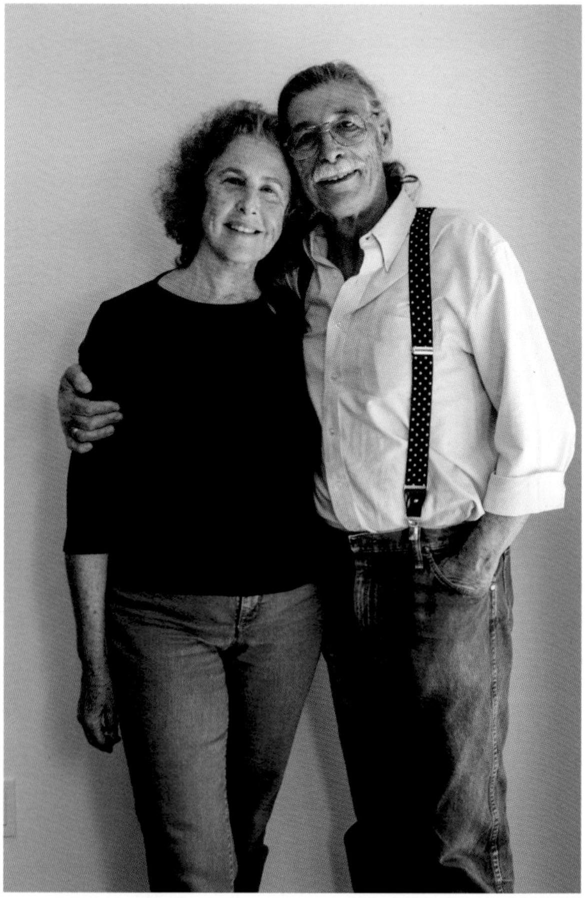

DAPHNA AND SHAMY NOILY

Daphna and Shamy Noily

Daphna: In 1968 my college roommate got pregnant. Abortions were still not legal. She had to go to Mexico to get an abortion and she came back very, very sick. She wouldn't go to the med center or to her parents, who were Holocaust survivors; they would never understand, she said. My role was being supportive. To witness what a terrible thing it is to have an unwanted pregnancy and have to have an abortion in that way, it always stuck with me.

After Shamy and I already had two children, I got pregnant unexpectedly. I was about to launch a program for preschool children and their families that I had created and was directing. My choice was to do this or have this third child. There was no way I could do both.

AT THE TIME OF MY FIRST ABORTION, I FELT THAT I WAS ONLY POSTPONING THE BIRTH OF ANOTHER CHILD, AND I KNEW THAT THIS PARTICULAR CAREER OPPORTUNITY WOULD NEVER BE POSSIBLE AT ANOTHER TIME.

Family and career are two important themes in my life. And I know that if ever push came to shove, family would take precedence over everything else. At the time of my first abortion, I felt that I was only postponing the birth of another child, and I knew that this particular career opportunity would never be possible at another time.

Shamy: For me it was very difficult to believe in the principle of a woman's right to choose, which I always believed in and still do, and to see your wife choose an abortion. I tried to talk her out of it, but she was determined to have it. I supported her physically but it was very hard for me to support her emotionally. I just had profound sadness about it. It was the first time in my life where something that was very rational to me, something I believed in, clashed with my emotions.

Daphna: We had a lot of discussions about it. I didn't have the physical strength or the emotional bandwidth to both have the child and run my program. And it was clear that my husband wasn't going to back me on this.

I finally told him I had decided to have an abortion and I'd appreciate it if he would drive me to the clinic and back, which he did. I was lucky that abortions were legal and I could go to our health care provider and have it done there. This wasn't an issue. My biggest issue was at home, dealing with my husband, who was really against it.

The next day, Shamy went off to work. I was completely a basket case. I went over to my friend's house and spent the whole day crying. I think part of it was the hormones, just the craziness of what's going on in your body, and part of it was that my husband wasn't there emotionally to support me in this decision I had wrestled with. I remember saying to Shamy, it's not like we aren't going to have more children. We are going to have more children, just at a time when I can handle it better.

Shamy: So, after the abortion, you go on and live your life.

Daphna: My third son was born in 1982, and a few years later, I unexpectedly got pregnant again. This time I told Shamy that I was pregnant, that I was going to Los Angeles to have an abortion and that he had nothing to do with it. It was very clear to me that he would not be supportive and I didn't want to deal with all the aftermath. By then, I had three little kids. It was clear I couldn't deal with another baby while our third son was still an infant.

My best girlfriend from high school lived in LA at the time. She had just had an abortion and she told me about the clinic she went to and how easy it was. I knew I would have the support of my mother and my close girlfriend in Los Angeles. This abortion experience was not at all traumatic. It was a non-event.

Shamy: The second abortion was less emotional. She took the decision away from me. It was not a conversation. It showed how strongly she felt about it.

Daphna: I have no regrets about having the abortions. In retrospect, a few years after the second abortion, our middle son got sick. I don't know how we would have dealt with another child through his illness and death. I really don't know how we would have done it. While I thought long and hard about my first abortion, I had no qualms about the second one at all. We just had to be more careful, use better birth control, because neither of those pregnancies were intended.

Shamy: Yes, we moved on. Very recently though, we were driving in the car with our 34-year-old son when Daphna brought up this abortion story project. Suddenly, I felt the sadness again, all these years later.

Daphna: That's when you said you didn't want me to participate in Roslyn's project. So I told Roslyn, I may not be able to participate. It was only months later when we talked about it that you said you wanted the other side to be told.

Shamy: Daphna and I had a young family. I think we both assumed we were going to have more kids. It just struck me as a very emotional thing to decide not to have a child because of work. And I'm a pretty stubborn guy. We're both strong people.

The abortion issue has two parts to it: one is cerebral, the idea that a woman has the right to choose is, in my mind, an absolute right. I went along with it. But the emotional part of it surprised me. An emotion just happens, it's not something you can turn off. You go beyond it. It's not something you live with every day. You survive it. But I was very surprised at how emotional I still feel about it.

I JUST HAD PROFOUND SADNESS ABOUT IT. IT WAS THE FIRST TIME IN MY LIFE WHERE SOMETHING THAT WAS VERY RATIONAL TO ME, SOMETHING I BELIEVED IN, CLASHED WITH MY EMOTIONS.

Daphna: I think if we had not gone through the death of our second son, it would have probably been a different feeling for Shamy. I think his sadness was intensified by the fact that we ended up losing our second son, who was almost 10 years old.

I think it's important that women do a lot of soul searching. For me it was not an easy decision to make, particularly the first abortion. Although I had to choose one or the other, career or more children, it wasn't a permanent choice. I feel that was the right decision. I don't have any regrets about it.

I think women have to look deep inside to figure out what they want so that they don't have regrets afterwards that they gave up things in order to have a family. When I look at some older women, I think a lot of them gave away their ability to have a very satisfying career because they felt the need or responsibility to raise a family. My mother is one of the women who gave up her career. My father in some ways made her give up her stage career, so that she could have me. I don't think she has ever gotten past it to this day.

Loretta Ross

AT 14, I became pregnant through incest when my married cousin raped me. This was 1968, so I had no choice but to have the baby. I was living in San Antonio, Texas. Perhaps there were girls going to Mexico to have abortions, but I didn't know about that.

I had hidden the pregnancy from my mother for a long time. I was like any other child who wakes up with a nightmare and goes to sleep hoping it'll be gone. When my mother knew I was pregnant, she stuck me in a home for unwed mothers. I was the only Black kid at this Salvation Army home. Going to a home for unwed mothers to hide is what people did in the '60s. The plan was that when I had the baby, I would give him up for adoption, and slide back into my high school life. I was totally in support of the adoption until the day my son was born. When that nurse put him in my arms, I couldn't do it anymore.

When my mother knew I was pregnant, she stuck me in a home for unwed mothers . . . Going to a home for unwed mothers to hide is what people did in the '60s.

I don't know if on my part it was mother love for my baby or teen rebellion. It might've been a little bit of both. I knew it was going to upend my life. I knew it was going to perhaps keep me from going to college, which was my biggest, dearest dream at the time. My high school balked at readmitting me. So my parents had to threaten a lawsuit for me to return to my high school. We didn't actually end up in court, but we were successful. We argued that it was sex discrimination because they weren't expelling the boys who made the girls pregnant, just the girls.

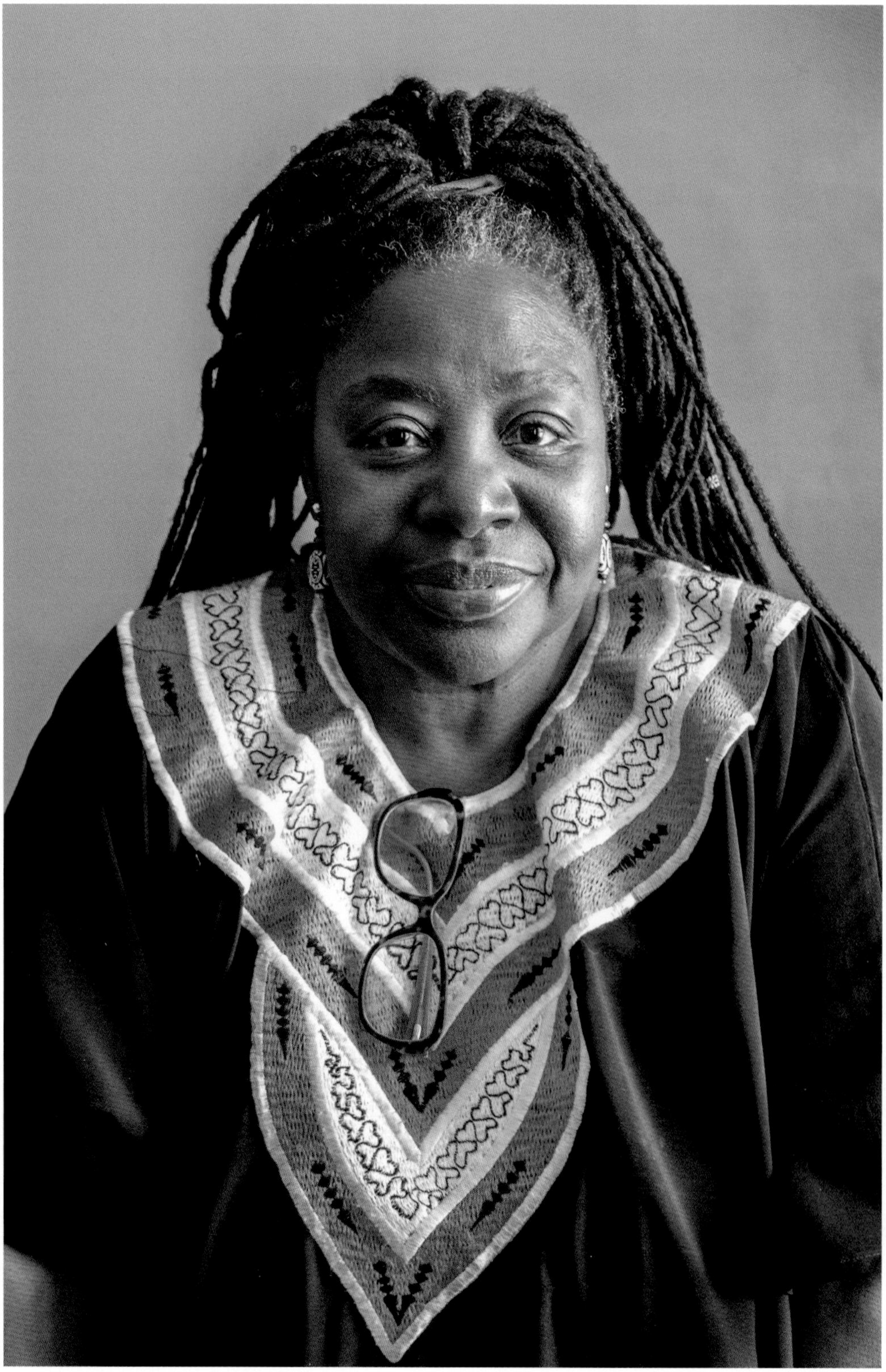

LORETTA ROSS

Many, many years later, I learned that my mother's overreaction to my confession that I was pregnant through incest was because she had been incested herself from age 8 to 16. She declined a chance to go to college in her hometown because it would've meant living with her uncle, who was abusing her. And so she had a lot of rage and unhealed hurt packed into her life around my childhood sexual abuse. She and I never talked about sex and sexuality.

Religion was a big part of my family as I was growing up. I became areligious at 14 with that pregnancy because one of the penances I had to do was stand up in front of my church and confess that I'd been a sinner. I was so unbelievably hurt by that. I had been sinned against. There was no censure for my cousin, who had made me pregnant; everything was heaped on me. Then my mom let me shop around, going to different churches in search of meaning and truth. Eventually I got baptized in the Baptist church, Church of Christ.

When I graduated high school, I received several scholarships including one to Radcliffe. But once Radcliffe found out that I'd had a baby, they couldn't rescind my acceptance, but they could rescind the scholarship. That put Radcliffe out of reach for my family. Instead, I took a scholarship from Howard University.

In 1970, I was a freshman at Howard University, one thousand miles away from home. In order to get birth control at age 16, I needed parental consent. I could not persuade my mother to sign the consent form. She just thought I would never have sex again until I got married. Needless to say, that didn't work. I became pregnant in my freshman year. My boyfriend at the time was in law school, and he was more than happy to pay for an abortion. But the question became how to get one. I was very lucky I was in Washington, D.C., which legalized abortion three years before Roe v. Wade.

My barriers to abortion in 1970 weren't financial or legal, but familial. Just like my mother wouldn't sign permission for me to have birth control, she wouldn't sign for me to obtain an abortion either. My older sister ended up forging my mother's signature for the permission form after months of delay and arguing. That's why I ended up having a late third-trimester abortion.

I celebrate the fact that I had an abortion. I'm frankly happy it was available to me. I think I had more freedom to decide in 1970 than people are facing now because of the increasing restrictions.

After I had the abortion, I got pregnant one more time and suffered a miscarriage. Apparently, nothing I was doing for contraception was working. I had tried condoms, and the pill. Finally, I went to Howard University Health Services, again forging my mom's signature, and had a Dalkon Shield IUD inserted. Its problems didn't manifest until I'd had it for several years, when I developed an acute infection and slipped into a coma. I went to George Washington Hospital and when I woke up I found out the doctor, head of OBGYN, had performed a hysterectomy without asking my permission. I woke up in post-op dizzy, drugged, and sterile. And this doctor was congratulating himself in my presence. That pissed me off. I mean, I'm 23 years old, and you're telling me I'm never going to have a baby again.

Now, I had been visiting this same doctor for six months with complaints of feeling ill. Even though there was research available, he never suggested my issues were related to this IUD. He kept diagnosing me with even more and more arcane-sounding STDs. He just refused to accept that the Dalkon Shield was the problem.

My reproductive career lasted seven years, age 14 to 21. Two years later we started the lawsuit against A.H. Robins, who manufactured the device. In 1976 we settled out of court.

In 1978, I started volunteering at the first Rape Crisis Center in the US and became its director in 1979. At that time I was much more of an anti-rape activist than a reproductive rights activist. I didn't start processing my sterilization abuse story in any real detail until the late '70s and early '80s.

Reproductive rights came into the conversation in the Black feminist community in Washington, D.C. largely through the agency of the Black Women Self-Help Collective. That's when my reproductive consciousness got stoked. It all crystallized for me in 1985 when I got the job at NOW as director of the Women of Color Program.

I remember when Ellie Smeal, president of NOW at the time, talked about organizing an abortion rights march. At the time, we didn't even say the A-word in the Black community. It was a clarifying challenge for me because that's when I started using the F-word for myself. I started calling myself a feminist. Up until then, I had denied that I was a feminist.

I think it is "respectability politics" that keeps the Women's Movement in general and Black people in particular from proclaiming our sex positivity the way we should for fear of being slut-shamed. That's an acute issue for Black women because we're already slut-shamed for being Black.

I began doing research on previous generations of Black women's activism. To my surprise, I found the large extent to which Black women were involved with Margaret Sanger and establishing birth control clinics in Black neighborhoods because they were turned away when they tried to go to the white clinics. All of this activism that had preceded us was unknown to us largely because of respectability politics.

The term "reproductive justice" was coined in June 1994. We were twelve Black women among 150 to 200 women who had come together in Chicago for a pro-choice conference sponsored by the Illinois Pro-Choice Alliance and the MS Foundation to discuss health care reform. The centrist Democratic politics of the day persuaded the organizers that if they omitted reproductive health care from health care reform, they could slide it by the Republicans. We were pissed off. They wanted to separate reproductive rights from social justice, which would leave out all these women who make their decisions about their bodies based on their social justice context. We spliced together reproductive rights and social justice, and that's where reproductive justice came from.

Our job at Sistersong is to lift up and amplify the voices of women of color, not necessarily to speak for them, but to create the spaces so they can speak for themselves.

White women for the most part were not facing the sterilization abuse that was visited on Native-American, African-American, and Latina women. We entered the movement at different vectors; we landed in the center of the states trying to deny us the right to control our bodies, whether it's preventing pregnancy, having an abortion, or preventing sterilization abuse.

Sistersong was founded in 1997 on the foundation of reproductive justice. I was one of the co-founders and, later, its national director. We brought together sixteen women of color organizations—Latina, African American, Native American, Asian, Pacific Islander—into a collective. Four previous attempts to organize a national coalition of women of color working on the sterilization of women of color and other issues had foundered for lack of money. What made Sistersong significant is that the Ford Foundation gave us $4 million to split among sixteen groups, an unheard-of level of funding to anything led by women of color in America.

Our job at Sistersong is to lift up and amplify the voices of women of color, not necessarily to speak for them, but to create the spaces so they can speak for themselves.

Communication and media organizing is a main thing. We create settings where people can come together. Our signature event is Let's Talk About Sex, a conference we have every two or three years on organizing women of color.

What keeps me going is my gift from the universe. I'm a quadruple Leo, which probably only means something to a child who was socialized in the '60s. That means that I have an inner sun, a well of inside energy. I blaze pretty brightly. And I don't mind others using my energy because the heat would probably consume me if I didn't share it.

There are movements in my footprints, right? I could no more not get up and participate in the human rights movement than I could hold in a fart after a bad meal. I just couldn't do that. When I was developing my feminist consciousness, I was privileged to stand on the shoulders and work with a lot of Black women who themselves have been active in the '30s, '40s, and '50s. And most of the time they hated me. I was a mouthy, dreadlocked, radical woman who would say motherfucker in the middle of the mayor's meeting. I did not sit there like a respectable Black woman. Nonetheless, they mentored me if for no other reason than to keep me from embarrassing them.

You build movements by bringing young people in. All of the places I've worked, the movements I've been engaged in are fueled by young people.

My son was amazing. I never regretted making that decision to keep him, though he did seem like a political changeling. The more feminist and radical I became, the more conservative he became. But also I attribute a large part of that to the fact that my mother had him for the first four to five years of his life. She was his biggest influence. She was ultra-Christian, he was an ultra-Christian. She was pro-family, he was very much into family. Those values were branded in his soul by my parents, which was good because a 14-year-old is not capable of raising a decent human being. So thank God I had co-parents.

Now I have one grandson and two step-grandchildren. My grandson, like my son, turned out intentionally and deliberately apolitical. When my son died two years ago from a heart attack at 47, it caused me and my grandson to become much closer.

I see incredible passion, resistance, and knowledge amongst young people right now. It does remind me of the way young people were recruited in the heyday of the Civil Rights Movement and put on the front lines.

Discomfort is a feature of doing political work in America. If being oppressed sucks, fighting oppression sucks even worse because all the power of the state is going to be turned against you. I've seen change happen, and I've been a part of it. I know more change is possible.

Erika Settles

ACTUALLY, IT WAS through listening to my mom's story one day that helped me come to terms with my childhood with her. Now when I think about my mother, I picture this young girl, 16, getting pregnant and just all the things that she had experienced, like abuse. It brought me into her world and for the first time I was able to have compassion. Gosh, I wish that I could've been there to protect her. I now realize why she made the decisions that she made when she was raising us. She did remarkably well considering everything that she experienced.

After hearing her story, I could make sense of my own story. So, when I was asked to tell my abortion story for the first time, it just resonated with me and I said, "yes."

Both of my parents are Mexican-American. My dad is first-generation American, and my mom's family has been here for many generations. I have a very large extended family. My ex-husband and I are divorced. We have four children together, three girls and a boy ranging from 8 to 14. Their dad is definitely involved in their life and he visits them every other weekend, but the majority of the time, I'm a single mom.

When I was growing up, because some family members had experienced sexual abuse, I was just determined that when I had kids, I would stay at home and not leave them with anybody. I needed to be present for them.

Internally I had always struggled with the belief in God. I knew about God and religion because of my grandmother. She was a very strict Baptist. She had converted from Catholicism and raised my mom and her siblings with that. They weren't allowed to go to dances. I was, for the most part, a child who did what she was told.

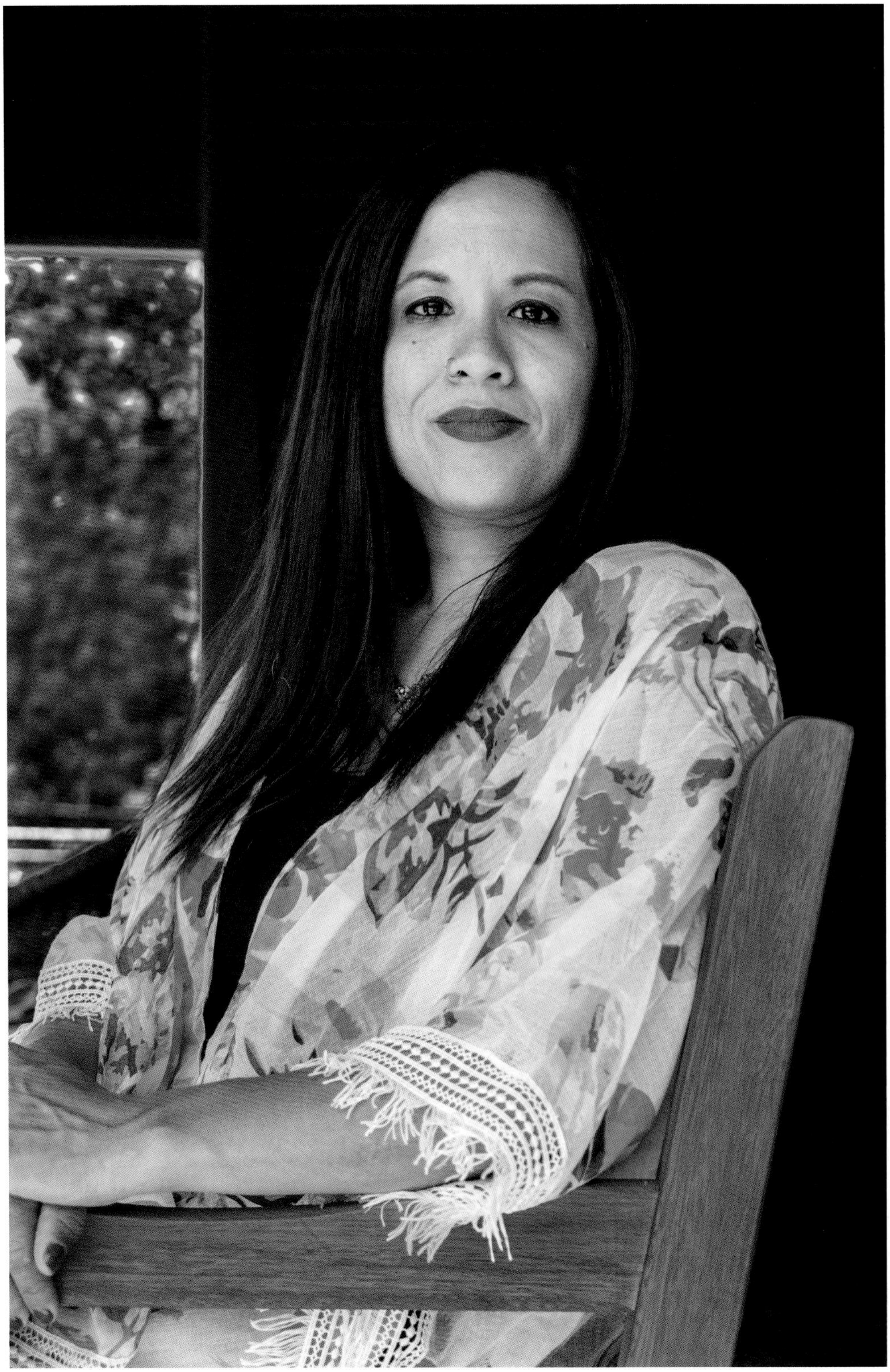

ERIKA SETTLES

In college, oddly enough, I had my own conversion experience. I just decided that I wanted to become a Christian. and I started going to church. On Friday nights we'd go to the university and we'd talk to people about Jesus, trying to convert them to Christianity. We called it witnessing. "If you don't believe, you're going to hell." And then, very staunch beliefs that sex before marriage is wrong, abortion is wrong, homosexuality is a sin as well.

It was during that time that I met my now ex-husband. I was 20. He had been raised with a religious background. I married him because he came to me at one point and said that he felt like God was wanting him to marry me.

At the time of my abortion, I had already been married for about nine years. We had been through fourteen moves by the time my oldest daughter was 8 years old. My ex-husband at the time didn't keep stable jobs. After so many moves, we finally had packed up all of our things and were living in our van in a Walmart parking lot. Feeding our kids became difficult. It was then that I realized things had to change.

So, we moved in with my mom. I got a job with Child Protective Services as a caseworker and a few months later we moved into our own house. For the first time we were financially stable, but it was at that point when I stopped living in survival mode that my emotions kind of caught up with me. My oldest child was struggling in school and I realized it was because of our instability and the turmoil we had been through.

It was during that time that I started to question God. Up until that point I had been making decisions based on, "What does God want me to do?" It was never a matter of what does Erika want? What does Erika think? I was experiencing religious conflict internally. I wanted to make decisions that were in line with my conscience. I was just emotionally kind of a wreck. And, instead of standing up and facing everything that I had before me, I ran away. I ended up having an affair.

My husband found out. I basically forced him to move out of the only house that we were stable in. I just pushed him away. After he moved out, I just came completely unraveled and I started going to clubs on the weekends, drinking when I didn't have my kids. I was doing awesome work at my job. I was getting raises and promotions, but on weekends I was just off.

It was at that point that I met a younger gentleman at a club; he was smiling at me and I smiled back. Then he pulled me to the dance floor, then we were dancing. It was just an escape, a fun time away from the reality that I was living at the time.

One time, literally one time, we had unprotected sex, and he asked, "Are you sure it's OK?" And I was like, "Yeah, I know my body. I know when I ovulate. I've got four kids, it's fine." And three weeks later I had headaches and nausea and on Mother's Day he brought me a pregnancy test. It was positive. I was in shock, of course. I was still technically married, even though we were separated.

He assumed that I was going to have an abortion and I was conflicted. He was angry and told me he was never going to be a part of a baby's life if I had it. I wavered kind of back and forth as to what to do. There was a conflict between my rational and emotional sides. I was thinking, "Erika, you've got four kids. You just got financially stable. You're finally able to provide for them. You know that you cannot take care of one more child." But emotionally I was thinking, "I love children and I love babies. You can do this."

I told my sister I was pregnant. My sister told me that if I wanted to keep it, that she could adopt it. I didn't say anything to her, but it didn't settle well with me because if I was going to have the baby, I would raise it. She meant well.

I was isolated. One day my now ex-husband came over and said, "What's going on? Are you pregnant?" I don't know what gave him that idea, but I admitted it. He even told me that he would help me raise it even though we weren't together, but I felt everybody was trying to give me solutions so that I could have this baby, but, in my mind, they weren't real solutions.

I kept hearing the words of the man who got me pregnant. "If you have this baby I will not be a part of its life." Because my own biological dad was minimally present in my own life growing up, I knew what that was like. Also, a lot of kids I worked with in my job did not have a father figure. I felt that no child deserves that kind of start in life.

I kept hearing the words of the man who got me pregnant. "If you have this baby I will not be a part of its life." Because my own biological dad was minimally present in my own life growing up, I knew what that was like . . . I felt that no child deserves that kind of start in life.

When I finally had to decide about the abortion, my rational side came out. I was able to choose what I thought was best for me, which is wrapped up in my children, and what I thought was best for them. I also thought about the fetus who would become a baby and what kind of life would that baby have.

Once I decided to have an abortion, I did a Google search to find a clinic. The man who got me pregnant took me to the clinic and he paid for it. I believe the abortion cost

$300 or $350. There were actually protestors outside of the clinic. The nurses were welcoming. I was given an ultrasound and they explained everything that would happen. I was six weeks pregnant. There was a waiting period. We had to come back in a few days for the actual procedure. They gave me medication and I believe it was the suction type of abortion. That was five years ago.

The Erika I am today isn't the scared one running away from her problems by having an affair. It is the Erika who believes in honesty and transparency and in the fact that we don't always make beautiful choices, but we can learn from them and grow and become our authentic selves. I think sharing our stories can lead to discovering who we are.

It took me losing myself to realize what my values and beliefs are.

YAMANI HERNANDEZ

Yamani Hernandez

WHEN I WAS an undergrad at Cornell University I took time off and did a year of public service here in Chicago and got really interested in the intersection between art and social justice. When I went back to school, I studied an individual curriculum that was a mixture of interior design, policy studies, design, and environmental analysis. The title of my major was Design as a Tool for Community Empowerment. I saw myself doing public art projects or some kind of socially responsible architecture work. I did end up going on to get a Master's in Architecture at the University of Washington, writing a thesis on activist architecture.

During a project with young people back here in Chicago, I met a young woman who needed an abortion, and that is how I moved from public architecture, art, design, education work to working on sexual health, rights, justice, and abortion. One project was teaching a class about wind-powered sculpture to a group of youth. One of the students, a 14-year-old girl, was already a mom. When the students got their final checks, she asked the rest of the people in the program to go with her to the check-cashing place, and offered to pay them $10 each to beat her up. She said it pretty much in front of me, so she wasn't hiding it. It was pretty shocking to me.

I asked her why she would pay someone to beat her up. She said, "I'm pregnant again. My parents told me that I cannot bring another baby home. If I do, I'll get kicked out of the house." She added that getting beat up was cheaper and easier to explain than an abortion. She was hoping if she got beat up, she would miscarry and wouldn't need an abortion.

I thought, this is an emergency. She just needs an abortion. Let me figure out how to help her pay for it. That's how I found out about abortion funds. I connected this 14-year-old girl with an organization that helps people who can't afford them pay for abortions—also rides, childcare, housing.

My own abortion happened when I was 19. I got pregnant the first time I had sex. I was very much in love. My partner was like a best friend. We eventually got married. At the time, I had a lot of ideas about wanting to be a mother and wanting to heal some of the wounds from my own childhood by becoming a mother. But when I got pregnant, I quickly figured out, after telling my partner and people in my family, including my mother, that I was pregnant, that nobody else was excited about this pregnancy except for me.

I felt a lot of stigma about being pregnant in college. I also felt a little coerced into my abortion. No one told me I had to this, but I didn't feel like it was my decision. It was a decision I made because I didn't feel like I had the support I needed to parent in a way that I wanted to.

I ALSO FELT A LITTLE COERCED INTO MY ABORTION. NO ONE TOLD ME I HAD TO THIS, BUT I DIDN'T FEEL LIKE IT WAS MY DECISION. IT WAS A DECISION I MADE BECAUSE I DIDN'T FEEL LIKE I HAD THE SUPPORT I NEEDED TO PARENT IN A WAY THAT I WANTED TO.

I had my abortion at Planned Parenthood here in Chicago. I was very emotionally disturbed going into the appointment. I went through the pre-counseling and, reflecting on it, I kind of wish somebody had told me to go home and think about it more, and come back. They did ask, "Are you sure?" and I answered, "Yes." It was my decision, but I definitely had mixed feelings about it.

I was in the first trimester and had a surgical abortion. The actual abortion procedure wasn't a pleasant experience. It was uncomfortable.

I wished I hadn't had the abortion, not because I have a problem with abortion. I remember my mom telling me that, whether I had an abortion or not, it was a permanent decision. I wanted her to be supportive of me bringing that first pregnancy to term. She said vehemently, "I'm not going to support you. I already raised my kids, I'm not trying to raise grandkids."

Mostly I didn't talk about my abortion. I don't remember anybody judging me or anything like that. It coincided with a time when I was leaving school to take a break for a year. It worked out in the sense that nobody ever really had to see me pregnant or know that I was pregnant. I remember losing weight after it, and people saying, "Oh my god, you look so good." I felt like, I can't look so good because I'm depressed.

Three years after my abortion I got pregnant with my first child. I wanted to get pregnant again. I felt I had made a mistake to have the abortion. I wanted to correct it. My partner and I had both graduated; I earned a Master's in Architecture at the University of Washington, writing a thesis on activist architecture. He had a job. It seemed like I had a viable career. We had made a home. Our relationship was clear. It definitely filled a desire to have a kid. We decided to get married.

So now I have a 17-year-old and a 12-year-old. They're wonderful, wonderful people. I love, love, love being a mom. Every child is going to have a grievance with their parents, so I'm not going to sit here and say that I've been a perfect parent and my kids will never have any criticisms of me. But there are some things that I tried to correct. One of the things in particular is, when my parents separated and later divorced, they had a lot of animosity toward each other. My marriage lasted ten years. Once I realized I didn't want to continue my own marriage, one of the things that I wanted for my children was that we would continue to be in a positive relationship with each other. It has worked out.

I never thought I'd be the CEO of the National Network of Abortion Funds. I just completely fell in love with the idea of a safety net of people that was predominantly thousands of volunteers helping people get their abortions. I was really touched at the commitment people have to supporting other people that they don't know.

In three years we have doubled our budget and tripled our staff. We've rebranded and built more of a movement around our work. We have seventy member organizations in thirty-eight states, and growing. I would say 90 percent of the organizations are volunteer run. Our people are leaders in strategizing in times of trouble and distress. They have direct contact with the people who are most impacted by the systemic barriers that prevent people from getting the care they need.

Storytelling is a huge, huge, huge piece of how abortion can be de-stigmatized. It's really important to hear a variety of stories to understand that, across race, class, age, and so many demographics, stories are all very similar, and also very different.

It's important to be able to say "abortion." I had a miscarriage just about six weeks ago, and I found the same thing even with miscarriage. People are like, why are you telling people you had a miscarriage? I'm like, because it's what happened to me. I feel injured, and I'm hurt, and just saying that I had the flu doesn't fucking capture it. I wanted that pregnancy. Saying miscarriage out loud is a way to honor what's going on with me. I think that's the same thing with abortion.

For my miscarriage I was in the Emergency Room. They called it a spontaneous abortion, a threatened miscarriage. I had to look it up, what do they mean, a threatened abortion? Do they think I tried to self-abort? They are just interchangeable words, abortion and miscarriage. But miscarriage was invented to make it softer and mean that it's not your fault. That is shame and stigma right there. The word abortion just means your uterus is emptying. That process is nothing new. It's never going to go away. We might as well just figure out how to accept it and talk about it, and treat people with compassion, and not judgment.

Both my children know what I do. We've had a lot of conversations about abortion, we've had conversations about sex, about sexism, about what it means to be a feminist, all of those things. They're not always nice, neat conversations. There have been times when they've asked me hard questions and we've had hard conversations. My older son sent me for my 40th birthday a list of forty things that he loves about me, and he talked about my work as one of them. It was sweet. I was very touched.

I think anti-choice people always try to make it seem like people who advocate for abortion are anti-family and anti-children. I always like to say that I come to this work because of a deep love of children, and because I really believe that children deserve to be with parents, in homes where they feel deeply, deeply loved.

Laurene Jauffret

I MOVED TO the United States with my mom and sister when I was 13. Up until then, I had lived in France. My mother is American. My dad, who was French, passed away when I was 3. My mom remarried and my step-dad lives in France. We came to the US because my mom wanted us to have more educational opportunities. I go back to France every summer.

Going from public school in France to a private French-American school in the US was very, very different. Academic-wise, it was really challenging for me. Friends-wise it was OK, and speaking English was not a problem because I already spoke English with my mom. I kind of went through a confusion, though: Should I be more French or should I be more American?

I definitely grew up in a very loving and supportive environment, very open-minded and accepting, respectful. I've always had a very nice trust with my mom because I was always honest and I told her everything.

My abortion happened a year ago when I was 19. I had just taken a semester off from college. I stopped birth control because I felt like it made me very depressed. I didn't feel like myself.

I had been in a relationship with my boyfriend for two years. I was two weeks late on my cycle. I had noticed that I was feeling different. I had a lot of interesting mood swings and I was extremely tired. I didn't know why. So I took a pregnancy test. But right before that my boyfriend and I had gotten in a huge fight. Then I had to call him to tell him that my pregnancy test said positive. I was freaking out. But he came right away to the house

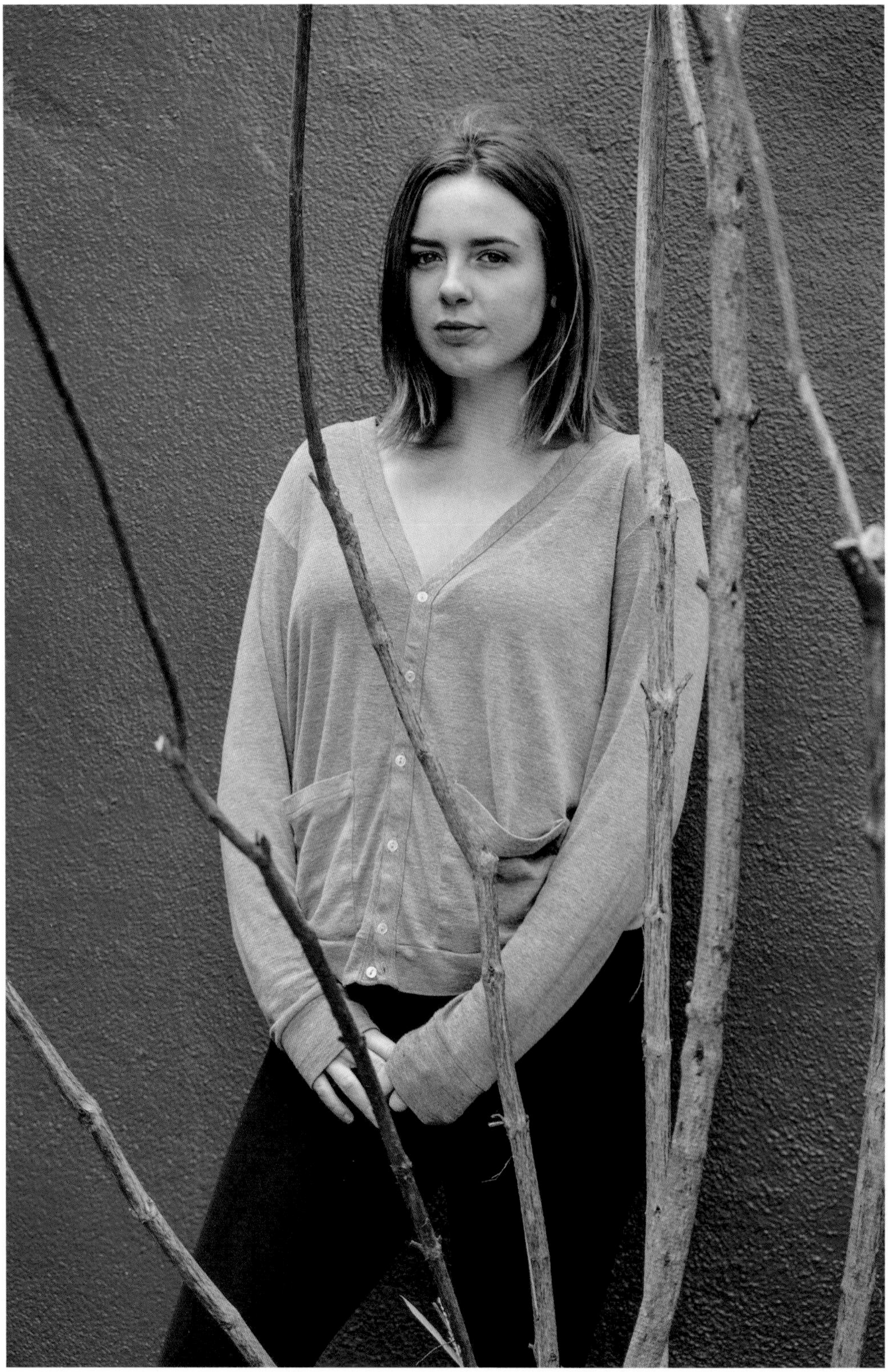

LAURENE JAUFFRET

and was very supportive. I told my mom and she was very supportive too. She said she would never impose a decision on me. She just wanted me to be sure of what I wanted to do. There was a time where she was like, "Well, if you do really want it, we could find a way to make it work." I was just freaked out about the financial part. That's what we all were most worried about.

The nurse at Planned Parenthood was really nice. She asked me what decision I wanted to make about the pregnancy. I chose to have the abortion because I couldn't financially support myself. It just wouldn't have been possible. So, I made the appointment to have the abortion five days later. I chose the pill, a medication abortion.

During the five days between the first appointment and the abortion, we went on a family trip to LA. My boyfriend came on the trip too. I felt very happy and comfortable, actually, really realizing that I was pregnant. It was empowering.

Apparently, my insurance wasn't working, so they were trying to charge me $800. I didn't have that money. The only job I was working was very part-time at Instacart. Finally, they sent me to this place to get Medi-Cal. Once I got accepted for Medi-Cal, I had to schedule an appointment a week later. During all that time that the abortion kept getting pushed back, I kept thinking maybe it was a sign that I should keep the pregnancy. After all, when I first found out I was pregnant, it gave me this feeling like I was doing something right.

When I was walking into the clinic to get the abortion these pro-life protestors followed me to the door. One of the three women shouted, "I hope you're not going to kill it. I hope you're not going to kill it. Think about it." She was talking about Jesus and all that. It was not the time to do that, so I got really mad and I flipped them off. My boyfriend just took me away, telling me not to pay attention to them. He came with me to all my appointments.

I was just really mad that they waste so much energy on trying to force their opinion on somebody else. If you're going to just stand there with a sign, OK. But if you're going to yell and follow people to the door and try to force your opinion upon somebody, that's not right.

Anyway, I went to the appointment, I took the first pill, and then I left Planned Parenthood to take the second pill at home. The first pill kills and the second pill sheds the lining. On my way to taking the bus back home I threw up the first pill right away, as I stepped out of Planned Parenthood. This person on the street was like, "Maybe you have morning sickness." I was just like, great. I felt like I was getting a bunch of signs. The second pill, I took at home. Then it was just a lot of bleeding and nausea.

I think I took three days off work. My boyfriend had to go to work but he kept checking on me. After the abortion I was kind of going through a very sad phase. I kind of felt a sense of numbness and emptiness. I felt very disconnected to my sexuality too. I wanted to be alone. I was not being affectionate. I remember being very worried about not being able to have kids after the abortion because I had taken the Plan B a couple of times. So, I was getting very paranoid about that. I do want to have children some time. I just felt so numb that I even went back to Planned Parenthood because I thought the abortion had damaged me emotionally and physically. They said that it was definitely a subconscious emotional thing going on. I wouldn't say it was traumatic but I would say definitely I did some emotional damage on myself.

AFTER THE ABORTION I WAS KIND OF GOING THROUGH A VERY SAD PHASE. I KIND OF FELT A SENSE OF NUMBNESS AND EMPTINESS. I FELT VERY DISCONNECTED TO MY SEXUALITY TOO. I WANTED TO BE ALONE.

If I had gotten pregnant in France, well, I lived in a small town, so the whole town would have known about it. Everyone knows my dad and my mom. Everybody knows everybody's business. My best friend in France had gotten pregnant when she was 15 and she had to stay in the hospital for a while. In France, whether it's the pill or the vacuum, it has to be in the hospital.

What I don't why get is why they can't just make abortion legal and whoever needs to get one gets it and whoever doesn't need to, doesn't get one. I saw that Texas was thinking about passing a bill about how if you give an abortion, you will face the death penalty. To me, it's so ironic how they call themselves pro-life but they're going to kill.

My boyfriend and I are still together. The abortion was really hard for him because he really wants to be a father. He was adopted by a single mother and he wants to be the father he never had. Every time we talked when I was pregnant, he would get very excited about having a baby. So for him, it was hard. I would tell somebody who got pregnant to listen to yourself, think about what would be the best for themselves and for the baby. Don't listen to anyone else. There are so many kids out there who are not supported or loved. You really need to think about, am I going to be able to give my full support?

Right now I'm studying trauma recovery and prevention, and sociology. I'm also working with survivors of domestic violence. Ever since I was little, I have had a lot of compassion and empathy for other people's pain. My dream would be to have an organization that works with holistic healing for any trauma and teaches self-care and things like that.

I remember when I was pregnant, the crazy thing is, I was just seeing babies everywhere. Pregnant women everywhere. Strollers everywhere. Maybe it was because I was noticing more, but they were just everywhere.

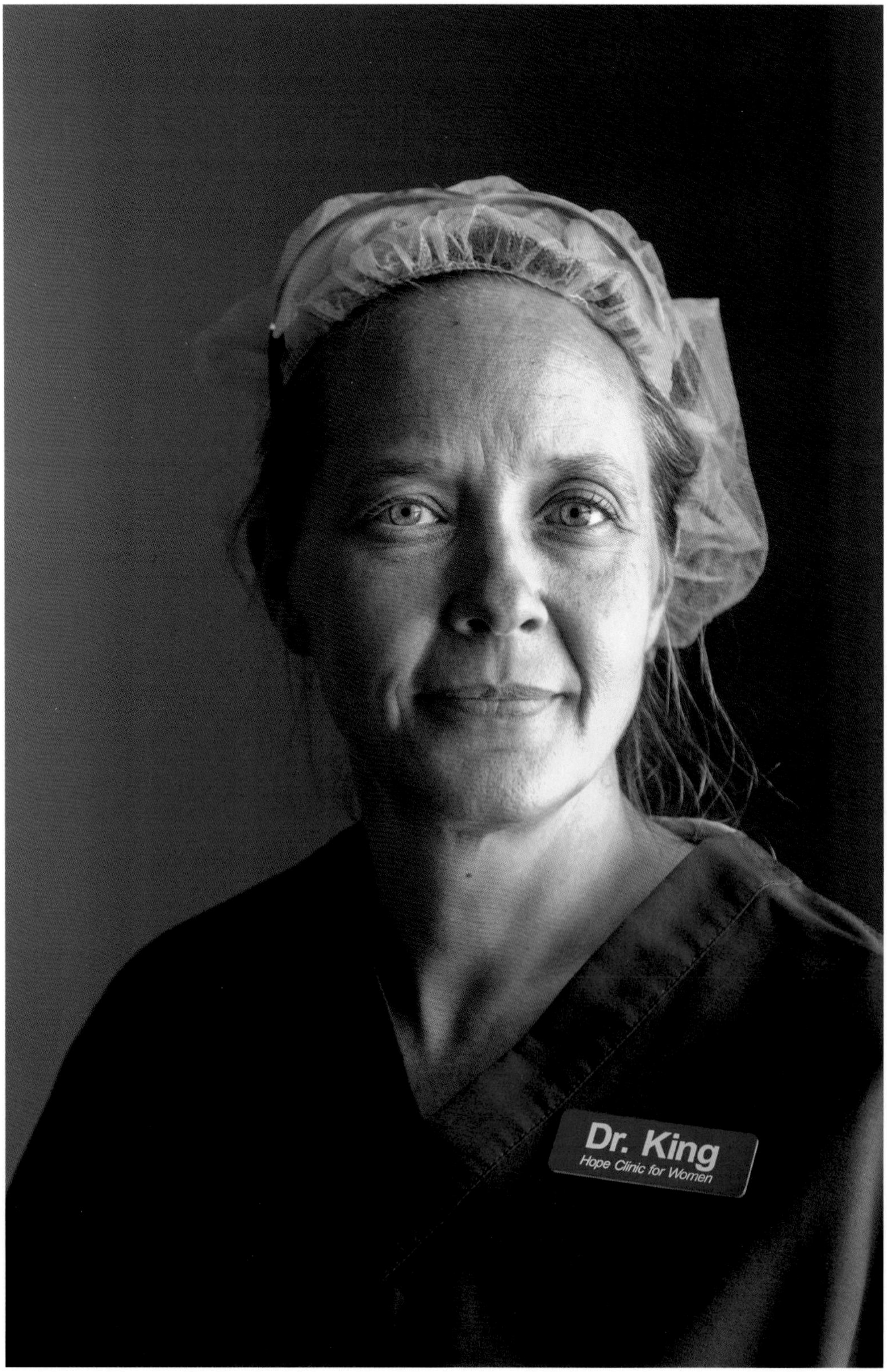

ERIN KING

Erin King

I GREW UP in this very liberal bubble, Northern California, for about half of my life, and the other half in the Washington, D.C. area.

Growing up, reproductive health care was one of the things we learned about in schools and in our families. It was like: People get pregnant, and here's the way to prevent pregnancy if you want to. If you get pregnant, here are the options you have. It was presented to me very equally.

In college I was part of a very naïve world where, of course, everyone could go to their student health center and get a whole year of birth control when they walked in the door. In medical school, where I trained as an OBGYN, the whole spectrum of gynecological care was presented to us, from different birth control methods and pregnancy prevention to sexually transmitted infections and treatment and who should have access, and then pregnancy. The pregnancy options were presented pretty fairly. I started to realize that access, not just to reproductive health care but to health care in general, really varies by where you live.

When I graduated from medical school and was looking for residencies, I still had this very naïve view that people who were being trained in gynecology would clearly be trained in abortion care too. I just randomly ended up at a program at Northwestern that did excellent training in abortion care. That's where I met my husband, who is an OBGYN too.

He knew a lot about abortion personally through his family. His mom had an abortion just prior to Roe v. Wade, in 1972 or 1973. She was a white woman who had means. Her gynecologist sent her to a psychologist and they agreed that her pregnancy was "psychologically harmful" and it was very easy for her to get an abortion. Their family talks very openly about that, and his mom's very vocal about access to abortion and other reproductive health care because of how important it was to their family.

My husband and I came to St. Louis after our residencies. I am working at the Hope Clinic in Granite City, Illinois, and at a hospital in St. Louis, Missouri.

In the part of Illinois where the Hope Clinic is located, there's no other abortion provider in the area, except for St. Louis. This area is pretty economically depressed, so we see a lot of patients who don't have great access to health care and have a hard time traveling very far. Besides local people, we see patients from Missouri, Illinois, Arkansas, Indiana, Kentucky, Tennessee, Iowa, Oklahoma, and Kansas. And because there's no gestational age cutoff in Illinois, we're able to see patients up to about the end of twenty-three weeks.

One day a week I see patients in my office in a hospital in downtown St. Louis. I do deliveries and surgeries there. However, at that facility, because of the funding the hospital receives, it's really difficult to even refer for an abortion, let alone see a patient for abortion care there.

I try to be very careful when someone's newly pregnant. I don't immediately offer congratulations. Instead, I say something like, "I see that you're pregnant. How do you feel about that? Is that a good thing for you right now? How are you feeling about being pregnant?" When someone says, "I'm so excited," I congratulate them. When someone is more, "I'm not ready for this right now," then I bring up abortion. I've had patients look at me like, "I can't have an abortion, that's illegal now."

When you're telling patients that you don't trust them to make a decision, that they have to wait a certain amount of time, and that you've put so much effort into making so many laws to restrict access to abortion, I think your patients know they are being told that abortion is wrong, you are bad, what you are doing is not right.

Every patient who comes here to Hope Clinic sees a trained educator who walks them through the procedure and does an informed consent, talking about risks and benefits, alternatives. Our staff is really good at talking to patients about the fact that we are medical providers, providing a medical service that we know you need to access. We know you have good reasons for being here; you don't have to explain yourself to us. This is a judgment-free zone.

A good summary of what's going on in Missouri and Illinois is laid out in two laws that were passed in 2019 in those two states. In May 2019, Missouri passed HB126, which essentially restricted abortion after eight weeks, and had a lot of other restrictions as well. It limits the reasons that people can have abortions. It put abortion from a provider perspective and from a patient perspective into the criminal code. It also has a lot of required information about how you make referrals, and then regulations for facilities that perform abortions.

If you look at the first three sentences of the bill, it sounds like you are reading the Bible: The Almighty God has given us life and is going to protect us, and the State of Missouri is under this God, and this God thinks that all children born and unborn have the same rights. This Missouri law went into effect on Wednesday, September 28, 2019.

About two weeks later Illinois passed the Reproductive Health Act. It's almost the exact opposite of Missouri's law. There's no religious language. Its first paragraph talks about how people who are pregnant have autonomy to choose what they do with those pregnancies, and that the state has no right to interfere from a medical or a legal perspective. It states that doctors have autonomy and the right to make medical decisions free of the state, but must instead adhere to evidence-based medical decision-making and be held to the same standards that other medical care providers are held to in Illinois.

I think what was happening in Missouri gave the final push to passage of the Illinois bill. I stayed up until almost midnight listening to the arguments the night the Illinois bill passed. The arguments the Illinois senators were making sounded like how I talk about medical decision-making: best medical practices, the patient's right to make decisions. A group of lawmakers from Missouri actually went up to Illinois to urge Illinois to pass the law. The Missouri lawmakers were saying, in effect, "This is bigger than our state. We don't want to have Missouri patients have to travel, but they need someplace to go for care."

The abortion restrictions in Missouri have grown over the last seven or eight years, for both patients and providers. Missouri added waiting periods and specific consent information that had to be presented. They started adding so many restrictions for providers that very few providers could comply without significant expense. That resulted in most of the clinics in Missouri having to close down. Today, the Planned Parenthood clinic in St. Louis is the only freestanding facility in the state that provides abortions.

I do try to have conversations with the other side. On an airplane, I had a seat next to a woman who was at the time president of Students for Life, an anti-choice student group. She's a beautiful woman. Super smart, really articulate. We had a pretty frank discussion about abortion. What I realized, unfortunately, was that she had been given a lot of misinformation about the medical risks for abortion. I said to her, "I would really want, at the end of this conversation, for you to have just a tiny bit of doubt about some of the information you've been given. It may never change your personal opinion about abortion. That is fine, but it might change some of the misinformation that you're giving out."

I think if you're anti-abortion, you've just got to say, "I'm personally anti-abortion, I personally think it's murder."

Many of our patients coming from a Christian background are concerned about what their God is going to feel. We advise them to ask their religious leader, because a lot of Christian churches are not anti-abortion. Rather, many are pro-forgiveness. In fact, I'm pretty sure the basic tenet of Christianity is forgiveness.

I don't think it's my job to decide when a life begins. My job is to give my patients high-quality medical care. They are capable of making their own decisions about their pregnancy, and I'm here to provide a medical procedure for them if they don't want to be pregnant anymore.

I think it's really important for patients to read and hear about abortion from people who have been here before them: You are not alone. You are normal. There are people who think you are making good decisions.

Many of our patients coming from a Christian background are concerned about what their God is going to feel. We advise them to ask their religious leader, because a lot of Christian churches are not anti-abortion. Rather, many are pro-forgiveness. In fact, I'm pretty sure the basic tenet of Christianity is forgiveness. If you've accepted Jesus and his teachings, then you are forgiven. That is the whole point of your religion, right?

I've had many people come up to me when I'm dropping my kid off at school, who say, "You don't know me, but thank you so much for what you're doing, and for helping patients." Then they ask me what they can do. I have two very good answers to that. First: Give money to organizations that are funding patients seeking abortion care. Second: Vote."

Nicole Stewart

GROWING UP IN Dallas, I was surrounded by people who didn't talk about what was actually going on. It was all, "We're great. Everything is just great. My goodness it's so good to see you." It was all just on the surface. That made me feel like it wasn't okay to have feelings, it wasn't okay to be confused or to not know. That is at the root of my desire to talk about things. It's so healing to give voice to our realities and the reality of the human experience, not what we think the human experience should be.

After a period in Los Angeles training and working as an actress, I got involved with a storytelling group. It was just people on stage, reading stories about themselves. Over a couple of years, I did several performances, took memoir-writing classes, and got good feedback about my work.

When I moved back to Dallas, NARAL Pro-Choice Texas asked me to join the board. I racked my brain wondering what I could do on the board to make a difference; I don't have legislative knowledge, I don't like fundraising. Then, I woke up one night and shot out of bed with this vision in my head of standing on a stage in a large theater, asking women in the audience to stand if they'd had an abortion.

In 2011, I had created a storytelling production company called Oral Fixation, based in Dallas, and had produced two shows on the issue of immigration for the Dallas Museum of Art. Abortion is probably more contentious than even immigration but that gave me the confidence to think maybe I can do this.

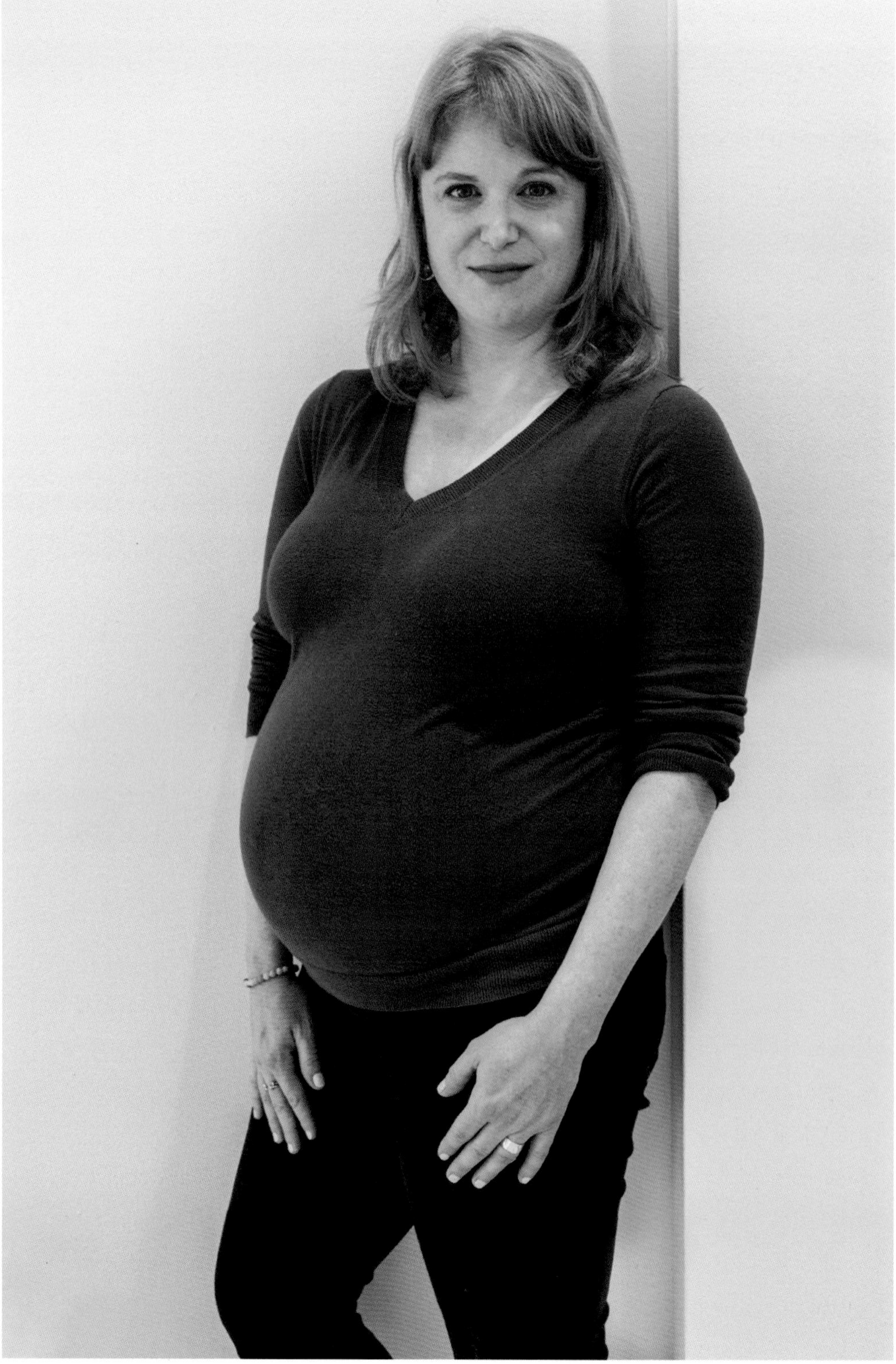

NICOLE STEWART

In the summer of 2015, I created "Out From Under The Rug: True Life Tales Of Abortion."

I ask participants to write their stories down. Putting your story down on paper is transformative. When someone sends me a story they've written down, it doesn't have to be pretty, I just need to know what happened and to have a sense of you and your voice as a writer. Then I start to meet on the phone with the individuals who will be in the show. Phone calls are a great way to create a private space, even better than being in person or on a video call. My intention from the beginning is to create a safe space of unconditional love so they feel wholly supported by me as a guide.

I get a lot of feedback that it's extremely cathartic because I help them process their story emotionally. Together, we create a "healing narrative," which is when the writer has achieved a degree of emotional distance from the experience so they can successfully recreate the experience on the page, so that someone who is listening or reading can feel like they're walking in their shoes.

And then in late June of 2013, I did walk in the shoes of women who have had abortions. I was working on the next season of Oral Fixation shows and had designed our season opener. The theme was "Bun in the Oven" and it was going to be a funny story around my own pregnancy.

I was 34 when I got married and felt a lot of pressure to get pregnant right away. We conceived quickly. We were nervous and thrilled.

We decided not to tell anybody for the first trimester. At our twenty-week appointment we had a sonogram and decided we wanted to find out the gender. The nurse told us it was a boy, and then she finished the sonogram in silence. She disappeared for a long time and came back to tell us we needed to meet with the doctor. The doctor told us some of the measurements were off, that his femurs were short. I didn't even know that they were measuring anything. Now, I come from a really tiny family, so I was like, "All right, He's going to be short." This was not shocking news to me.

But then the doctor said she would make an appointment the next day with a maternal fetal specialist for a higher-level ultrasound. At that appointment, a very matter-of-fact doctor looked at the ultrasound and told us she saw a constellation of markers indicating abnormalities in the baby, particularly in the development of the brain. Within the first ten minutes of the appointment, she said we might want to consider terminating the pregnancy. If so, we didn't have much time because the gestational limit on abortion at that time was twenty-four weeks, when a baby is viable outside the womb.

Ten days later, the results of an amniocentesis showed that the baby didn't have Down syndrome. Another ultrasound showed that all of the problems we had seen two weeks earlier were aggravated: They referred me for an MRI of my pelvis to look at the baby's brain. The radiologist told us not only was the rear part of the cerebellum missing, but the entire brain was abnormal.

My husband and I decided to have an abortion. I was twenty-one-and-a-half weeks pregnant. The procedure was a D&E, dilation and extraction. The first day was the consultation for a mandatory ultrasound and a recitation of these lies, basically, from the state of Texas about how abortion may cause breast cancer and all that stuff. Then they make you wait twenty-four hours so you're sure before you can actually start the abortion.

During that mandatory ultrasound I had this amazing connection with my doctor. She was this really beautiful woman, probably a few years older than me, and she took a lot of care and spent time showing me the abnormalities on the screen. I knew that every day that passed his situation was getting worse. The fluid was building up in his brain and in his lungs. The doctor put her hand on me and she said, "One of my friends had this happen to her, and now they have three healthy children." That was the best thing anyone could possibly say.

A HUGE MOTIVATOR FOR ME TELLING MY STORY IS HONORING THE LEGACY OF MY FIRST PREGNANCY THAT WAS ABORTED; BEING ABLE TO HAVE HIS LIFE MAKE A DIFFERENCE FOR OTHER PEOPLE.

The second day I went back and they inserted Laminaria, which is like seaweed, into my cervix to expand and open it up. It's pretty painful. The third day they replace it. On the fourth day, they take it out and give the baby a shot to stop his heart. That was really hard. That is when I knew I lost him. It was also hard to carry him for another day after his heart stopped.

We elected to have an autopsy, which showed nothing, then cremated his remains. We had a death certificate issued. On what would have been his due date, we scattered his ashes around a tree we had planted on the day of our wedding on my in-law's property.

I started off by telling people we had lost the baby. Then I started to say we terminated the pregnancy because of fetal abnormalities. Finally I started to say we had an abortion. The feedback that I got was unbelievably illuminating. Many people shared with me their stories of lost pregnancies. I started to feel like I wasn't alone out there.

The first time I told my story was on stage at a TEDx talk in front of 750 people. It was a twelve-minute talk, and the first ten minutes I talked about storytelling and how I came into it. Then I said "Okay, I'm going to tell you a story now and I want you to think about how I must feel telling you and how you're feeling as I tell you." I told a short version of my abortion story in two minutes, then went off stage and collapsed into a puddle. My husband gathered me up in his arms and took me out to the lobby, where for about an hour after that I received appreciation. Most memorable were men coming to thank me for helping them understand why a woman would need an abortion after twenty weeks. That really made an impression on me. I thought, "wow, this is opening people's minds."

A huge motivator for me telling my story is honoring the legacy of my first pregnancy that was aborted; being able to have his life make a difference for other people.

After the abortion I wanted to get pregnant right away. Instead, I had these bloody periods that, on an unconscious level, I associated with being punished for having an abortion. When I finally sought medical attention, my OB found a fibroid that was corrected with surgery, followed by a devastating miscarriage.

It was a very challenging time—to be a public face of abortion and also suffering these reproductive issues. We waited, and happily, I got pregnant with my daughter, who is now 2½. I did a lot of therapy. I did a lot of work with counselors, including a maternal fetal specialist. Throughout the pregnancy, I kept telling myself to be calm, serene. We named our daughter Serena. We really prayed for her to have a countenance that was peaceful and it came true. She's an absolutely confident, fearless, beautiful bright light.

It's not easy to get people to write or speak about abortion. For example, in my current *Out From Under the Rug* show, it was essential to have at least one male voice, because so frequently abortion is talked about as a women's issue. I also felt it was really important to engage the LGBTQIA community because they often feel left out of the abortion conversation.

Being a white woman in the abortion rights space is also tricky because women of color are disproportionately affected by abortion restriction laws and usually lack access. They really need support and they need a voice. There is a lack of trust that comes from the history of being oppressed. I understand it. I respect it. I just hope that we can all find a way to come together.

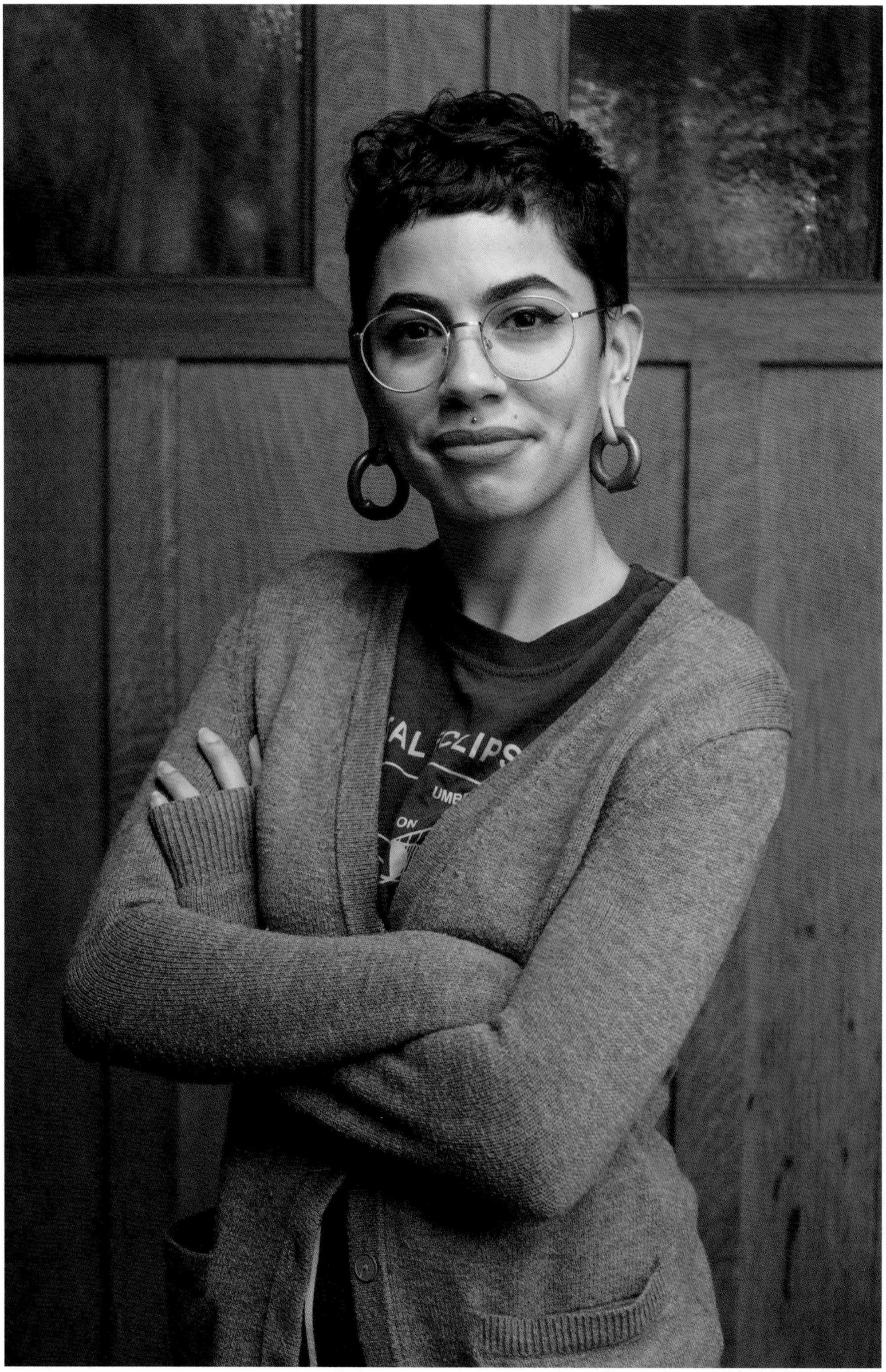

JACK QU'EMI GUTIERREZ

Jack Qu'emi Gutierrez

IT DEPENDS ON the audience, but the way I like to describe my job is, "I sell dicks for a living." I manage an erotic boutique in LA . . . so, sex toys. I run the first erotic boutique *Hustler* ever opened.

I used to teach Sex Ed for Planned Parenthood and then it turned into this job. It's very on-brand for me. No one was surprised when I told them about my new job. They just went, "Ooh! That's gonna be a fun time." And it has been. It's a good time because it's educational.

I spend most of my day educating people about their own bodies, and I can focus on the pleasure aspect. When you teach Sex Ed, especially in schools, they don't let you talk about that at all. You can only talk about function. My customers are mainly couples, mainly professionals, who are usually very open about what they want. We also get a lot of dancers and entertainers. They get a discount. And military get a discount because we care.

Gutierrez is my dad's surname, Caribbean. He is a Black and my mom's a white Puerto Rican. I have an older sister who lives with my mother in Miami. We were a military family. We landed in Miami and just stayed there. My parents split up when I was 12.

I had an abortion when I was 20, when I was still living in Orlando. I had a long-term partner; we had been high-school sweethearts in Miami. We ended up going to the same college and all that jazz. We made terrible partners. We argued all the time. We were mean to each other. He did not want to be a parent. Getting pregnant was the big thing that kind of ended things. Funny enough, we're still friendly.

I tried to be safe and that didn't really work out. The condom broke. I took a Plan B, thought it should be fine. Then May rolls over, I celebrate my birthday and I'm like, "I don't think it's fine." We thought that taking Plan B would be the end of it, and we would just move on with our lives. But it turns out that sometimes Plan B doesn't work.

I got a pregnancy test and found out I was pregnant. I was not excited about that. I knew immediately that if pregnancy ever happened, it was getting terminated. Even now, the idea of being a parent grosses me out. I don't like children. I don't want to be pregnant for a lot of reasons, my gender being a big one.

It's very important to acknowledge that cisgender women aren't the only people that need reproductive health care, or access to abortions explicitly, and that other identities should be respected and acknowledged just as much.

I guess the thing that makes my story interesting is that I'm not a cisgender woman who's experienced an abortion. I identify as non-binary. I don't identify with any particular gender. My pronouns are they, them, theirs. I definitely identify as a transgender person, because I feel like that is home. But I also enjoy being vague about it. I reserve the right to change my mind at any moment. I'm like the Trans power ranger.

I've been very out and forthcoming about this for almost a decade now. One of the main reasons why I share my story is that I didn't know any other Trans people that were open and visible about having had an abortion. Now I know one other and that's it.

I feel like the narrative around reproductive health and access focuses mainly on language that only really includes cisgender women. When I tell my story, it's very important to acknowledge that cisgender women aren't the only people that need reproductive health care, or access to abortions explicitly, and that other identities should be respected and acknowledged just as much.

I haven't had a sit-down-in-person conversation with my family about the gender thing. I tried with my mother when I was in college. It didn't go badly, but it didn't go well.

I hadn't been out very long when my abortion happened. So I didn't really have the language to express to the people at Planned Parenthood how to speak to me. The forms at the clinic didn't have a space for pronouns, or a preferred name. I get why you may need a legal name for insurance purposes and all that jazz, but mind you, I didn't even use my insurance. So what's the matter? For me the pronouns were the biggest issue. I mean, they were trying to be nice, but they kept going, "Okay, miss, miss, miss." And I'm like, "No." It just makes me so uncomfortable.

I decided to have a medication abortion, not a surgical one. I thought, "I can go home and deal with it privately and not have someone's face up my crotch, right?" I was five weeks and three days pregnant at the time of my abortion. It cost $500. I was terrified. And they had protesters outside the clinic at eight in the morning with signs, like "Abortions hurt fathers too."

I had never been inside the Planned Parenthood before, even though I was advocating for them. And I walked in, and I immediately just felt comfortable, because the first face I saw was this sweet woman in the front smiling at me. "Good morning, how are you?" And I'm like, "Oh! She's a human being, thank God." I remember, *Maid in Manhattan* was playing in the lobby. So Jennifer Lopez is intrinsically tied to my uterus at this point.

For a medication abortion, you are basically inducing a miscarriage, and everybody's body is different. They give you anti-nausea medication and painkillers too, but for me, it was so much pain, so much nausea. I didn't leave bed for a week. I didn't get my appetite back for months.

I don't think my abortion was sad. It's a relief, it's definitely a relief. Like leaving there, I felt nauseous obviously, but just peace.

Having my abortion made me hyper-aware of my uterus. Something in my head keeps saying, "Oh! You don't want that." I've tried to get sterilized and the doctors won't do it. You know what the doctors' reasons are? Ridiculous. One, you're under 30, or two, you haven't had a child yet. I don't want them, that's the whole point, honey. Right now, I'm utilizing a hormonal IUD and enjoying a life where I don't have to think about having a uterus. A lot of my dysphonia stems from having a uterus, not so much the being femme and boobs and all that. I've got great boobs, I'm loving that. It's just, the inside. I had periods that upset me.

I want a hysterectomy. Take that shit out. Good-bye, give it to someone who wants it. I don't want it. I'm good. Like give me menopause at 30. I'm cool with that. I've accepted that. I mean, look at my face. I have piercings all over my face. I've got holes everywhere and I stretch my ears and stuff. You can't see, but I have tattoos everywhere too. I'm saying, taking out my uterus, maybe it's just another form of body modification for me, you know?

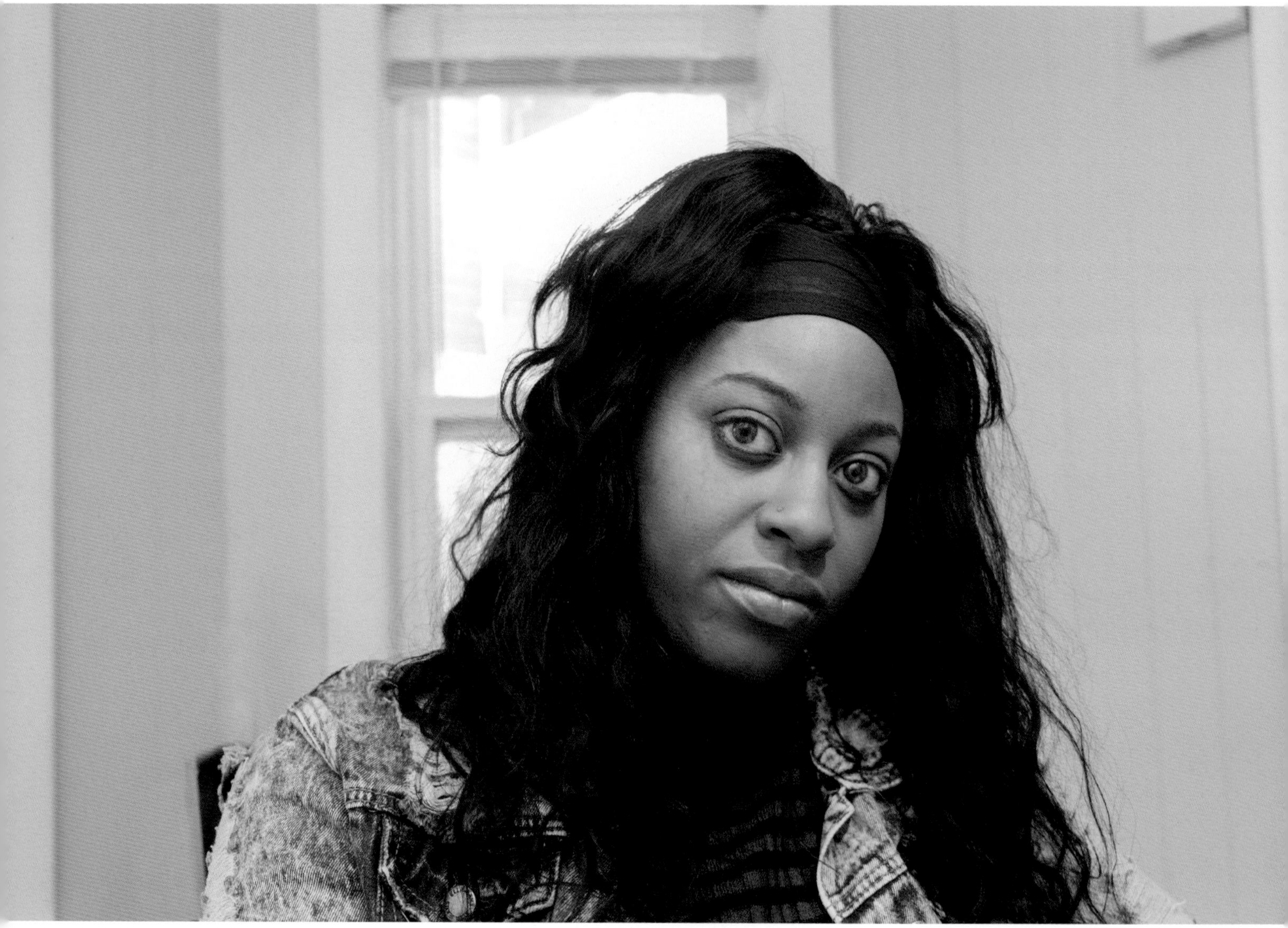

KAYLA MOYE

Kayla Moye

THE LONG STORY short is that I found out I was pregnant while I was incarcerated. I was incarcerated for almost ninety days. That was the loneliest time.

I found out I was pregnant in a horrible way. When you get admitted into a county jail or a prison, during the intake they do health questions. Because I'm allergic to the TB test, they gave me an X-ray screening, and before they give you an X-ray screening, they have to give you a pregnancy test, because if you're pregnant, you can't have an X-ray. They shouted out that I was pregnant from another room. That's how I found out. It was like, super embarrassing and very unethical.

I asked for an abortion about a month into incarceration, and I was denied. Denying an abortion in prison is not legal. You cannot deny anyone an abortion since Roe v. Wade. The prison officials were probably thinking I wouldn't be there long enough, that I could make the decision to have an abortion when I got out. But it didn't work out that way. After ninety days I got released. In Ohio there is a ban on abortions after twenty weeks, and I was over twenty weeks pregnant when I got out. So that's how I ended up having my son.

I always worked full-time jobs. I always took care of myself and handled my responsibilities, But birth control was never my friend. I have tried every birth control possible. I had a complication with the IUD. It dropped down into my uterus and caused a major infection. We tried to use condoms and stuff like that.

My son is now 3 and I live with him and his father. We're together in a successful relationship. We're buying a home together, but I want to get married first. That's the goal.

We've had ups and downs, times we felt we were ready to have kids, like we do now, and times when it's been hard for us. That's when we mutually made the decision that an abortion was fair and the right thing for the both of us.

Having my abortion after my son was born was hard because I already had a child, and I knew what it was like to love this little human being. I felt more guilty about it. But if I hadn't had this abortion, I wouldn't have been able to finish school. I wouldn't have been able to get approved for this loan to buy a house. There have been many accomplishments since.

My spouse's thinking overall is he will support my decision as a woman, which really is all I ask. If I want to have the baby, we'll have the baby. If I want to have an abortion, he'll go to the clinic with me. But, his first choice is not going to be an abortion. I'm human, so I understand where he's coming from. I also understand that I know when I'm ready, and I know when I'm not.

He's not really verbal about it, but he is my other half, so, you know, at this very table, we have sat across and had conversations about having a baby, delivering a baby, having an abortion, being incarcerated, having another abortion, and expecting again. That's a hell of a journey.

My spouse thinks a lot differently than me, which I think is why we're so compatible. We come from totally different households, so that plays a huge part in our lives. I didn't grow up in poverty, at all. My parents were always wealthy. My high school was 98 percent Caucasian, so it was only me and one other girl who were African-American, out of a population of like 1,000 kids. And so I know how to fit in. I know how to prove who I am and try to dodge the stigma.

If we could talk about abortions like we can talk about pizza, or about watching the news, or any other conversation that we would normally have, then he or anybody else who is kind of uneasy about it wouldn't have those feelings. Before he met me, he never even experienced having to support someone who's had an abortion. It's unnatural for him, and I understand that.

It comes around to stigma, which is why I try to speak out on my story. That's why I like to include my boyfriend in my story. Even though I have had support from my spouse and my family, it's not because they love abortions. It's because they love me. They support me, so I have to support abortion for them, if that makes sense.

Me, being a young, Black woman, I want every other young Black woman to hear my story. I definitely want someone to take away that if an abortion is necessary, it's necessary. It's safe. I want people who look at abortions in a negative light to hear my story. I have been incarcerated. I have been, almost, without a home. I had to drop out of school, and I had a lot of barriers, and yet I never let that hold me back from anything I want to do in life, from getting my degree, to everything else. I want people to really know that abortion is available. I wish everyone could have the support that I had. I wish I could be that support for everyone, because there's a lot of people who don't have that support.

Race plays a huge part of my life, you know. It's not easy. People look at me and think here is this young, Black, irresponsible girl with all these tattoos. Then they hear my story and they're like "Wow. She's really inspirational."

Race plays a huge part of my life, you know. It's not easy. People look at me and think here is this young, Black, irresponsible girl with all these tattoos. Then they hear my story and they're like "Wow. She's really inspirational." When I get that response, I know I'm impacting someone, and that's my goal.

My mother and father are both African-American. As a kid, I always had to fit in: an African-American girl, living in a predominantly white neighborhood in Houston. But I also felt like I didn't fit in with my own people. Now I can fit in with anybody.

The house I am buying is in a Cleveland suburb, near where my mother now lives. It's about 60 percent white, but it has all different ethnicities, and that is what I like. I like to be in the midst of a broader community of all different nationalities.

My mom is like my best friend. We're very close, probably the closest person in the world, and she's a phenomenal help with my son. I'm very independent, so it's hard for me to ask for help, but she's always been that one to help me regardless of if I ask or not.

Everyone supports me. Everyone is pro-Kayla, but not a lot of people are pro-abortion. I kind of deal with that, and me being okay with it, because like I said, I'm doing the work for them. I think about how normal I want abortions to be, and it makes me speechless because of how abnormal it is.

I am expecting a baby in two months, so a lot of things have just been put on hold for a while. But I am working in business management and I plan on becoming an entrepreneur as an event planner. I already have a name for it. Give me about a year and I should be where I want to be.

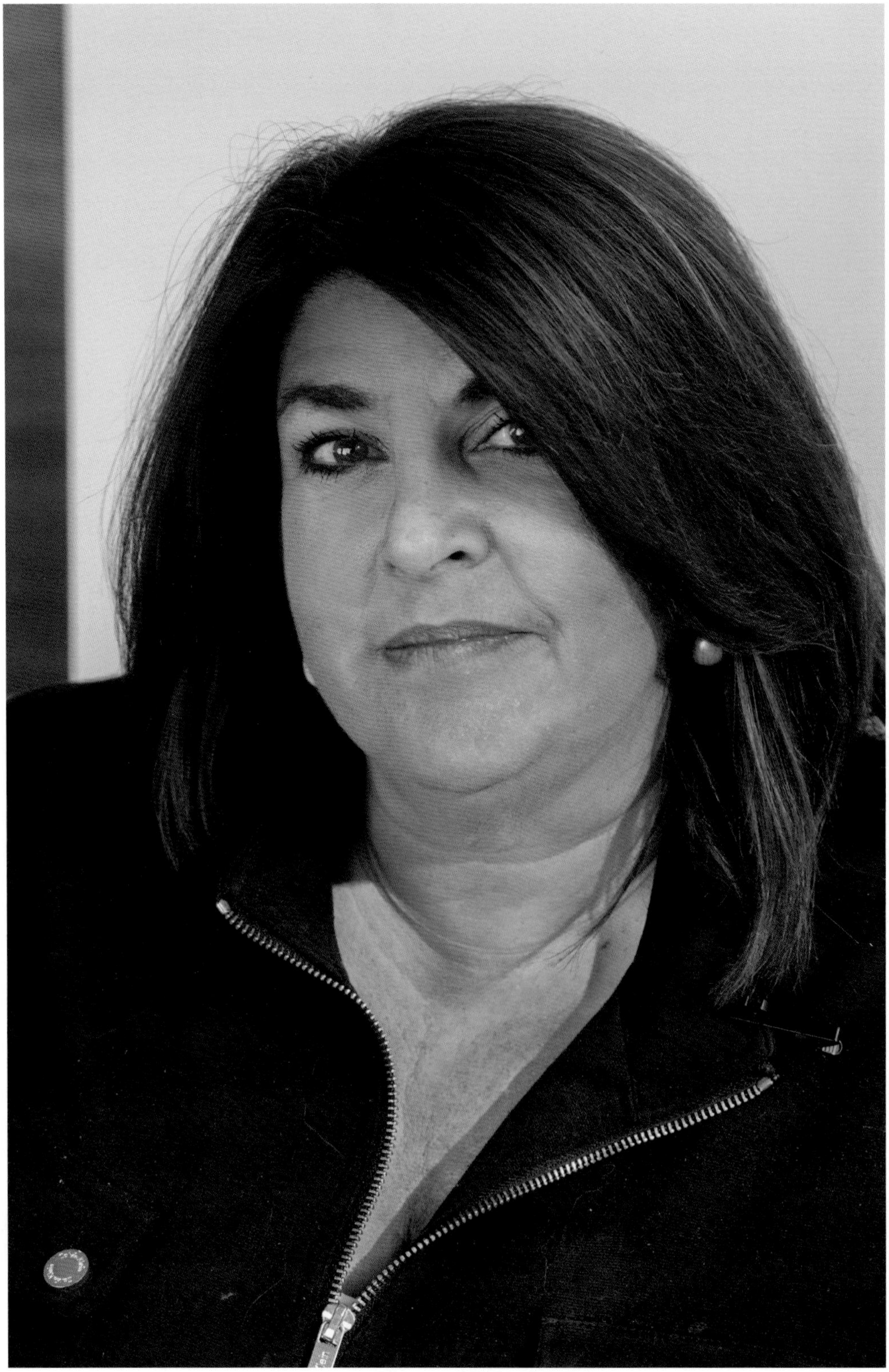

DEBRA HAUSER

Debra Hauser

MY FAMILY WAS fairly progressive, so I did not grow up with a lot of shame or stigma around abortion or sexuality or any of that. I was raised in a family that had money, and that drew me to do work for people who didn't have it. After college, I went into the Peace Corps and was sent to Paraguay. In the first couple of weeks after I arrived, I was told not to do any family planning work because the Peace Corps had been thrown out of Bolivia for having done some family planning work.

My role in the Peace Corps was to do health education and childhood vaccinations. And I did a lot of teaching about family planning. Within maybe two weeks of being in my town, people started to knock on my door and ask about contraception. Although abortion was illegal in the whole country, there were a couple of people in the town who did abortions.

Whenever I'm talking about why I do the work I do, I tell about this one very, very poor family in Paraguay. They lived between two towns that I would walk back and forth between. The wife was a young woman, probably my age, 23 or 24 at most. She had four kids and she was very pregnant. I had a lot of trouble communicating with this family because although Spanish is one of the official languages of Paraguay, they also speak Guarani, a completely different language. One day when I was passing through, I realized this young woman wasn't pregnant anymore, but there wasn't a baby there either. It turns out she had given birth, but then she starved the baby because she couldn't afford to feed the children that she already had. That was really life changing for me. I thought nobody should ever have to make that decision and be put through that. That's why I did my grad work in population planning and international health at University of Michigan, with a very strong focus on family planning.

Today, I'm president of Advocates for Youth. Our goal is to work with and for young people and young people's allies, to champion programs and advocate for policies that recognize their rights to honest sex education and confidential sexual health services. We do that with an eye toward those most marginalized or disproportionately impacted by sexual health morbidities. We have programs that are, for example, working at the intersection of homophobia and Islamophobia. We teach advocacy skills to raise awareness and how to mobilize their peers. We work with them to hone their story of self. In short, we give them the skills to make change in their communities.

My own abortion took place in 1995. I was married to a man who was later diagnosed with a mental illness, but at the time I was oblivious. I was 35, was working full-time, and had a 6-month-old baby when my husband went to work one day and didn't return. He called to say he was on his way home and then he didn't show up for days and days. At some point I realized I was pregnant again. Three, four weeks went by, no word from him. The money was disappearing.

There was no question in my mind what I was going to do about being pregnant. I had a child in my arms that I had to get to daycare. I had to be able to go to work every day. There was no way I could possibly have another child under these circumstances. My responsibility to my child was the most important thing to me. I understood instinctively what I had to do and I did it.

I had worked at an abortion clinic between college and my Peace Corps assignment. It was on the border of Washington D.C. and Maryland. I just never thought twice. I just did it. People were lovely and I had enough money. I took my child to daycare and went by myself to the clinic. After the abortion, I went home.

At the time I didn't tell anyone my husband was missing. I would go to work every day, do my work, pick up my kid, stop in Old Town because it was a good place for him to play, and then go home, put him to bed, and do it again the next day. I mean the abortion was the smallest part of this. As far as I was concerned, my life was in total turmoil.

My husband showed up three or four weeks after the abortion. He continued to come in and then disappear again. He got a diagnosis and the psychiatrist warned me that us staying married was unlikely. Shortly after that we got a divorce. A couple of years later he committed suicide.

I didn't talk about the abortion probably for another fifteen years. A few people knew. My mom knew because she was in the courthouse when we talked about it in relation to the divorce. Obviously my ex-husband knew because it was one of the things he tried to throw at me during the divorce.

YOU'VE GOT TO SHIFT THE CULTURAL NARRATIVE TO ONE THAT EMBRACES BODILY AUTONOMY, ONE THAT RECOGNIZES THAT PEOPLE WHO HAVE ABORTIONS KNOW BEST FOR THEMSELVES, THEIR BODIES, AND THEIR FAMILIES . . . IF YOU DON'T WANT TO HAVE AN ABORTION, I SUPPORT THAT TOO.

It wasn't that I was ashamed of that abortion or that I had any question about whether it was the right thing to do. None. But the cacophony of noise around abortion, the judgment, the shame that people want to spew onto you, keeps people from talking. If I believe you're going to judge me, or if I believe you're going to think differently about me because of an abortion, I would need a really good reason to tell you about it. There was no reason to tell my story.

Storytelling can be used as a tool to build empathy. At Advocates for Youth, we're doing that with our '1 in 3' campaign. Started in 2011, it was the first of this generation's storytelling campaigns, with the goal of combating a culture that was allowing abortion restrictions to flourish across the country.

If you can break through the silence and have people share their stories, the next person will also share their story. The more of us that tell our stories—those of us that are privileged enough to be able to do so—more and more people will tell their stories. This breaks the silence and the stigma related to abortion. It takes away others' ability to shame us into silence.

If I tell you that what you do is immoral and wrong, whether you think it is or not, you're not going to tell me that you did it. So if you're not telling me that you did it and the next person isn't telling me that they did it, and the person after that isn't telling me that they did it, I'm left to think that I'm the only one who did it. The stigma and shame grow exponentially. There's no way to break through that silence until somebody owns up and says, "I did it and I don't think it's immoral. In fact, I think what's immoral is you telling me that it's immoral." And then the next person says, "I thought that too, but I was afraid to say it." And then the next person says me too, and then you realize that in a room of ten women, three of them have had an abortion.

Stigma not only works on silencing those of us who have had abortion, it also works on silencing politicians that might stand up for abortion. If you're afraid that more than half your constituency may walk away, even if you stand up for something that you believe is morally right, you're not going to do it.

Underlying all of this, including the controversy about sex education, is the idea that if you empower us to have bodily autonomy, that we will become too powerful. That worries the people who would like to stay in control. There's a real cultural war about whether we move forward or backward. And backward wasn't so good for a lot of people. I had a friend who used to say culture sets the ceiling to which policy can reach. If culture says we only believe in abortion in certain circumstances, that's the ceiling that policy will hit.

You've got to shift the cultural narrative to one that embraces bodily autonomy, one that recognizes that people who have abortions know best for themselves, their bodies, and their families. And they should have full access to those options. If you don't want to have an abortion, I support that too.

About 30 percent of young people say they're both pro-choice and pro-life. If you ask whether they support having abortion access in their community, upwards of 70 percent will say yes. So it's a different question. Asking what you personally believe is very different from asking if you believe other people should have access.

Stephanie Sanchez

I WAS BORN and raised in Southern California. I grew up in a single-mother household, just my mom, my younger sister, and me. My mom came from Mexico. She really struggled a lot raising my sister and me alone, especially financially. She told us to get an education, to go to college so we could get good jobs and not struggle the way that she struggled.

My sister and I both went to college. My sister is getting her PhD in Sociology. My BA is in Public Administration. I have my own business as a political treasurer, controlling the money that goes in and out of candidates' electoral campaigns. My first job out of college was on a political campaign and I kind of fell in love with the work and stayed in it.

I grew up in a very Caucasian neighborhood rather than a Latino community because my mom wanted us to go to a good school. When I got to high school, a lot of people, especially the Latinos, would make fun of me. Some kids in high school said that I wasn't Mexican because I didn't speak Spanish very well. I started taking Chicano Studies courses in college and learning more about the culture and the community's struggles. Maybe in a way it was me trying to claim my identity, stuck in between these two worlds, not really knowing who I was. Now when asked how I identify, I always say Mexican American.

I had my abortion seven years ago when I was 26. My boyfriend and I had been together for like five years when I got pregnant. At that time, we were just not in a good place. When I found out I was pregnant, I was devastated. I knew that I wasn't going to keep the child because I just didn't think it was right to bring a child into this world when the father and I are just not going to work out.

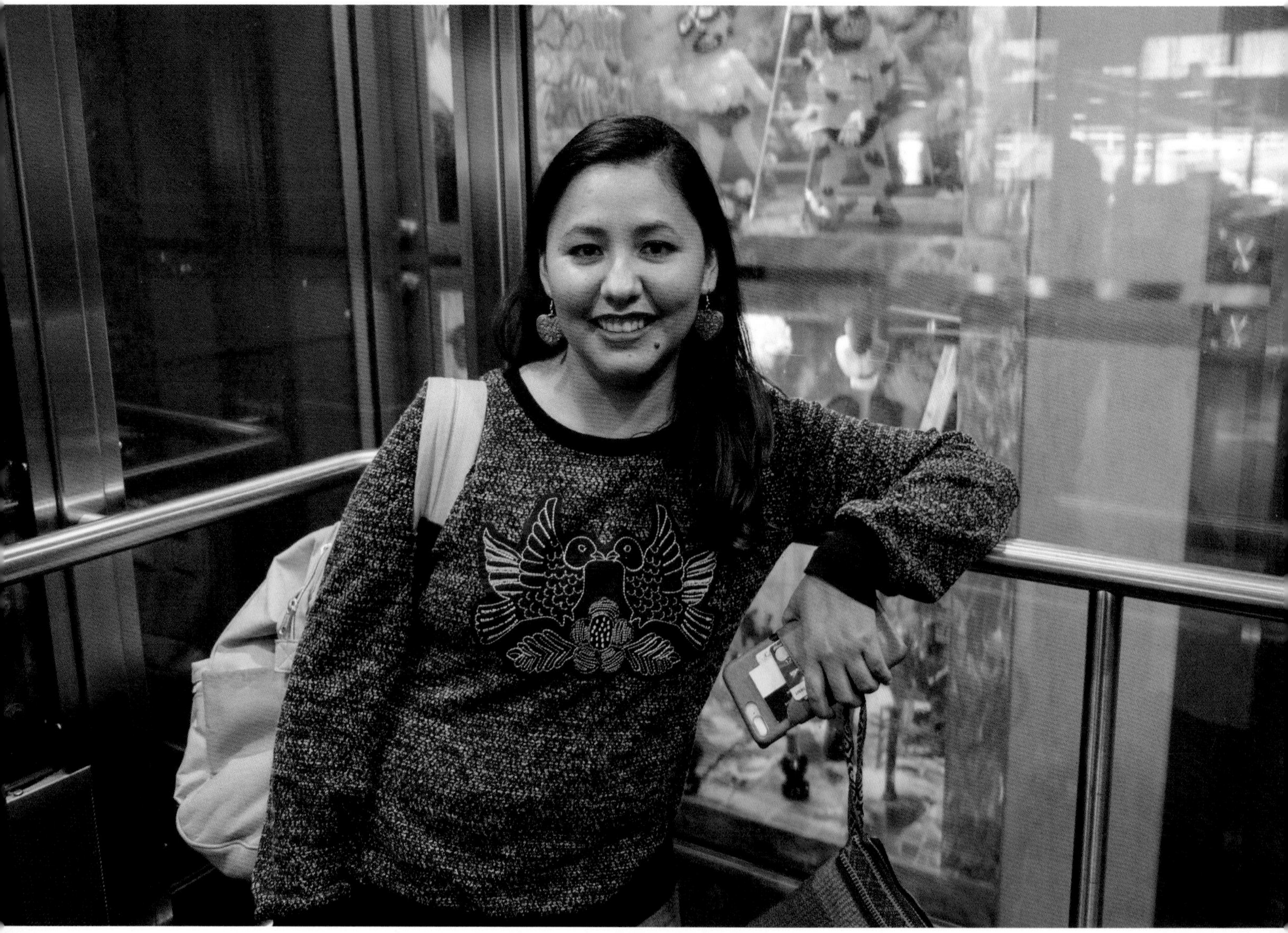

STEPHANIE SANCHEZ

I think another reason why I made that choice was seeing my mom struggle so much with my sister and me. I didn't want to have to go through the same experience, bringing a child into this world and not be able to raise a child in a good environment.

My boyfriend wanted to keep the child. I told him, "You're either with me or not." Even though he didn't want me to have an abortion, he supported my choice. He ended up being by my side. I made an appointment at Planned Parenthood, and just went in and got it done. He paid.

I've always been pro-choice, so leading up to it, I was fine. Then after I got the abortion I ended up feeling so guilty. I just went downhill and entered a very dark space, very depressed. I think that we don't really talk about that part of what happens after the abortion. How is it going to affect you mentally or physically?

I remember my mom telling me as a teenager something like, "If you ever get pregnant, I'm going to make you have that child so you can know what it's like to suffer like I suffered." That kind of stuck in my head. Years later I told my mother about my abortion. I didn't tell her face to face. I wrote her a letter. She wrote back. Although I don't remember much about the letter, I do remember her writing that she also had an abortion when she was younger. There was compassion in her letter and some motherly tough love I guess. I think I even told her about my not wanting to have a baby because I didn't want to be in her shoes.

I WENT TO CONFESSION AND I TOLD THE PRIEST THAT IT'S HARD TO COME TO CHURCH WHEN I KNOW THAT THE CHURCH IS PRO-LIFE.

Today is the first time I have told my story. Hiding it is part of the shame that I've felt. Speaking out, I'm no longer letting this part of my story hold me back. This is a choice I made and I learned from. I can't let it stop me from living my life.

After a while, I ended up going to therapy. I went in cycles. I would feel well and it would hit me again. Then I did two post-abortion retreats, the first was through the Catholic Diocese here in San Diego. At that time, I didn't have a relationship with God. I wasn't going to church. I didn't really understand how God plays a role in all of this. At the second retreat, which was in Peru, they said basically God forgives you for this choice you made. A lot of the women there blamed God for being pregnant. I couldn't relate to that because I never blamed God. It was my decision and my choice.

I started going to church again because it felt like a call. But I also wanted to get more involved and I think maybe it's going to redeem myself. Two days ago, I went to confession and I told the priest that it's hard to come to church when I know that the church is pro-life. How do you think it makes us feel to come to church and have that thrown in our face?

The priest was very compassionate. He was telling me that he's known a lot of people who've had abortions. He asked that I connect with another lady who also had an abortion so that I'd have someone to talk to within the Catholic community. He recommended that maybe I should become a mentor in the Catholic Church for women who've had abortions.

THE PRIEST WAS VERY COMPASSIONATE . . . HE RECOMMENDED THAT MAYBE I SHOULD BECOME A MENTOR IN THE CATHOLIC CHURCH FOR WOMEN WHO'VE HAD ABORTIONS.

We didn't finish the conversation because there were others waiting for confession with him. But today I actually went to Mass before coming here. The same priest was leading the Mass and during his homily he started talking about our discussion. I wondered if I had prompted his homily because I went to confession.

As kids, we grew up thinking God was going to punish us for all these things we did. It's the first thing parents would say when their kids did something wrong, any wrong choice you made. As I started going to church as an adult, I realized it doesn't teach that. It teaches Jesus came here to die on the cross for us, for all of our sins, because God is compassionate and forgives everyone.

I know God has forgiven me and now, it's just like the guilt or the shame that I still hold.

For the longest time I felt that I couldn't be in a relationship or feel worthy of having kids. I guess that's another guilt that I have. But now I think I have moved past that and I do hope to eventually be in a relationship and have a family.

Yes. I want to become a mentor to young girls in some way. I'm still not sure how. I think that this whole past year, not only did the whole abortion thing come back, but I started doing more healing with myself and my childhood traumas: having an absent father, growing up in a single-mother household without a lot of resources. I'm just doing the healing work and trying to understand the deeper things that are within me, and learning about intergenerational trauma and how it carries on. Especially people of color, we don't have the resources or mentors. To younger girls, starting at a very young age, we can tell them that you're loved, you have so much power within you. It definitely is a growth journey.

Shelley Sella

WHEN I WAS 2 years old, my parents moved from Israel to New York City. My mother was born in what was then Palestine. My father fled from Poland to Palestine in 1939. My parents weren't religious, but sent my siblings and me to a Yeshiva because they wanted us to learn Hebrew. After seventh grade I went to a secular school.

I first got interested in women's health at the University of Wisconsin in Madison, where I went to college. I fashioned an independent major that included women and health, women's studies and science. That was during the '70s, a time when the women's health movement was in its heyday.

When I was about 20, I spent a summer volunteering at a feminist clinic in Los Angeles. That was the first time I saw an abortion. I still remember counseling a woman, being there with her while she was going through the abortion, and my experience of this very intimate and powerful process.

That motivated me to learn how to provide abortions. My friends in Madison encouraged me to go to medical school, as did my parents. I attended medical school in Israel and returned to the US to start my family practice residency in Madison. I was very drawn to birth at that time, however, I was shocked by how birth was viewed in the hospital, as a medical problem to be managed with many interventions. I wanted to see what birth would be like without all the interventions, if it could just be allowed to unfold naturally rather than sticking to a time schedule or this intervention or that one. I thought the only way I could really see what this process would be like would be by attending home births.

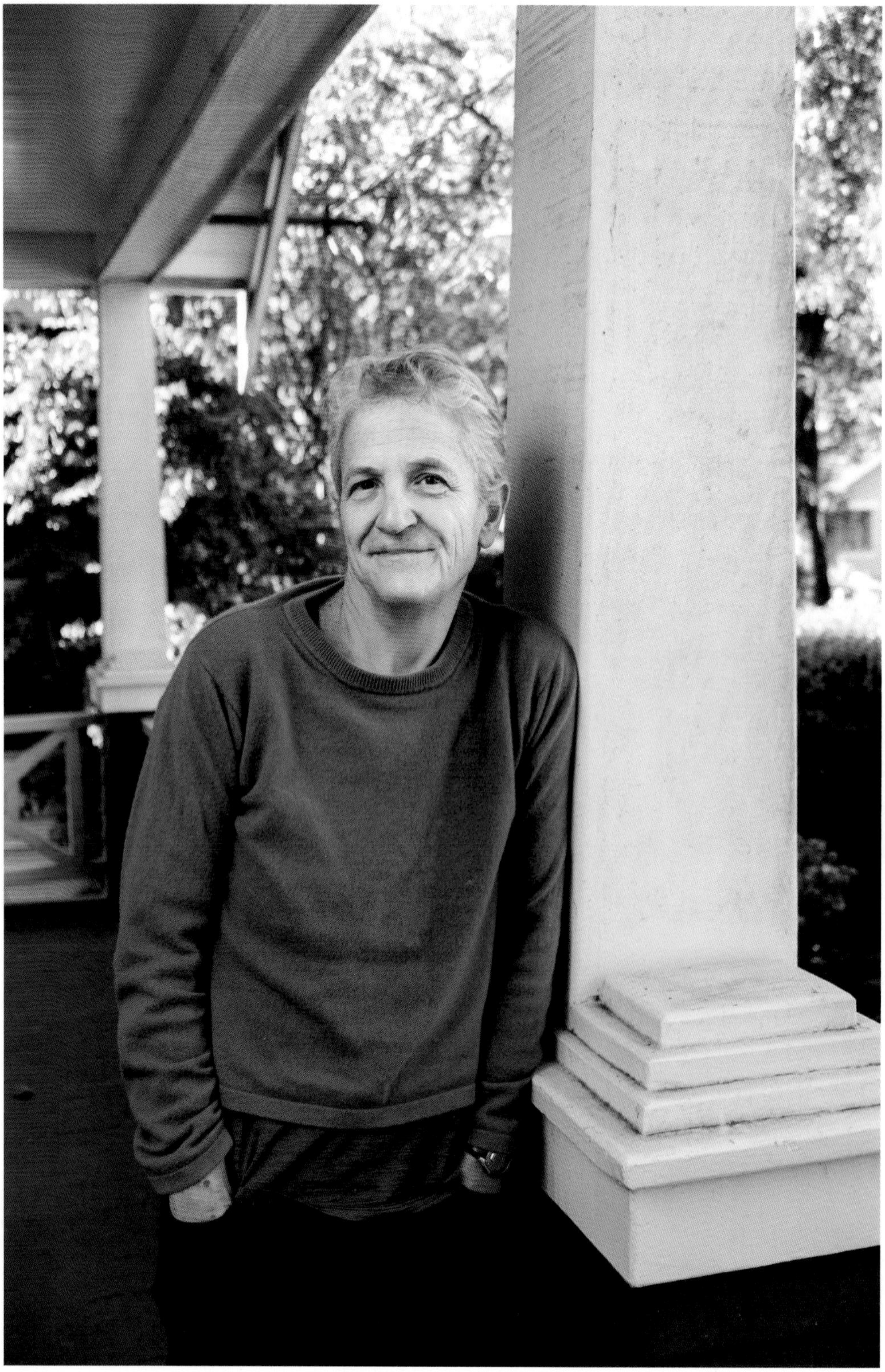

SHELLEY SELLA

I wasn't sure what I'd be getting into and I wondered if people would be sitting around and eating placentas and who knows what? Lighting candles and chanting? But I still wanted that experience. I had an introduction to a midwife in Santa Cruz, California, who was looking for an apprentice. I took a leave from residency and moved to Santa Cruz to work with her.

After two years in Santa Cruz, I moved to Oakland, California, to complete my residency training, this time in OBGYN at Kaiser Permanente. Following residency, I worked as an OBGYN for a few years, becoming more and more frustrated with the field. Obstetrics seemed to focus on doing C-sections, and gynecology was centered on giving women hormones.

At the time I asked myself, "What parts of being a health care provider for women feel meaningful and useful to me? What am I drawn to do?" I realized that I was most drawn to home birth and abortion. Being a physician, it didn't make sense to be a midwife, so I focused on being an abortion provider.

My initial training in abortion care came in bits and pieces. As a resident, I heard about a third-trimester abortion provider in Los Angeles, Dr. Jim McMahon, a deeply creative and innovative doctor. I was able to meet him and spend time at his clinic. We really connected, and started talking about the possibility of my working with him. Sadly, he died from a brain tumor before that could happen.

Dr. McMahon told me about Dr. George Tiller in Wichita, Kansas, who was also providing third -trimester abortions. Many years later, at a National Abortion Federation meeting, I actually met Dr. Tiller. He was at the conference showing a running clip of a third-trimester abortion procedure, which entailed induction, labor, and delivery of a stillborn. He was talking about the process and said, "The woman's body is smarter than the doctor. Time, patience, and the baby will come." He emphasized that the key was not trying to fit a woman's birthing process to the schedule of the doctor or clinic staff. After listening to his words, I said to him, 'That's midwifery!" And really, within five minutes, he had offered me a job. I started working for him in June 2002.

Dr. Tiller was very smart, psychologically astute, and a complicated person. One of the ways he trained me was just having me be with him all the time, watching and listening. When he was talking to patients and conferring with them, I was there. It was just amazing to see how he could zero in on what was going on with the patients.

I don't know Dr. Tiller's deepest motives for doing the work he did. I do know some of his story. His father, mother, sister, and brother-in-law were all killed in a plane crash. He was a young doctor at the time and had been planning to go into dermatology. However, his father had been a family physician. So Dr. Tiller decided to become a family physician too. To his surprise, when he began to practice, women came to him and asked if he could help them the way his father had. He had not realized that his father had quietly provided abortion care to his patients who desperately needed that help before Roe v. Wade.

At first, Dr. Tiller said no to these requests. But women kept asking him, and he eventually began to provide abortion care. Exactly how he got into third-trimester abortion, I don't know.

I AM DRAWN TO THE YOUNG WOMEN I SEE AND TO THEIR INCREDIBLE POTENTIAL, WHICH WOULD BE SORELY DIMINISHED, IF NOT COMPLETELY EXTINGUISHED, IF FORCED TO CONTINUE A PREGNANCY. DR. TILLER CALLED THIS "THE DUNGEON OF MANDATORY MOTHERHOOD."

I worked with Dr. Tiller for seven years, commuting to Wichita from California. I'd really been looking for a mentor in abortion, and I didn't have one until I met him. My training with him was very systematic, learning abortion techniques step by step. The opportunity to work with Dr. Tiller was like a dream come true. He was very patient. He was amazing. He stood by me, always. He was really a father figure, in the best sense of the word. He was a great mentor. I am very, very grateful and really lucky to have worked with him.

Dr. Tiller was assassinated in church, May 31, 2009, and his wife, Jeanie closed the clinic the next day. Dr. Tiller knew that the clinic would close when he died. He didn't have succession plans. There were two other doctors at the clinic, Drs. Susan Robinson and Leroy Carhart. After the clinic was closed, Susan and I decided to look for work together.

We were invited to visit Southwestern Women's Options, a clinic in Albuquerque, New Mexico, owned and run by friends of Dr. Tiller's, Drs. Curtis and Glenna Boyd. They wanted to expand to provide third-trimester abortions to fill the void left after Dr. Tiller' s death. After visiting the clinic and meeting the staff, it felt like the right place for us.

The Boyd philosophy is to meet the woman where she's at and to satisfy her emotional needs, not just her physical needs. There's a huge emphasis on emotional support and how to help someone get through this experience. Dr. Tiller's clinic was also a very loving place. The warm and supportive environment in both clinics is remarkably distinct from most health care institutions.

I think that abortion is absolutely crucial for women's lives, and because of that I view my work as deeply pro-life and pro-family. Abortion is sometimes a matter of physical survival; for example, for women who are abused and trapped in a dangerous situation, or for women who have conditions that threaten their health and lives by continuing a pregnancy. Sometimes abortion is about financial survival, making it possible for a woman to make ends meet. And sometimes it's about pursuing a better life by finishing high school, going to college, seeking a career, and following a dream, whatever that may be.

The women who come to the clinic are from all situations, from all over the country and the world. But they all realize that if they were to continue their pregnancy it could be a disaster for them, the child, and their family. Women care deeply about what their children's lives will be like and often decide to have an abortion in order to save their child a life of suffering. For example, I see many women with deeply desired pregnancies who have learned that there is something very wrong with their baby and decide that, hard as it is, the best decision for them and their child is to end the pregnancy. Similarly, I see women who are addicted to drugs or alcohol who have grave concerns for the health of their child and the life that it would have.

I am drawn to the young women I see and to their incredible potential, which would be sorely diminished, if not completely extinguished, if forced to continue a pregnancy. Dr. Tiller called this "the dungeon of mandatory motherhood." I mainly see women who do not come from privilege and do not have unlimited resources. These young women have many dreams: of finishing high school, going to college, being doctors, lawyers, athletes, and of having a better life. I don't know where life will take them, but I strongly believe that for these young women, an abortion may help them along their path.

Having been in vulnerable, powerless situations myself, I know how important it is for women to be able to control their bodies. I sometimes feel such deep, deep empathy for what these women are going through. I understand. And I think that's what drives me, remembering the feelings and wanting to be there for someone in a way that I would have wanted.

The women who come to the clinic are from all situations, from all over the country and the world. But they all realize that if they were to continue their pregnancy it could be a disaster for them, the child, and their family.

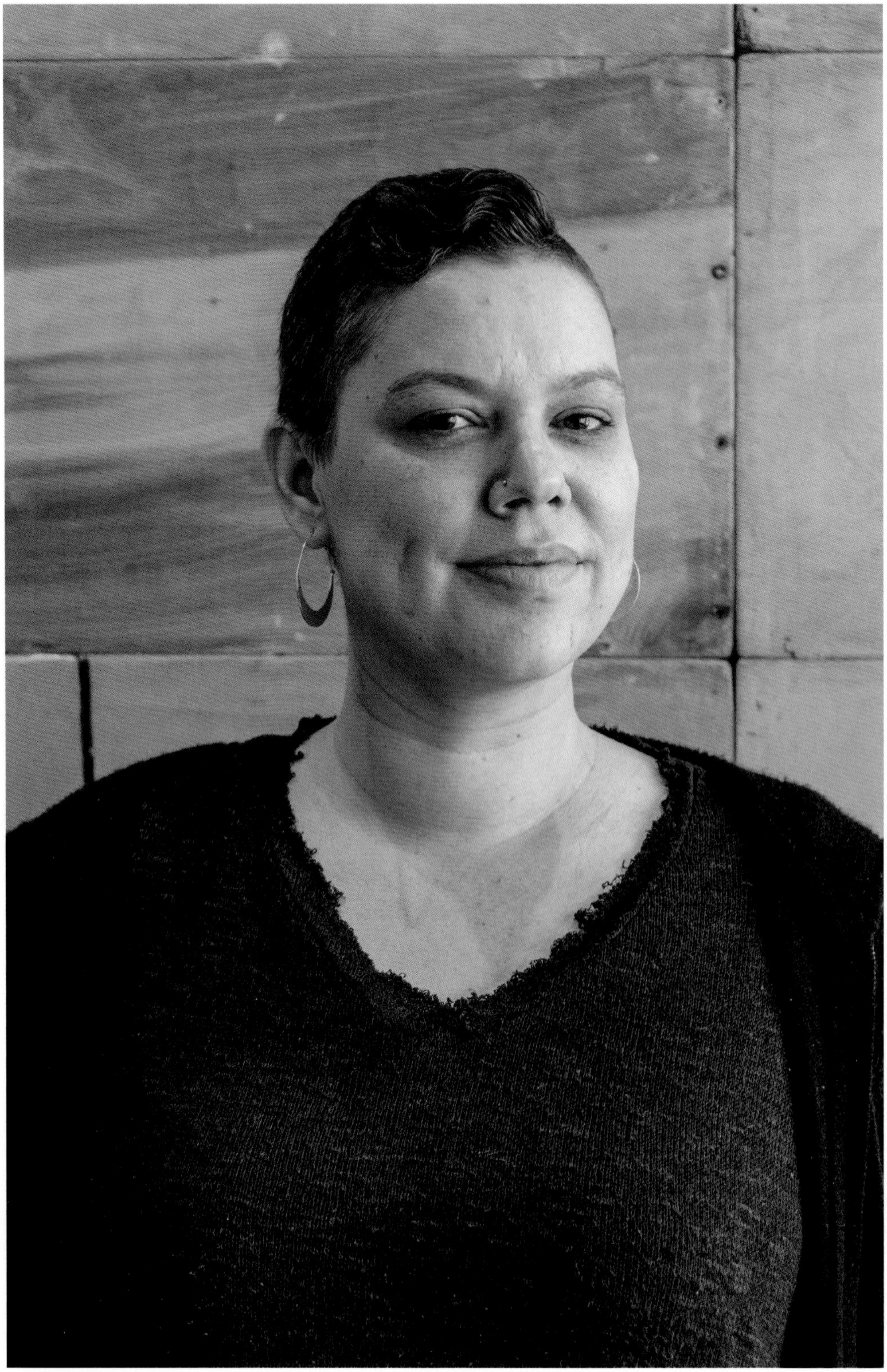

MEGAN JEYIFO

Megan Jeyifo

I'M 35 YEARS old. My first abortion was twenty years ago. Last year I sat down and decided to write out what I remembered of having my first abortion when I was 15.

A lot of what I wrote about in that moment were things that I hadn't remembered, details I had forgotten about. I remember being very proud of what I wrote when showing it to my husband. Then I presented my abortion story for the first time to friends and family. I did this in an effort to raise money for the Chicago Abortion Fund, where I am now a board member.

I grew up in Milwaukee and lived in the one integrated neighborhood. I took a bus to a private Catholic school. I don't even like to look at my pictures of myself in that time period. I was so miserable. It was the summer after my mother died at age 43. That's when I found out I was pregnant. After leaving school my sophomore year, I had been doing a combination of an alternative school and home schooling. That was because I was really struggling with being in school and the trauma of losing my mother.

When I didn't get my period, I took a pregnancy test, and it was negative. I could feel my body changing, but I ignored it. Then six or eight weeks later, I took another test. I remember thinking that I had spent so much money on the first test — it was $13 — and it didn't work. In my mind that justified stealing the second test from Walgreen's. Somehow in my 15-year-old brain I was like, "Yeah. This is owed to me." The second test showed I was pregnant.

In Wisconsin at that time you needed parental consent. Planned Parenthood referred me to an independent clinic that was pretty close to my house. They did a sonogram, and I was twenty-two weeks pregnant. They told me I needed to have an adult with me, a parent, when I came back. And they told me how much it would cost. I think it was $600. I went back to the clinic with my friend's boyfriend, who was in his 30s. We looked nothing alike but I said he was my brother. The clinic said fine. He signed the paper and left. There was a twenty-four-hour waiting period, so I came back the next day to begin the actual abortion. I was so lucky. I just made the cutoff for a legal abortion in Wisconsin. The abortion I had would not be legal now.

I had to ask my father's partner for money for the abortion. It was really difficult to ask her because I didn't particularly like her. Then I had to pay her back, slipping money underneath her door, which was crazy.

Even with that familial, liberal, pro-choice background, I still felt this terror about my abortion. I just couldn't tell my dad. Part of it was he's trying to hold his family together. These kids, they don't have a mom.

It was a two-day procedure. I went in alone on the first day. It was a surgical procedure, but they had to first use laminaria, a seaweed which dilates the cervix. It was absurdly painful. I remember them telling me when they were sending me home after the first day that if I didn't come back in twenty-four hours they would call 911 because "this is dangerous. You could get hurt. You could be really sick." I remember the nurse who inserted the laminaria was awful. I didn't have a word for it then, but she was a slut-shamer. She made me feel really ashamed and bad. Then the next day when I came back the doctor was very nice.

On the second day my father's partner dropped me off and I took a taxi home by myself. Now, as a parent and as a human being, that is mind-boggling.

My dad found out about my abortion because my little brother and sister knew. My brother and I got in an argument and my brother, in front of the whole family, yelled it out. My dad was vehemently feminist and pro-choice. He later helped me when I needed a second abortion when I was 19. He helped me financially and was very supportive.

I came from a family that was extremely liberal and very open about abortion rights. My mom, who was a clinic escort, sent me to a YMCA summer camp wearing a shirt that had a child drawing an American flag on it and a family standing in front of the flag. In a child's writing around the flag it said, "Pro-choice, pro-choice, pro-choice." I remember it. I wore it until it got holes in the collar. I gave my eighth-grade presentation at a Catholic school on choice. I don't think I knew the words "abortion access" then. I don't think I understood what that really meant, but I knew "My body, My choice." My mom probably had a bumper sticker that said that.

Even with that familial, liberal, pro-choice background, I still felt this terror about my abortion. I just couldn't tell my dad. Part of it was he's trying to hold his family together. These kids, they don't have a mom. I don't want to put this on him.

After the procedure, they had given me some pretty hardcore pain pills. My friends must have come over afterwards. I remember taking a walk around my neighborhood to smoke a cigarette or something. I didn't want to take the pain pills. I lived in a neighborhood where you would see people on crack or whatever. I had friends whose parents did drugs. So when I decided not to take the drugs, one of my male friends was like, "Oh, well, just give them to me." I remember thinking, "No, I'm not going to give you my abortion pain pills."

I'm wondering if I felt stigma at the time of my abortion. I do know I felt no guilt. I remember very clearly as I fell into sleep the night it was over, just thinking to myself, "It feels so good to be relieved. This is past me."

I never told the person who got me pregnant anything until four or five months later. I saw him with a friend of mine he had started dating. I told them both at the same time, and they were both really sad and really nice. He was like, "I'm sorry that I wasn't there for you." He was a drug dealer. He was someone that didn't stay in one place.

From the age of 13 to 17, I really made poor choices. I wouldn't be the person I am without going through these experiences. By the time I was 18, I was completely self-sufficient. I'm very happy with how everything turned out. It's mind-boggling to me that my husband is a neuroscience PhD at a university and I did not finish high school. The biggest bump I had was trying to get pregnant when I was 29. I tried for a year. Finally after a lot of tests and drugs, I got pregnant with twins.

Looking back, I think a lot of girls in my peer group had babies because they thought that it would save them. They thought they'd magically become responsible or they'd have somebody to love them. That's not what happened in a lot of instances. I guess it sounds so corny, but you know your own life. I knew the minute I saw a positive sign on a pregnancy test that I was in no position to become a parent.

Up until recently I was only vocal about my first abortion experience. I didn't talk about the second abortion because I did feel stigma about having two. I don't think I feel that anymore. I'm starting to talk about it publicly. The second time was much different.

I was living in Saint Thomas. I was working full-time, I found out I was pregnant right away, and I called a doctor. I asked my dad for money. It was the last time I asked my dad for money. I think he took it out of a trust fund that mom had left for us. She left us $25,000, and I think I asked for $600. I flew to Puerto Rico for the abortion with my boyfriend. "It was just like, I've been here before. I know what this is. I know this is what I'm going to do."

Maite Salazar

ABORTION IS A very serious health issue, and it's the key to so many other issues: poverty, not having enough food, not having a job. It especially affects women of color because if they're stuck with a bunch of kids it's hard to get yourself out of that situation. Denying women rights to the autonomy of their own bodies is a way to control populations. Morally and ethically, I'm against that.

I had my abortion 15 years ago, when I was 18. I was newly married to someone who was not very nice to me, in the simplest of words. When I got pregnant, like two months after we got married, I had already kind of realized my mistake in marrying someone I hadn't really known for very long.

I had grown up in a home with very little love, so I needed it. When you're that young and some boy comes along and says 'I love you,' you're like, 'Oh, good. We'll get married and this will be it the rest of my life.' Looking back on it, that was hilariously naïve, but my intentions were pure at the time. When I got pregnant, I knew that I couldn't raise a child with this man. I didn't want my child to grow up in the environment of fear and anxiety that my husband had created for me. I decided I wanted to have an abortion. My husband was supportive of it.

He even agreed to come with me. He was in the Army, and the night before my appointment, he told me that he had to go to a mandatory barbecue at his unit. He couldn't get out of it. So I had to go to my procedure by myself.

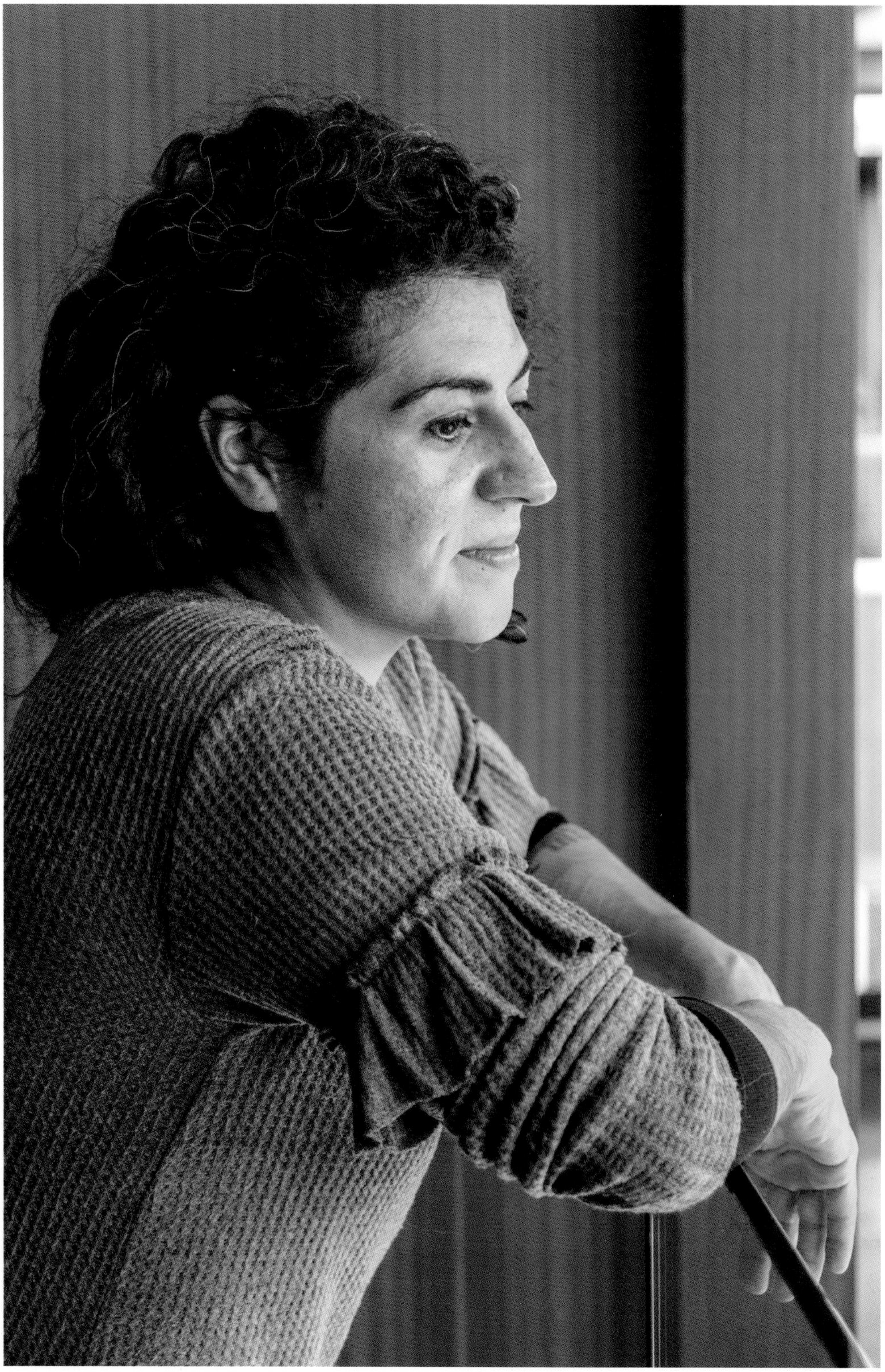

MAITE SALAZAR

I went to Planned Parenthood over in Kansas because of the 72-hour waiting period in Missouri, where we lived. I went in for a kind of counseling session to tell them why I wanted the abortion. Then they took me for an exam and an ultrasound. All of that was fine. The actual abortion itself was like weird. They took me back into a room and everyone was in gowns. They usually give you anesthesia, but in my case since I was driving myself home, I couldn't get any of the twilight anesthesia. Basically, they gave me two Tylenols and a Valium. And that was not enough.

I originally went in to get the medication abortion where you take the pills and expel at home. But when they did the ultrasound they told me I was too far along. This is how ignorant I was in terms of my own body. I had no idea when they started counting the pregnancy—from your last period, right? I had no idea. When I scheduled the abortion, I told the lady on the phone I was two weeks pregnant, when really I should've been telling her six weeks.

Anyway, I had to drive myself home afterwards. I threw up on myself on the way. It was bad. It was just an all-around not-good experience. When I got home, I had to walk in my house covered in puke. It just sucked. Nobody was there either. I was just like by myself forever.

Afterwards my husband said I wasn't really supposed to talk about my abortion. I wasn't supposed to cry about it. It wasn't until 12 years after I had my abortion that I started talking about it.

I think my abortion and my silence that followed it led to me having alcoholism. Like just drinking all the time to try to forget about how much it sucked. The abortion itself was traumatic, but it was the abandonment, really. I understood I would be alone for the rest of my life, even in the hardest of times. That led me to drinking more and more and more until seven years ago, I got liver cirrhosis. I'm told I'm going to die, that I'm not going to walk out of the hospital. Well, I got sober and put myself in an outpatient rehab and I have been sober ever since.

My family has lived in New Mexico since the dawn of time, basically. Both of my parents, like most people in New Mexico are a mix of European and Native. We have indigenous relatives from the Pueblos and Diné (Navajo) people. We also have Basque ancestry. We moved to Kansas City, Missouri just before I turned seven. I've been here ever since.

When we moved to Kansas City, my parents wanted to be white. They wanted to fit in. They got really nice jobs and were starting to make money. We lived in white neighborhoods. I went to white schools. It was an incredible culture shock, coming from New Mexico where I was used to the majority of the people looking like me. But here, I have spent 95 percent of my life as the only brown person in the room.

NOW THAT I'VE DISCOVERED MORE ABOUT MY CULTURES, I REALIZE THAT A LOT OF MY VALUES ALIGN WITH THE CULTURES FROM THE ANCIENT TIMES . . . HONESTY, INTEGRITY, TAKING CARE OF NOT ONLY YOURSELF AND YOUR FAMILY BUT THE ENTIRE COMMUNITY.

It was not a very good household to grow up in. It was abusive verbally, emotionally and physically. I was expected to be perfect at all times, so like I would get hit if I didn't get straight As. That type of thing. And every week we went to an evangelical church called the Foursquare Church. It's like one of those churches where people pray with their hands in the air and they speak in tongues and faint. I considered myself a Christian until about 13, when I decided none of this made sense to me. I had my own moral and ethical values.

Now that I've discovered more about my cultures, I realize that a lot of my values align with the cultures from the ancient times. What was important to them was honesty, integrity, taking care of not only yourself and your family but the entire community. And being a warrior not by going out to fight, but by making sure that everyone in your immediate area is fed, clothed, and happy.

In college at University of Missouri-Kansas City, I took a class called *The Politics of Sex and Gender* with, Dr. Harris Mirkin. He influenced me a lot, especially on feelings of morality and sexuality. Coming from my parents and from the church, I saw sexuality as, 'You don't go there.' Making out was a sin. Going from that to acknowledging myself as a queer person and as somebody who is allowed to own that sexuality was very game-changing for me.

It's really hard to define myself. The smallest most compact identity that I could give you is I'm mixed indigenous Latinx person. I say "Latinx" because I was raised in Latinx culture. And then I'm pansexual, so anything goes. And I'm non-binary trans person, so I don't identify strongly with a gender. I sort of go in between them. And then "artist." I'm a starving candidate at the moment, but I have worked for many years in TV and film production. I've been an author, small business owner, cultural reporter, editor, performer, bartender, server, manager, producer, musician, artist, and finder of odd-jobs. I look at life like it's an art piece.

I also do a lot of social activism. I went to Standing Rock twice and I just got back from the Mexican border about a month and a half ago. I stayed in an indigenous resistance camp there. My philosophy is to experience things firsthand. I like to talk to other people who've experienced things firsthand.

I'm a candidate for Missouri's Fifth Congressional District. Reproductive rights are a big reason that I wanted to run for office, to actually protect reproductive rights instead of having all these states making legislation that basically bars us from having our Constitutional right to abortion.

On the campaign trail, when people want to talk about abortion, I say our reproductive rights are under attack. As somebody who's had an abortion I think that this is ridiculous. I'm running for office in the Bible Belt. There are many, many conservative people here. Abortion is not talked about. So for me to sit here and be like, "I've had an abortion. It was the best decision and I stand by it."

I tell people that I too want to prevent abortion. The way we do that is to educate our children on sexual education, on their bodies, starting at a young age. Then we make birth control available without a prescription.

I haven't really gotten a huge amount of flak about this particular issue. I've never really had somebody come up and say, "I think this is wrong." I think most people are on the page that abortion is necessary and it needs to be safe. And you know, I always say to people that they don't have to have an abortion if they don't want to. It just needs to be there for people who do.

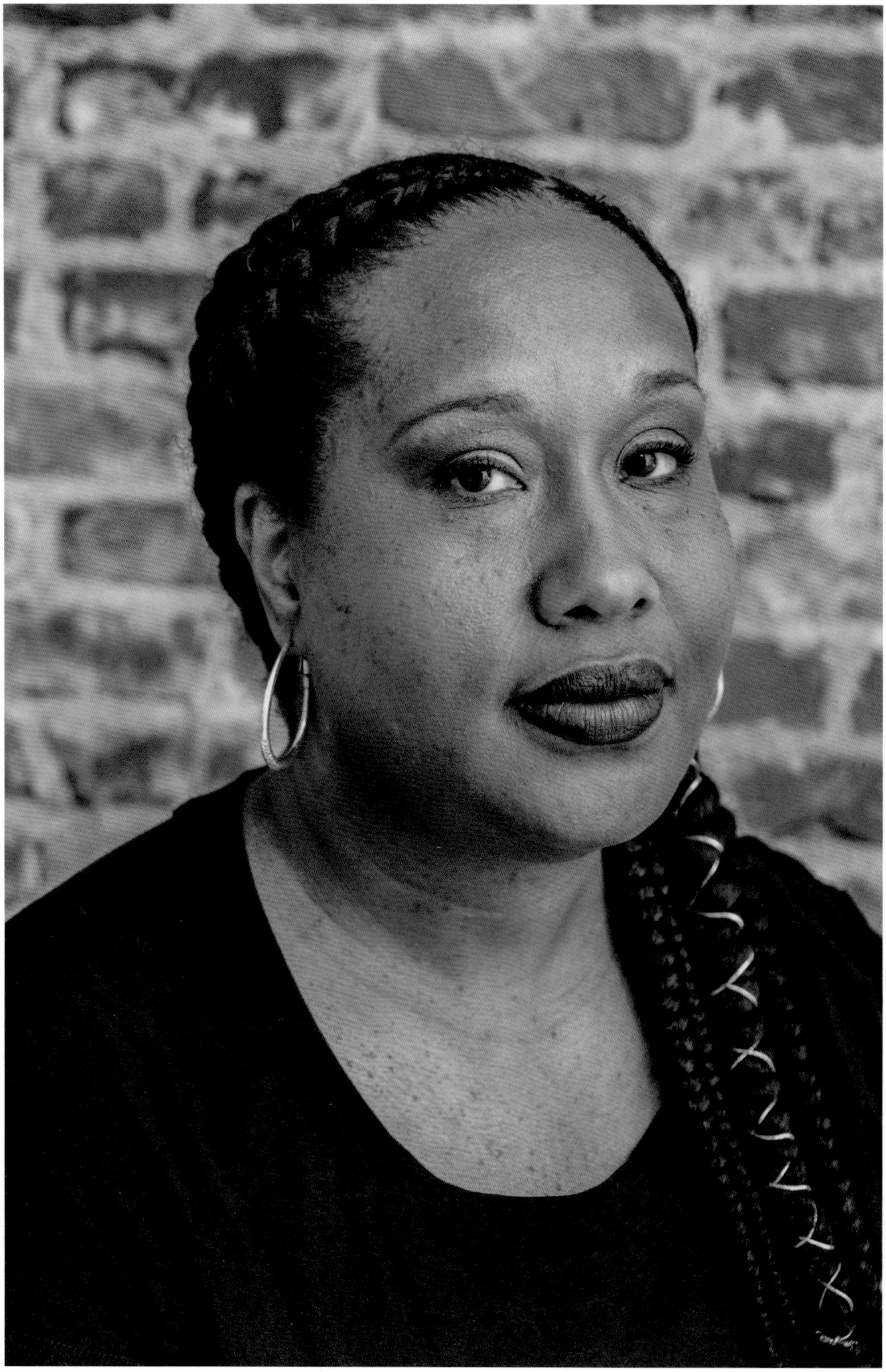

SUKARI OLAWUMI

Sukari Olawumi

AT THE EARLY age of 6 I knew I was called to be in the medical field. It was 1980 and we had moved from Chicago to Atlanta. My father had pulmonary sarcoidosis and the doctors said that the climate would be better in the South. The nurses at Georgia Baptist Hospital took such good care of him and inspired me to want to help people. After I graduated high school and went on to college, I wanted to pursue nursing, but having children stopped that dream from happening. Instead, I became a medical assistant and then went to school to be a scrub tech. From scrub tech I pursued ultrasound. That's what I've been doing since 2004.

After working in multiple hospitals and private practices, I found my place in abortion care. I have been in reproductive justice work for about ten years, and have been on the board of ARC (Access Reproductive Care of the Southeast) for a year now. It is a nonprofit that helps pay for abortions and provides practical support like lodging, transportation, and childcare.

I knew about reproductive justice from a personal experience. I had a termination when I was 25 years old. When I had my abortion, I saw the passion of the workers helping me with a difficult decision.

I already had two kids when I got pregnant with a gentleman who had other children. I knew he was not going to be able to help me financially with the child because of his other obligations. I was already struggling with my own two children and I wanted to give them the best life that I could possibly give them. I knew that I wasn't going to stop my schooling again due to pregnancy. I wanted a career to give them a better life. You hear about the stigma of abortion. I have to say that being a single parent with two kids, I faced stigma every day. The world was looking at me like I was lesser as a person because I had two children out of wedlock. In fact, when I had gotten got pregnant earlier with my son, I remember the pastor of my church telling me, "Nobody can judge you. You hold your head up in whatever decision you make." I used that same strong foundation in the church when I made the decision to end a pregnancy later on.

When I told the father that I did not want to keep the pregnancy, he agreed that it was my choice, but he didn't agree with it. He did not speak to me anymore afterward. That hurt, but I used that hurt as a building block, a powerful tool or weapon, to get me where I am. It gave me the motivation, the drive, the determination, to provide a better life for my kids. I couldn't just sulk and feel sorry for myself. I felt like abortion was the best decision for me and I don't regret it!

> **Because ultrasound is the first stop at the clinic, I deal with so many different waves of emotions . . . I know I make a difference with these women because I know how I felt when I was faced with that decision.**

When I got pregnant, I was an ER tech, doing three twelve-hour shifts a week and going to school at night. My mother kept my kids while I was at school. My mom has always been my biggest supporter. She said whatever I decided to do, she would help in whatever way. Unfortunately, I had to pay for the abortion out of pocket,. But I had emotional support from my family and friends. My kids were my cheerleaders also. My daughter always made me put my school report card on the refrigerator and she would tell me C's were unacceptable because that's what I told them about their grades. In my work in ultrasound, I see so many different anomalies in pregnancies, so many different ages and so many different scenarios. Because ultrasound is the first stop at the clinic, I deal with so many different waves of emotions before people see a counselor.

Some people want to continue their pregnancy, but due to anomalies choose termination because the fetus won't have any quality of life. Others can't afford another mouth to feed. Some are struggling with addictions and don't wish to bring a child into the world with an addiction. Others have been sexually assaulted. Some just say "now is not a good time." I know I make a difference with these women because I know how I felt when I was faced with that decision.

I tell them, "It's okay. Hold your head up. You have to do what's best for you in your situation, nobody else." Every day I reassure them, "You're not alone. I've been where you are." I become somewhat of a storyteller in the ultrasound room. I let it be known that my room is a safe space for them if they want to talk. Most important, I tell them that nobody can judge them.

When they arrive, some are crying, some have a blank face, or some just want you to listen. Most often, they're afraid of not knowing what to expect. Not only do I do the ultrasound, I am that big sister or mother figure, hand holder, hugger, Kleenex giver, until they get to the counselor.

It's hard when I have to tell someone that she is too far along in the pregnancy for a termination. In Georgia the law prohibits abortion after twenty-one weeks and six days. Sometimes women arrive thinking that they're twelve weeks and they're already eighteen weeks and they have already had to use the rent money to get to the clinic and can't afford the higher fee for a later abortion.

I'm able to tell them about the various organizations that can help with funds. I tell them not to be discouraged. We'll put our heads together collectively and see what we can do to get this done.

It gives me so much joy when I see women bond and exchange telephone numbers or they hug each other before they leave. Seeing these acts of kindness helps me at the end of the day to say, hey you did a really good thing today. She's walking out and her head is held high because she took your words of affirmation and used them throughout the day to get herself through.

I remember one particular patient who had been molested. She was 12 years old and her whole world had been flipped upside down. Before she was put to sleep, she asked me to say the Lord's Prayer with her. My mind went blank. I couldn't remember a prayer I have said a thousand times, Finally, the words of the prayer began to flow from my mouth. Everyone in the room repeated it with me until she was asleep.

When she woke up, I was in the recovery room with her. She said she wanted a strawberry sundae from McDonald's. I went to go get that baby that strawberry sundae from McDonald's. I cried all the way there and cried all the way back because I knew they were about to take her back to a world where she would need years of counseling and faith to help her suppress the trauma she had encountered.

The smile on her face from something as small as a $1 sundae was radiant. I wanted nothing more at that moment than to help her forget that her innocence was taken, even if it was only temporary. If I could have taken her home with me that day, I would have without hesitation. This is why I work so hard to help eliminate the stigma against abortion, why I use my voice for people of color who are shamed or are made to feel insignificant.

My work with ARC involves me with the community. That is why I am a member of the board. ARC is made up of people who look like me, who can identify with the same issues I face. It is dedicated to erasing stigma and lowering barriers for people of color in the abortion arena. We aren't out barking about abortion, abortion, abortion. We talk about abortion in a way that women will say, "thank you for the work that you do, even though I don't believe in this way." That counts as a win, because they see what you're doing.

Geoffrey Harris

THINKING ABOUT WHEN I was 15, so far your life has been completely perfect, and you kind of see this pathway for yourself, where it's like, I'm going to go to this high school, go to this college, marry this girl, and have kids. Nothing like I'm going to have to have an abortion at 15. It was like the craziest slap in the face I could've gotten.

My girlfriend was 16 when she got pregnant. We had already been dating for like a year. We just hooked up, and we didn't use a condom. Afterwards we got Plan B and used it, but then she still was pregnant, which is kind of weird.

She took a pregnancy test and it came up negative, but she still didn't get her period. By then a week had passed, so we went to Planned Parenthood to get a 100 percent conclusive result. She got a positive result. We were completely devastated, and then we walked out and found out her car had been towed. You can't write a worse day.

I WAS WITH MY GIRLFRIEND IN THE PROCEDURE ROOM AS IT WAS HAPPENING . . . I WAS HOLDING HER HAND, GOING THROUGH THIS EXPERIENCE, AND I NEVER FELT SO ALONE.

I didn't want to sway her choice either which way, because it's her body and it's ultimately her choice. I didn't want to pressure her. She wanted to get an abortion. She was 16. She was from really strict Chinese parents, and she didn't even really let them know.

Going to Planned Parenthood for the abortion was a surreal experience. I wasn't old enough to drive, so my mother had to drive us. She had interned at Planned Parenthood during college, so for her to re-engage with Planned Parenthood with a completely different experience must've been tough on her.

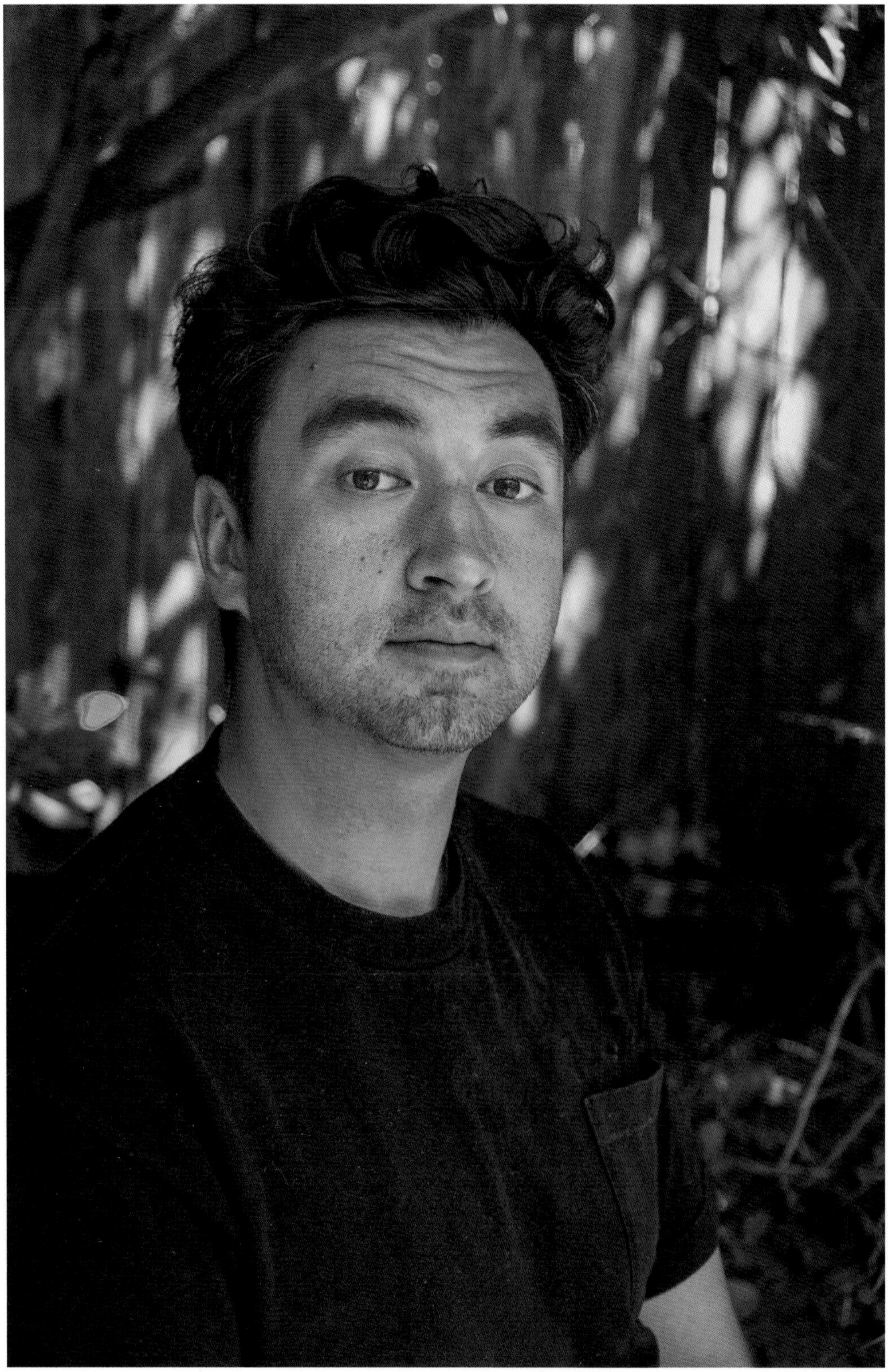

GEOFFREY HARRIS

I was with my girlfriend in the procedure room as it was happening. I'm just going to be real with you, completely candid. This is what happened. Before the procedure, they gave her some sort of narcotic, and she was just super loopy during the procedure. Like almost in a giggly, playful state. I was holding her hand, going through this experience, and I never felt so alone, because she was just in and out of consciousness, almost like laughing. It was just hard for her and hard for me. It was really intense.

That whole day was like a David Lynch movie or something. There's so many different emotional layers on top of every scene. As we were driving out, there was this protester lady. My eyes locked onto her eyes, and she could just see that I was completely heartbroken from what happened. She kind of put down her sign a little bit. I don't know. I was kind of just trying to protect my girlfriend from seeing that lady.

It was just hard for her and hard for me. It was really intense . . . That whole day was like a David Lynch movie or something.

After the abortion, we really didn't really talk to anybody about it. We were trying to keep it under wraps. We dated for another year after that, and then she went to college, and then we broke up. That was kind of hard to be a little young'un and see your girl go off to college.

I'm half Filipino on my mother's side. My dad's side is just good old-fashioned white, like from the Revolution. My grandmother's German-Irish from St. Paul, and my dad's English-Irish from Chicago or somewhere. Growing up mixed race is a really hard thing because you don't identify with any race and instead you're kind of your own race. It's a gift and a curse. It's just weird being mixed race. You don't feel comfortable in any sort of social situation.

Buddhism was very present in my family. We're all pretty devout. Buddhism is more of a philosophy than anything else. It's subjective. There's no real passage that says don't get an abortion, but if you were to read certain sutras, I don't think abortion would be supported necessarily. It's touchy. The Buddhist organization that we subscribe to, Soka Gakkai International or SGI, is very progressive and probably would support abortion for sure.

At the time of the abortion, I was pretty devout. My girlfriend came from a Christian-Chinese background. I think she went to a Christian middle school. She was a really smart student. She ended up becoming a doctor, and she definitely had her own life path that she knew since she was a little kid. What we did was the right thing because she's in a better place now because of it, and I would've never wanted to take that away from her. But, yeah, it's just unfortunate.

I kind of had a falling out with Buddhism in my early twenties where I tried to read different religions—the Old and New Testament and the Quran and all this stuff. But now, my Buddhist practice is everything. I consistently chant and meditate throughout the day. And I read different Buddhist scriptures. Buddha wrote eighty different sutras, and all that practice just led me back to the same exact sutra, the same exact practice that I've been practicing as a kid. For me, the lotus sutra is the greatest story ever written.

I worked in tech for eight years, starting at age 18. When I was 26, I just felt I was in front of a computer all the time. Now I'm 30. I have done some artist management, including TLC, the '90s R&B group, and an indie rock mega icon superstar act, Christopher Owens. Now I work in the cannabis industry. This gives me the ability to be outside. It's such a beautiful concept and it's kind of fun. Growing up in the city my entire life, it's kind of suffocating, and there's just something beautiful about getting outside of the Bay Area.

And here's my second abortion story. I call it the Tinder abortion. I only tell a few people about my past, and especially because that first abortion was really traumatic. While I was dating a girl for a few months on Tinder, I told her about the abortion. We broke up and then got back together at a Halloween party. At the end of the party, she was just like, "Oh, so you know, I found out I was pregnant when we broke up, and I had an abortion." Hearing that resurfaced a lot of stuff from the first one, and kind of emotionally wrecked me for a good three to four months. The first abortion was so traumatic, and to think that something like that happened twice, so much later in life, it was really heartbreaking for me. Ten months later, she called me and said she had lied. She didn't even really have an abortion. She just wanted to get back together. I guess she was trying to bind me to this traumatic experience. We did not get back together.

When I think back fifteen years after the abortion, it's difficult. It happened so young. It's like something that I usually keep down, super buried, so it's good to let it out. If you think about it for too long, it could definitely ruin your day. If I completely think about it, it's devastating. I try not to think about it too often.

Karen Thurston

I NEVER TALKED to another person about my abortions until I was 40 years old. I met a woman through church. We hit it off and we were at her house when she started talking about an unintended pregnancy when she was young. Her parents had sent her away to have the baby and put it up for adoption.

It was the first time anybody had ever talked to me about an unplanned pregnancy. I just started telling her everything about me. It was a flood of relief to finally tell someone. She was compassionate.

My parents married young, just out of high school. As my dad moved up in his career, we moved from Texas to New Jersey to Georgia. My parents were very loving, very committed to their marriage. My sister is four years older and my brother is eight years younger. I was a classic middle child, which had a big influence on how my life unfolded. My sister has a lively personality, outgoing and confident. In her teens, she was difficult for my parents to manage. When my brother came along, my mother was focused on taking care of him.

I had no education about my body or sex. It wasn't available in school and my parents didn't talk about it. There was no internet, no access to information. We didn't have books in our home at all and didn't go to the library, so I had really no resources at my fingertips. The resources that I had were basically my sister and her friends.

When I hit puberty I didn't understand what was happening with my body. I remember getting my period. My mother gave me the pads and told me to wear them. It was like,

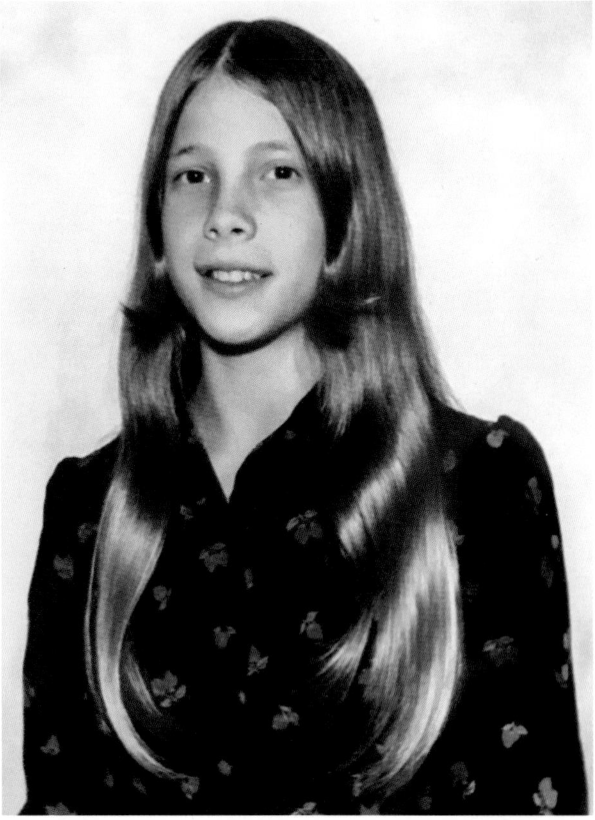

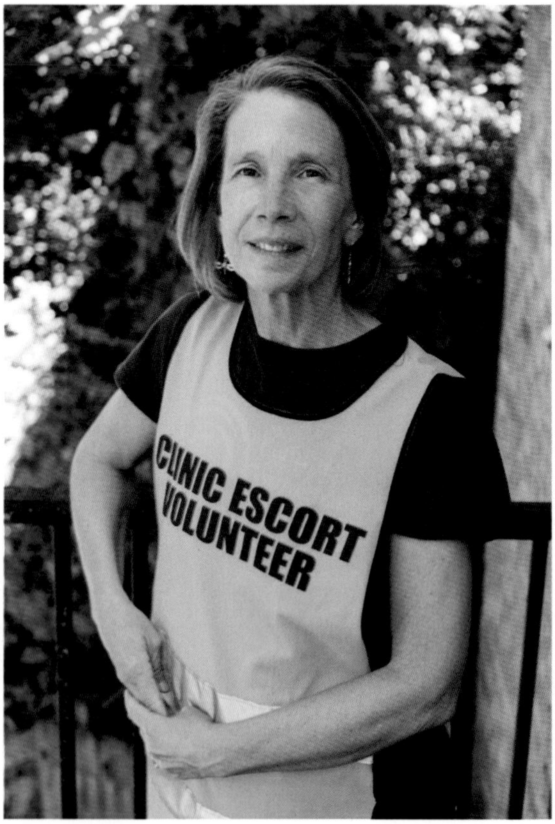

KAREN THURSTON

"This is a woman's lot. This will happen every month." One day we ran out of pads, and my mother told me to use one of her tampons. She explained what to do with a tampon. I was horrified. I didn't even know there was a place in my body for something like that to fit.

All of this led up to my abortion when I was 13. We had moved to Georgia, where my outgoing, sparkly sister had made friends quickly. I looked up to my sister very much and wanted to be just like her. My mother thought that my sister would behave better when I was with her, so she sent me out with my sister. Her friends were partygoers. They were older and had long hair. One guy started paying attention to me. I felt like he was a friend. Soon he started putting pressure on me to have sex. I didn't know how to handle the situation. I was taught to obey and to not hurt other people's feelings. I was easily persuaded into things that I didn't understand. So, we had sex.

I found out I was pregnant because I was throwing up all the time. I thought it was the weirdest sickness, the flu or a bug. My mother finally asked me if I was pregnant. I said, no, because I'd only had one encounter. It had been painful and unromantic and terrible. You're taught that you get pregnant when you're married and in love and it's all beautiful and it's the best thing in your life.

I could just tell by my mother's tone that being pregnant would be a terrible thing. She drove me to a doctor. In the doctor's office, it was just this old man doctor and me. He was feeling around inside of me and it hurt. I was scared. I was pregnant, of course. My parents and I had only one conversation about the whole situation. It boiled down to, "We're going to take care of this and you must go along."

MY FATHER WAS ASHAMED OF ME. HE TOLD ME NEVER TO TELL ANYONE. EVER. NOT EVEN MY HUSBAND WHEN I GREW UP AND GOT MARRIED. I JUST BURIED THIS SECRET FOR TWENTY-SEVEN YEARS.

This was in 1973, just after Roe v. Wade. I don't know how they arranged the abortion. But I do know it felt punitive. My father was ashamed of me. He told me never to tell anyone. Ever. Not even my husband when I grew up and got married. I just buried this secret for twenty-seven years. I internalized the message that this is so horrible that no one can know this about me.

Later, in college I was in a long-term relationship with a guy I thought I might spend my life with. He was studying to be a pilot. The relationship started out fine, but then he treated me terribly. I was using a diaphragm and I got pregnant. I was devastated. I thought, wow, I bet there's no one else on this Earth who's gotten pregnant twice. I was 19.

I was fortunate that he arranged for the abortion and paid for it. I was still living at home with my parents. Having to see my parents every day, knowing how horrible they thought I was when I was 13, I couldn't imagine what they would think if they knew about this. But they didn't find out.

It took a long time, but eventually, I felt like I needed to come out about my abortion, and like people coming out on the gender scale will tell you, "It's a process." But I could still hear my father saying, "Don't ever tell your husband."

One day it just all came out of me in tears. My husband was so loving, he embraced me and held me. He cried with me and he became my greatest supporter. Fourteen years later I found the courage to tell our two sons. They too were compassionate and loving. One son helped me get online and I discovered there was a whole group of people working to solve this problem of stigma and abortion. I knew I had to get involved.

I am so grateful to have this opportunity to try to end this problem of stigma. We're all quiet about the reality of our lives. The only people talking are the ones who don't experience abortion, don't understand it, and just pile on the shame.

I became a volunteer as a clinic escort here at the Feminist Women's Health Center in 2015. The antis who picket outside clinics are daunting and cruel. It's emotional violence. I try to be a comforting presence for a person coming for care.

My first escorting experience was in Louisville, Kentucky, at a clinic on a busy city street. They have hundreds of protesters, many of them very aggressive. One of the protesters was a preacher man. He got right up in my face with his bullhorn, telling me I'm evil, I'm going to hell. I stood there with my chin up, my head high, and just looked at him in the eyes. I never looked away. It was very empowering for me. I was terrified, but it was really the first time that I held my head up high. I had spent a lot of my life literally looking down at the ground. Here I was facing the worst of it. I thought I am going to do this as long as I'm physically able.

When a patient drives up to our clinic, I try to wave them up past the protesters. I tell them I'm here because they deserve to feel loved and respected for coming to get care for whatever reason they are here.

All kinds of people come through our clinic, all of humanity, from different ethnicities and economic backgrounds. It's a parade of the human condition. The protesters are also a variety of humanity. One woman regrets having had an abortion when she was young. People from the nearby Catholic church stand there with their rosaries—an image of public shaming for the women coming here.

The demonstrators sometimes bring their children. One boy who looked about 9 years old just glared, looking angrily at me for a few minutes. I was crushed to imagine this young child being taught to hate a stranger so intensely.

Just a few years ago, I actually talked to my mother about my volunteer work. I thanked her for getting me abortion care when I was young. I said I knew it must have been hard for them as parents, but it saved my life. Her response was, "Well, it's just something women have to do and we just shouldn't talk about it."

Abortion care saved my life. It's why I have a wonderful husband, two great sons, and two awesome grandchildren. I trace everything good in my life back to being able to get care. I have so much love in my heart for people who provide abortion and for the organizations that are trying to help people access care.

I recognize that I'm a privileged white person who did not have trouble accessing care. It's my duty to do what I can to help others get care. Fighting the stigma is part of that process. Even my being silenced for so long was a gift because it taught me not to judge people you don't know. Everybody deserves compassion and love. My experience has given me a wide-open heart for other people. My biggest dream is that the words of my story will float out there and meet the person who may be helped by hearing them.

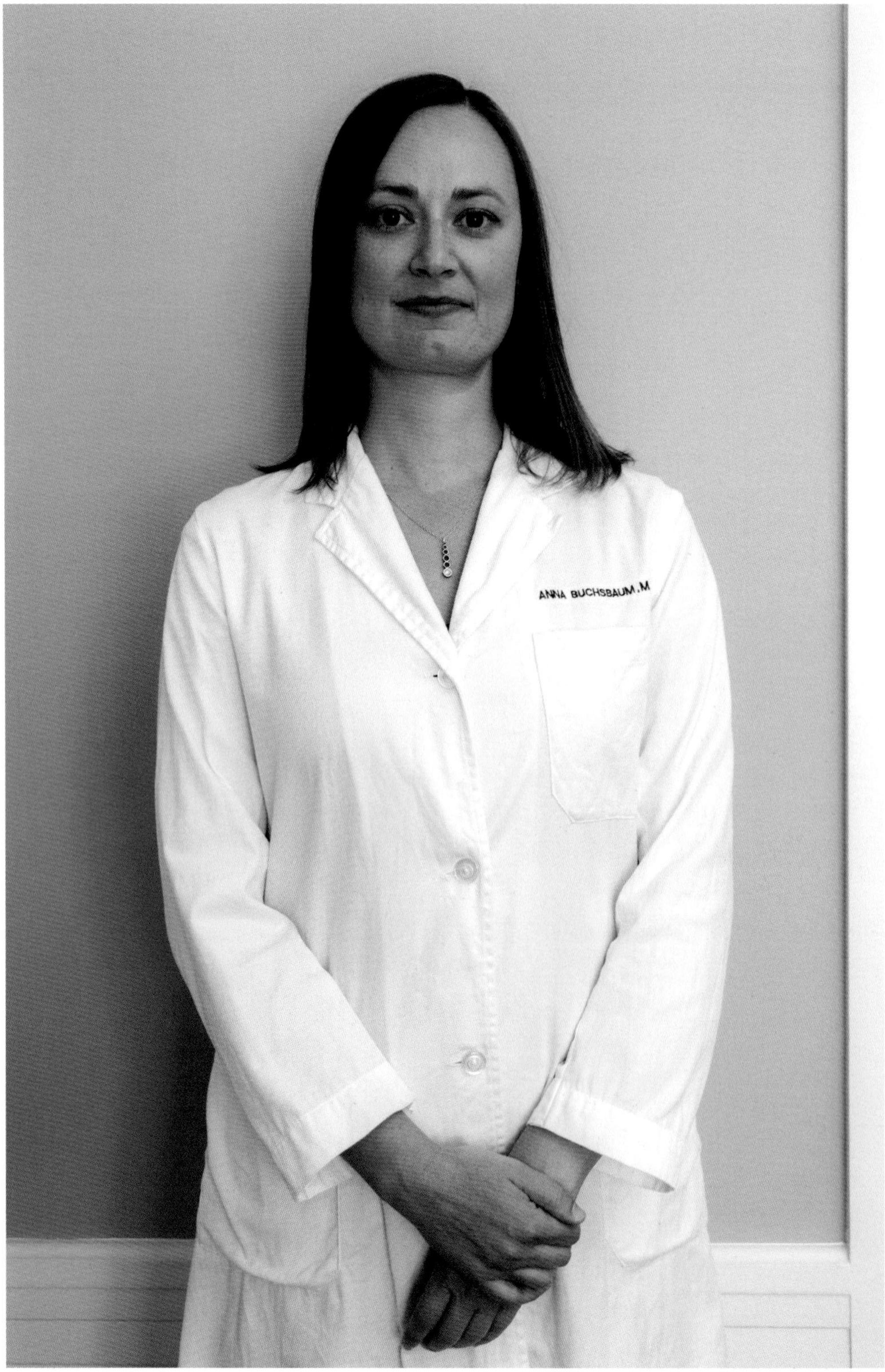

ANNA BUCHSBAUM

Anna Buchsbaum

GROWING UP IN San Francisco, it was a known value in my family that my parents were pro-choice. As a teenager I remember going to pro-choice protests with my mom. And, of course at that age, your world is so small, you think everything is like your own family.

When I got to medical school in Buffalo, New York, I realized that is not the case. There was one abortion clinic in the city of Buffalo, and its primary provider, Dr. Barnett Slepian, had been killed for his abortion work in the '90s. I hadn't really put any of that together before I got there.

Being in a community where people felt very negatively, or were just apathetic about abortion made me realize that abortion was not accessible to everybody.

In medical school, I joined Medical Students for Choice. We had, maybe, three members out of approximately 130 students. That piqued my interest to get more involved. I knew I could help make it accessible by training as an OBGYN and becoming an abortion provider.

At Buffalo there were one or two practicing OBGYNs who would do abortions if they were medically required, and they would do them in an operating room setting regardless of the gestational age. So I got to see one abortion when I was a medical student during my OBGYN rotation in the university hospital. But really, abortion is one of the procedures all OBGYN residents are supposed to learn and do.

After graduating in 2007, I did a residency in OBGYN at a medical group in Oakland, California, which was a totally different situation from Buffalo. They have attending physicians who have done the Fellowship in Family Planning, and who ran a Ryan Residency Training Program, which I went on to do myself.

The Fellowship in Family Planning is an amazing two-year fellowship where you learn to do clinical abortion up to twenty-four weeks of gestational age. You learn how to take care of medically complicated patients who are seeking contraception. You get a Master's in Public Health.

I did my fellowship at Emory University in Atlanta, Georgia, in a high-volume abortion clinic. The patient population was generally low income, with no insurance or under-insured, primarily African American. I performed "elective abortions" where there was no medical reason for the procedure.

Now I work for a medical group in San Francisco where the patient population is women who primarily are aborting highly desired pregnancies that, using genetic testing, have been diagnosed with fetal anomalies. They tend to be upper-middle class women, highly educated, a very different patient population than Atlanta.

In my mind, all reasons for choosing an abortion are equally valid. That is why abortion has to remain legal and accessible.

By the time these women get to me, they have pretty much made their decision. The genetic counselors have talked with them extensively about what the diagnosis for the fetus means. The patient will make the decision about whether to continue the pregnancy—and more often than not, these decisions to terminate are devastating. The women are often tearful in my office and I have to be very sensitive about the way I handle that. I'm not counseling them about their decision. I'm trying to help them be more comfortable with their decision.

Often I get people who come to my office and say, "I'm pro-life, I don't believe in abortion. But my situation is different. My baby wouldn't survive. Therefore, I have to have this procedure." This is an emotional challenge for them and for me.

To hear someone come in and say she doesn't believe in abortion but is forced to be doing this is frustrating. To me, these upper-middle class women who have chosen to terminate a fetal anomaly are in a very similar situation to the low-income women I met in Atlanta who couldn't afford another child. Neither group of women would say they are frivolously choosing to have an abortion. In my mind, all reasons for choosing an abortion are equally valid. That is why abortion has to remain legal and accessible.

At Emory University, we didn't have a clinic devoted to abortion care. We did our abortions in the Labor & Delivery operating room, which has its own complexities. It was hard for a woman to abort a pregnancy amongst a lot of women delivering babies.

In addition, at Emory we had a lot of what we would call "pushbacks" from other staff members who disapproved of and would not participate in abortion procedures. Because we could only do abortions in a hospital operating room under anesthesia, we had to deal with anesthesiologists who did not agree with doing the procedure. Many anesthesiologists refused to be part of an abortion. In that case, we might have to wait for the next shift. Our patient would be waiting, without anything to eat or drink, for the eight hours until the next anesthesiologist would come on and be willing to participate. The nursing staff who may not have wanted to help us, or the staff who checked a woman in for her procedure may have said something judgmental to the patient.

As the abortion provider trying to protect your patient from all of that, you try to fight those fights out in the hallway, but inevitably the patient would know what was going on. And that made me feel horrible. It made the patients feel horrible.

Also, there certainly are challenges for women everywhere who have to travel a certain distance to have an abortion. Even here, I have patients who travel three and four hours to have an abortion in San Francisco because it isn't available in their hometown in the wider Bay Area.

Here in San Francisco I will perform an abortion up to twelve weeks in the office setting. It is integrated into my daily life. For example, I can do a pap smear for a patient, then an abortion, then see a prenatal patient and then another abortion. After twelve weeks I perform the procedure in the operating room, keeping in mind the safety and comfort of the patient.

Personally, I have never felt threatened. I also have never been in the public eye. I'm very open with my friends and family about what I do. My colleagues know what I do. But none of that feels risky or scary to me. Perhaps in Arkansas or Louisiana it would feel scarier.

I do feel conflicted. I have a strong desire not to care about that risk, to be out there and to be very clear that I am an abortion provider. This is what I look like and this is my name. I am proud of what I do. It seems very important to me not to hide it.

Women have to be able to make the best choices for their individual lives without politicians or grandparents or neighbors judging them. That decision should be between that woman and her doctor. It's unfortunate that the decision has left the doctor's office and has gone into the political realm. I wish people would stop being judgmental.

I also wish that abortion would be funded as all other health care is. Not all insurance companies provide coverage for abortion care. Many states, many Medicaid programs, do not pay for abortion care, Georgia being one of them. Many of the women I saw in Atlanta wrangled up enough cash somehow from friends and family, and it took a long time, so they were in their second trimesters by the time they had the money. Or they could get funding through the National Abortion Federation. If we could document a medical problem like a seizure disorder or a cardiac anomaly that would make carrying the pregnancy to full term risky for the mother, Medicaid Services would pay for it.

Federal dollars cannot be used to pay for abortions. Even here in San Francisco, I've had patients who work for the federal government whose insurance will not pay for their abortion regardless of their reasons, even for a fetal anomaly. That just singles out abortion and contraception in a way that no other medical procedure is singled out. In an ideal world that wouldn't be the case.

One-third of women have an abortion. Women have abortions for all sorts of reasons and it's my job, no matter what, to provide that service. It is a really routine part of reproductive health care.

I want to normalize abortion. Along with gynecological and prenatal care, abortion is part of treating women as a whole person. It rounds out women's reproductive health care.

Ashley Underwood

I GREW UP in Youngstown, Ohio. It was a very tight-knit middle-class Black community. Most families owned their homes and raised their kids there, and by the time I came along, they were raising their grandchildren. Everyone was college educated

My extended family is huge and extremely tight-knit. Thanksgiving at my aunt's house would be two-hundred-plus people every single year.

I grew up very religious: church every single Sunday, Bible school, vacation Bible school, Sunday School revivals. My grandpa is a minister, and for a while my mom and I went to his church. It was this really small Pentecostal church, extremely religious. For children's church, we used to watch on Friday nights "Left Behind." It was the scariest dystopian thing about when the rapture comes and people are left behind, if they haven't accepted Jesus in their hearts. I felt scared! I felt like whenever I did anything wrong, which was a sin, I just felt like, "Oh God, this is going to cause me to go to hell."

After high school I went to Tennessee State University. It's an HBCU, which stands for historically Black colleges and universities, institutions that came about during the time when African Americans weren't allowed to go to other schools. Since they've been around for so long, it's kind of a cultural thing. It's like a really cool thing to go to an HBCU.

Going to school in the South, especially an HBCU, it had that same type of conservative middle-class Black social norms. Even if you did party Saturday night, you were on the bus that came to pick us up to go to church off campus.

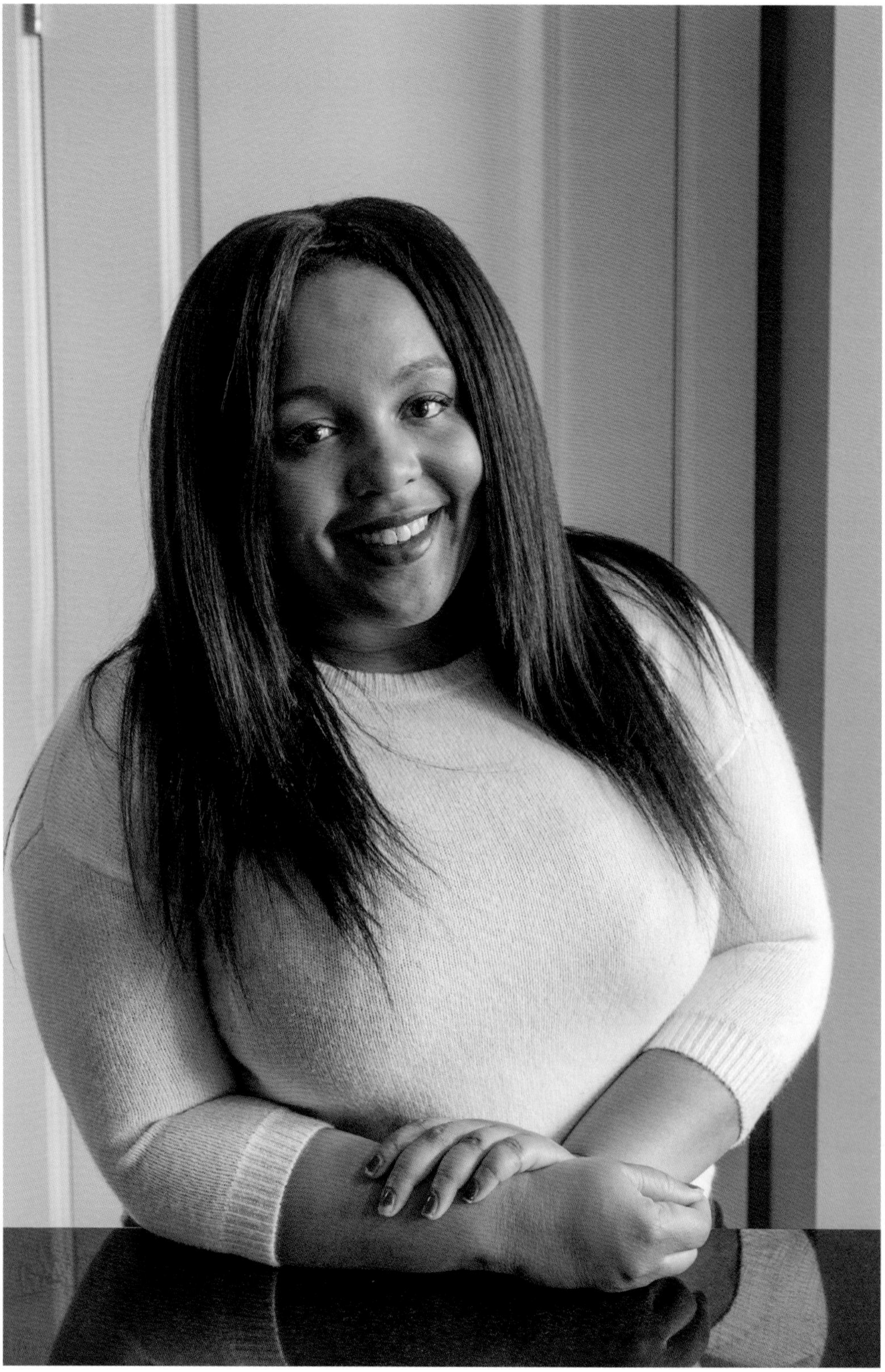

ASHLEY UNDERWOOD

Prior to going to college, I never drank, I never smoked, I never had sex. I was super virginal. When I got to campus, I started partying hard, but I was able to keep up my grades. What kind of kept me a little bit on track was being selected for the Miss Black and Gold pageant; pageants are really big on HBCU campuses. I placed third runner-up. It was great.

At college my social circle still went to church pretty frequently, but over time it waned for me to maybe twice a month, then only once a month. But I never felt like my connection really changed. During that time, I was able to get to know God for myself. Just living on campus, experiencing the world for myself and not what my mom or my grandparents would tell me. I really started to know a lot more about myself.

When I graduated, I was really depressed. In that dark moment is when I really formed my relationship with God, trying to figure out which way to go, what I wanted to do.

I got my Bachelors in biology because I thought I wanted to be a doctor, but in my junior year I realized that being a physician in no way fit my personality or the lifestyle I wanted to live. So I started thinking outside of the box. I knew I wanted to be in health and to help people. The led me to the world of public health. I ended up getting a Master's degree in public health from Case Western Reserve University in 2015.

I had my abortion when I was 26. I had a year's experience as a community health worker, working with teen moms, talking to them about how to have a healthy pregnancy, and how to prevent future pregnancies. I also did birth control demonstrations in high school. And then, guess what? After all that experience, I ended up with an unplanned pregnancy. That was when I realized, it can really happen to anyone.

On paper, I was a good match with the guy I was dating. Here I am: I'm young, I have my degrees, I'm starting to work, I've traveled. I'm feeling good. And he's this very handsome, Ivy-League-educated guy. He played football. I'm like, "Oh my God, we could be the next Michelle and Barack!" Really, we were just two dummies who thought that we were smart enough to know when to pull out. And we weren't.

When I was hired to work at the abortion clinic, I had never been in an abortion clinic before. I knew I had so much to learn about reproductive rights and women's history and reproductive justice. I was fascinated. I wanted to do everything! Around the same time, I went on a bus to the rally outside of the Supreme Court for Texas v. Hellerstedt. I have a picture of me outside the Supreme Court wearing a Statue of Liberty headpiece, and my little pro-choice pins, and I'm grinning. When I look back on it, that's the day that I had my first pregnancy symptoms.

After waiting a week, when I was a full seven days late, I got myself a pregnancy test. It was positive. I was really, really stressed out, and I just broke down. Luckily, everyone I work with and everyone at the clinic was just so nice and supportive. I remember, I was boohooing on a couch upstairs and someone just came and rubbed my shoulder, didn't even say anything, and left.

When I told the guy I was dating that I was pregnant, he didn't respond the way I wanted him to. I knew I was not going to have a baby. I felt like I had worked too hard, that I was finally breaking ground in a career and a life path that I was really happy with, that I could see myself advancing in. I just refused to be a single mom. I refused. I knew I was going to have an abortion. I didn't need to talk to him about that.

I wanted to keep things as normal as possible, because I felt my life was spinning out of control. I'm not a crier. My reaction to everything is to smile or laugh, even when I'm feeling so uncomfortable. I was afraid to tell my mom. When I called her and she heard the tone of my voice, I just broke down. She just said, "Either I'm going to be a grandma, or you're going to get an abortion, but either way is OK for me." That was the best thing I could hear. I just didn't want to disappoint her. She said, 'There's nothing you can do that won't make me proud of you." That warmed my heart and it was what I needed to hear.

All these years I've been a Christian and going to church. I felt God's presence when it was time for me to make that decision.

During the week of waiting for the procedure I just spent a lot of time by myself, a lot of time praying, a lot of time crying. And I just felt this sense of peace that I'm okay. All these years I've been a Christian and going to church. I felt God's presence when it was time for me to make that decision.

I also felt connected to the fetus, but not in a way that it was my baby. I feel like I'm a very spiritual person, and so I felt like it was a spirit that had visited me. And I kind of felt that I was grateful for it, because I do think that I do want to be a mom, and that when that time comes, that spirit will return to me.

I feel like my pregnancy was a wake-up call. Like, there is a life that you want, and there is a life that you're living, and there are steps that you need to take to get that life that you want. After the abortion, I just reevaluated myself.

I feel like my abortion was really meant to be, and honestly, I'm grateful for it. I feel like it was the first adult decision of my life. It was the first time that I took control and took charge of my body and thought about my future and made that decision for myself. Having my abortion is when I lost my sense of being naïve and a goody-two-shoes type of girl. I feel like it's when I became a woman.

I want other people to know that having an abortion is okay. It is a powerful experience and it was scariest thing I had done. Once I did it, I'm like, well, everything else is going to be a breeze.

I want to debunk some of those myths that having an abortion is going to make you less of a Christian or will separate you from God. Any trial is going to bring you closer to God.

I WANT TO DEBUNK SOME OF THOSE MYTHS THAT HAVING AN ABORTION IS GOING TO MAKE YOU LESS OF A CHRISTIAN OR WILL SEPARATE YOU FROM GOD. ANY TRIAL IS GOING TO BRING YOU CLOSER TO GOD.

If you're a Christian, people automatically assume that you are pro-life. The things the protestors outside the clinic say are disgusting, and it pisses me off to no end that they are using the God that I worship, taking His name in vain, trying to shame the women who come here. And I'm just like, "Show me in the Bible where Jesus shamed women. Show me in the Bible where Jesus is telling you to wake up on a Saturday and harass people trying to get to their medical appointments." That's not Christ-like at all. I want to reclaim that term Christian and showcase what an authentic Christian looks like. I want to say that it is OK to have an abortion and still call yourself a Christian.

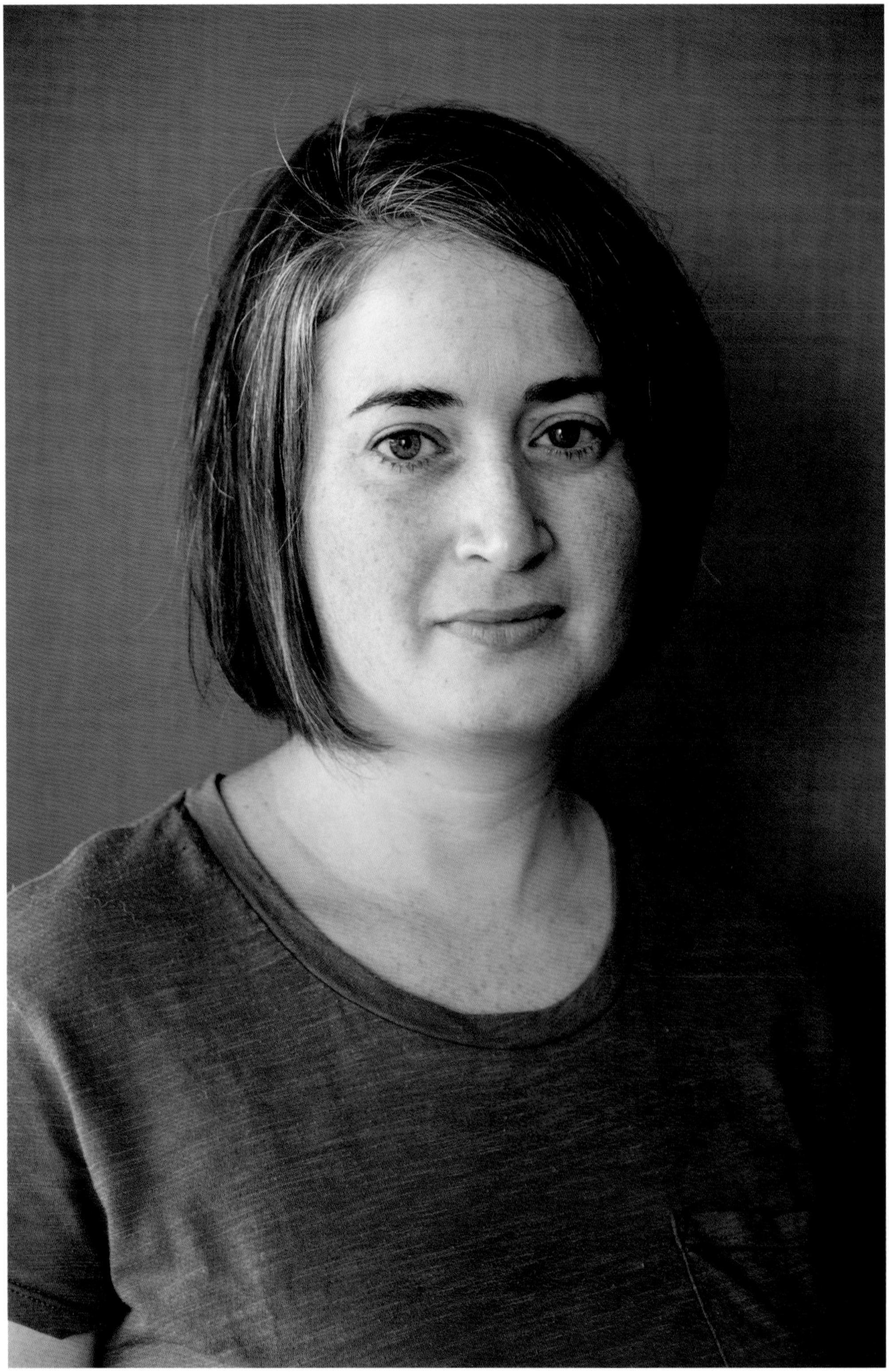

RACHEL GOLDBERG

Rachel Goldberg

BECAUSE HALF MY family is Jewish and half is Protestant, I have learned to navigate the differences. I've always existed in different spaces. Like now I have my activism community and my farming community and then there's the other world of my family community.

My husband and I wanted to start a family right after we married in 2015 and we wanted to be close to family. We also wanted to farm, so we moved to Missouri, where my husband's family lives. We raise wool sheep, heritage breeds that are endangered. I love my sheep. They're really sweet; they're a lot of fun. I work with the wool, knitting, spinning, and dyeing.

Our rural community in southwest Missouri has 417 people. I think the biggest culture shock for me has been living in a small town in Missouri. It's a pretty conservative area, and there is a lot of fear of outsiders.

I had been feeling weird and decided to take a pregnancy test. I was in the bathroom brushing my teeth while the pregnancy test was waiting to show. When I saw the little, "yes," I started screaming with joy. My husband was on the other side of the door asking if I was okay. I had to slip the pregnancy test under the door because I was so excited I couldn't get the door open to show it to him. The next day, I made an appointment and my doctor confirmed the pregnancy.

At about ten or fifteen weeks, my blood work noted an elevated risk of a genetic anomaly. We repeated the blood test and the second test came back all clear. We hadn't told anyone we were pregnant, so at our twenty-week ultrasound, we were really excited to get ultrasound pictures and make cute little gifts for our parents. But at the twenty-week ultrasound, the tech was really quiet. Then she said she was going to get the doctor.

The doctor told us the ultrasound showed some abnormalities. We were referred to a high-risk doctor for more tests. I was twenty-two weeks pregnant by the time the high-risk doctor could see us. At that appointment I had an hour-long ultrasound. I just started crying in the middle of it because it was really obvious that something was not right. The technicians were talking quietly to each other, but I could hear what they were saying. They couldn't find his stomach and they weren't sure if he had all four chambers of his heart.

The doctor explained that they suspected some form of skeletal dysplasia, which is dwarfism. I thought, "Oh, dwarfism, that's a survivable condition." It was scary, but it seemed like if he could have a good quality life then that would be fine. The doctor asked our permission to send our ultrasound to a specialist in St. Louis for more of a prognosis. He also recommended an amniocentesis test.

Essentially, we had learned that there was a potential to lose the baby and also me during delivery. If we both survived, the baby would basically have to have surgeries until complications from one killed him.

Over the next couple of weeks, the more we learned, the more obvious it became how serious our son's condition was. It boiled down to the doctor basically saying he couldn't tell us that he's going to survive.

Our rural hospital didn't have the capacity to handle a high-risk pregnancy. If we chose to continue the pregnancy we would have to deliver in St. Louis or Kansas City. We realized this was not a viable pregnancy and discussed the possibility of an abortion.

While waiting for the amniocentesis results to come back, we visited my family in Connecticut over Thanksgiving. I was twenty-four weeks pregnant and showing. We had to tell my family of our situation. My family was really understanding, and they were mostly concerned about us.

We met with the doctor the day after we got home from Connecticut. The amniocentesis really didn't give us any new information. Without a confirmed diagnosis, the problem was that, under Missouri law, at that stage of my pregnancy the doctor could only do an abortion if there was a clear risk to my health. The doctor told us that he could not perform an abortion. He then told us about a doctor in Colorado, one of four doctors in the US who will perform late-term abortions.

I phoned the Colorado doctor's office and talked with someone who was so understanding. She talked me through everything, told me exactly what would happen with the procedure and just what I would need. She said they could get us in as soon as we made the decision.

My husband and I talked it over. Essentially, we had learned that there was a potential to lose the baby and also me during delivery. If we both survived, the baby would basically have to have surgeries until complications from one killed him.

The clinic fit us in the following Tuesday. We drove to Colorado on Sunday, a ten-hour drive. Because of the violence at the clinic, you can't take anything in with you other than your ID. The clinic has all bulletproof glass because at some point someone had fired a gun at the clinic. Fortunately, there were no protestors the day we got there. It was a multi-day procedure. They start dilating over a couple of days, and the last day you go through labor and delivery. I was in labor from 8:00 in the morning and until I delivered at 4:00 in the afternoon.

After the delivery, the doctor rested him on my belly for a minute or two, and I chose not to see him. They offered to take photographs but I chose not to. I have one ultrasound picture of him. He was clearly seriously sick and I just wanted to remember the way that I think of him in my head, you know? It was heartbreaking.

At 6:00 that night, it's probably the weirdest thing that's ever happened to me, but I just left the clinic without a baby. I can't describe it. I had been pregnant for twenty-seven weeks, spent eight hours in labor and delivery, and then just left without a baby.

I went back to the hotel and ate a hamburger. Actually, I'm a vegetarian. I don't know if that tells you about how weirdly emotional an experience it was. We got cleared to leave at 10:00 the next morning, and my husband drove me the ten hours back to Missouri. I went back to work on Monday.

Because it wasn't considered a delivery, I had to use paid time off. My boss was probably one of the most supportive people during that whole experience. She checked in on me every day. She cried with me when I told her that it doesn't look like he's going to make it, and this is the decision we have to make. My insurance did not cover the procedure because even though my insurance covered abortion, they would not cover this Colorado doctor who did late-term abortions. It was not a really great time in my life, so I didn't have the energy to contest the decision. I put half the cost of the abortion on my credit card and took out a loan to cover the other half. It cost $10,000, plus travel and hotel and all of that. We're still paying on that loan. It's not like we had a lot of extra money at the time.

I think it was the following week when I heard on the radio that Missouri was trying to pass a law saying that you couldn't have an abortion for a Down Syndrome diagnosis. I was appalled. I emailed the executive director for NARAL describing what had happened to me and asking what I could do to help. She suggested I go testify in Jefferson City. Honestly, most of my healing was just taking all my anger and frustration at what Missouri had put me through, and testifying. I got involved in a lot of advocacy work.

During that time we wanted to get an autopsy done to see if we could get any more answers about whether the same thing would happen again in another pregnancy. I wanted to transfer his remains back to a pathologist in St. Louis, the one who was an expert in skeletal dysplasia. Well, we couldn't do that because we weren't patients of the hospital in St. Louis. Missouri was telling us we couldn't terminate because it was a baby, but we couldn't bring the remains back from another state because it wasn't human remains, it was medical waste.

About a year after my abortion, I got pregnant. I have an amazing 2-year-old son now. It's just so wonderful to have him. At my six-week follow-up I got an IUD because I just was like, I can't be pregnant again. It was just so traumatic the first time; the second time got a little scary at the end too.

I would like people who read my story to take away the importance of voting. Get involved in local politics, because state politics matter. They are making the laws that are impacting your life every day. Vote for a politician who is going to protect people's right to make medical decisions for themselves. Vote for a politician who is putting money and research into making this a safe place for families to give birth in. Vote for a politician who's not going to take food out of hungry children's mouths and put it into fake clinics. All of this is a form of control. It's a way to keep poor people poor, to keep women in their place. It's a way to control populations of people that they dislike.

Daniela Diaz

I'M ORIGINALLY FROM Caracas, Venezuela. In 1994, when I was 9, I immigrated to the United States with my aunt and my mom. My American hometown became Philadelphia. The three of us lived together in a tiny space. In my mind it was fun, it was like living a playful dream.

I went to college in Pennsylvania. This opened so many doors for me. I studied abroad, I participated in Engineers Without Borders in a rural indigenous community in Honduras. I was the only Spanish speaker in the program and was responsible for performing our needs-based assessments. While working there I met a 14- or 15-year-old girl. I was holding her child while doing the assessment, having a really good time with her 9-month old. At the end of my trip she told me I should take the baby with me because it would have a better life. I didn't take the child with me, but I understood the importance of reproductive health work in all its interdisciplinary forms and the need for it to be seen from the lens of economic and reproductive justice.

I came back to the US and tried to do similar work. I earned my Master's in international relations and finally got to bring reproductive health into my work doing an analysis for the Organization for Economic Cooperation and Development in Paris. That led to access to birth control and education around family planning, and stigma around condoms in Latin American culture.

In 2013, I returned to the US and started doing temp work in Bethlehem, Pennsylvania. One street over, there was an abortion clinic. I saw the protesters out there, and I thought,

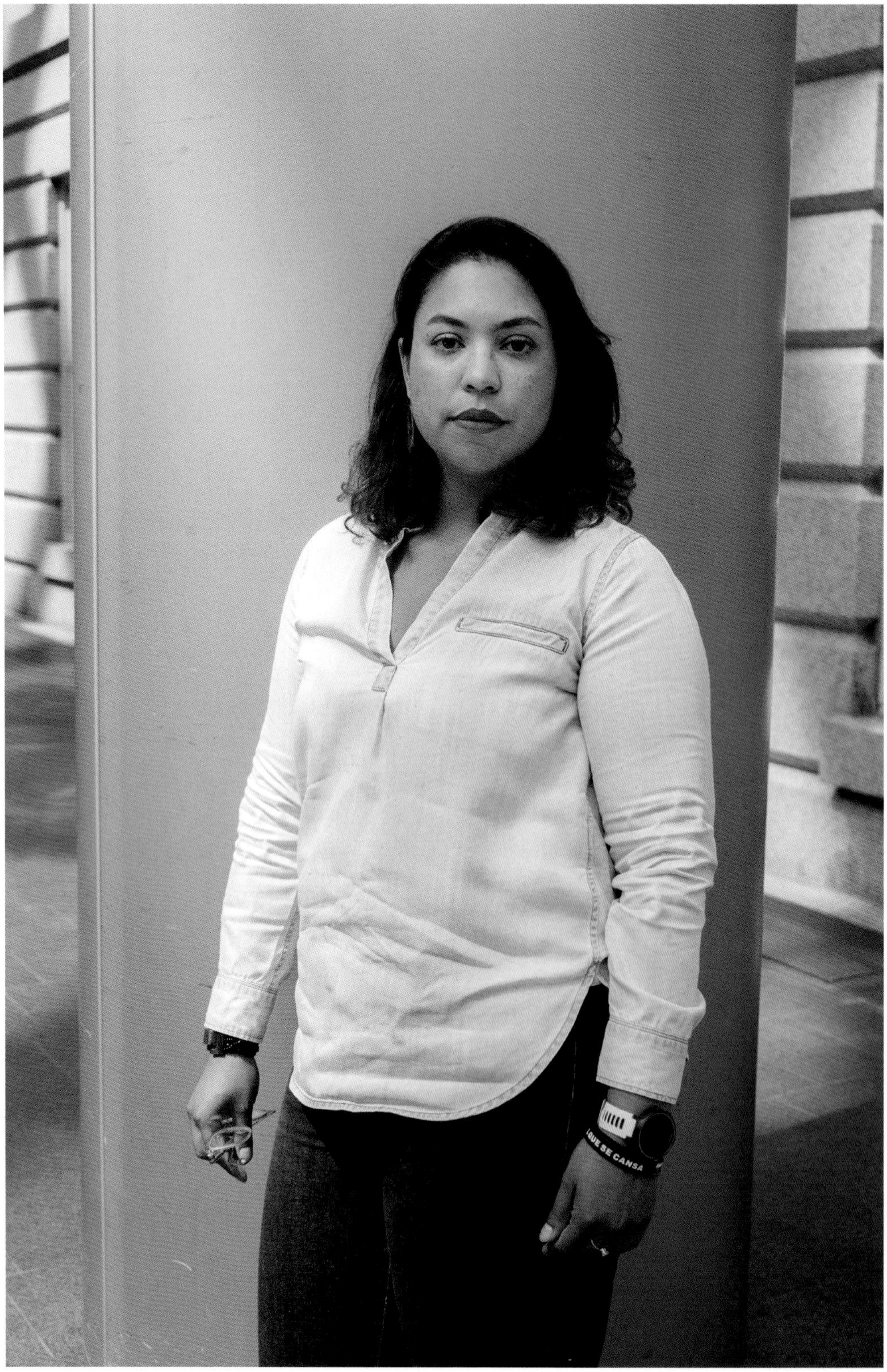

DANIELA DIAZ

"I need to go work there!" After volunteering for a while, I was hired as a patient educator, working with their non-English speaking patients. I know what it's like to look at a doctor and not have any idea about how to talk to them about what you're feeling.

I wanted to do work on a national level, so I moved to Washington, D.C.. After the move, I wasn't feeling very well. I thought I was having acid reflux, caused by eating fruit nonstop, plus stress from the move and needing to be "on" for my new job.

I had been using NuvaRing for birth control. It's a progesterone-based ring that you insert in the vaginal canal and it stays there three to four weeks. At the end of February 2015, I removed the NuvaRing and waited six days for my period. I thought, this isn't normal. I called a girlfriend who told me to buy a pregnancy test. I stayed in a state of denial for about twenty-four hours, replaying my sexual encounters from the past month. I bought a pregnancy test and ate half of a cantaloupe! I called my friend, placed the phone on the sink, and took the pregnancy test. The first test came back erroneous. The second one came back positive.

I burst into laughter, what I used to call "the midnight giggles." I knew immediately that I needed to schedule an abortion because I was not ready for parenthood. I knew what my options were. I had counseled so many pregnant people in this process. Here I am with all of this information on my side to feel safe and secure in making this decision.

I had scheduled my appointment for a Thursday at a Planned Parenthood clinic in Washington D.C.. Everything was in order. I was ready to have the procedure. But that Thursday the entire city of Washington, D.C. was closed due to a snowstorm. Less than an inch of snow got in the way of me accessing my abortion. I couldn't believe it.

When the clinic called to tell me they were closed, that's when I called my mom. I told her the whole story, including the snowstorm closing the clinic down. The big deal for me was the fact that the clinic was closed, not that I was pregnant. My mom sounded okay as she heard me out. She was present in that moment with me. I called my aunt too.

I got another date for the procedure the following week; the wait made that the worst week of my life. It felt like—the word in Spanish is *incertidumbre* —the same level of insecurity or uncertainty of not knowing what's about to happen with your future. It's akin to waiting on immigration where you don't know if they are going to give you a visa or not.

Due to my work in the abortion field I held a lot of privilege in my abortion experience. I didn't have to go to different states, I didn't have to go to multiple facilities because of gestational age, and I was fortunate to work at a place that provided me the health insurance to cover the surgical abortion, although I did have to pay additional for sedation.

My mom and my aunt both came down the weekend before my procedure. They wanted to know that I was sure about my decision, and to reassure me that they would support me regardless of what I chose to do. I loved having them there.

LAWS, BORDERS, AND IMMIGRATION ARE OBSTACLES THAT DIFFER WORLDWIDE, BUT THE EXPERIENCE OF UNCERTAINTY WHEN WAITING ON A PREGNANCY TEST IS THE SAME ALL OVER THE WORLD . . . WE SHARE THE SAME EXISTENTIAL EXPERIENCE OF WHAT IS HAPPENING IN OUR LIVES, OF THE PEOPLE WHO CAN SUPPORT US, OF THE OBSTACLES WE CONFRONT.

My mom wanted to take me to the clinic for the procedure, but I knew there would be protestors. I told her not to come. Instead, a good friend walked me to the clinic and stayed with me the whole time. I wore my Planned Parenthood shirt to show support. They gave me medications both to calm me down and partially sedate me. They put in an IUD afterwards. It was a very loving environment. The procedure was over quickly. I felt intense waves of cramps that quickly subsided once the aspiration abortion was complete. Then I was off in the recovery room and my mom came to pick me up.

I was really happy that morning because I knew that I had the power of choice over things in my life. In Venezuela I wouldn't have had that choice. Abortion is not legal back home, yet they still happen everywhere. People who can afford it cross the border to Colombia. Some middle-class or upper-class people who have a US visa might come here or Puerto Rico or Mexico City.

We came back home from the clinic. I laid down, watched TV, took naps with my mom, which was lovely. She made me some delicious food, although I wasn't very hungry. The next morning, when my mom asked me how I was feeling, I burst into tears. I had never understood the value of my being here at that specific juncture of my life. I had a new understanding of freedom, the freedom of bodily autonomy.

Trusting your body and feeling hormonal normalcy after an abortion can take time. Your body thinks that it's pregnant for six to eight weeks after a procedure. The color of my areolae had changed. They got much darker and I was really happy to see them go back to their usual shade. Getting used to a new birth control method was challenging, and with the IUD I didn't have any periods.

When I think back on my abortion, I feel just as sure of my decision as I did when I made it. Inevitably there's a part of me that thinks of Venezuela and of many places, where people don't have the freedom to control their lives. Even here in the US, only eighty counties have abortion clinics. There are people here in the US who can't afford an abortion, can't access it, and are intimidated. Many have grown up in a society that has told them this choice is wrong. It's important for people to see that abortion is normal.

Laws, borders, and immigration are obstacles that differ worldwide, but the experience of uncertainty when waiting on a pregnancy test is the same all over the world. The decision-making process is unique to every individual but we share the same existential experience of what is happening in our lives, of the people who can support us, of the obstacles we confront.

My experience is full of specific forms of privilege that I know other people will never see. I wish people could make the decision regarding abortion with the same understanding and access that I was given, or greater if possible.

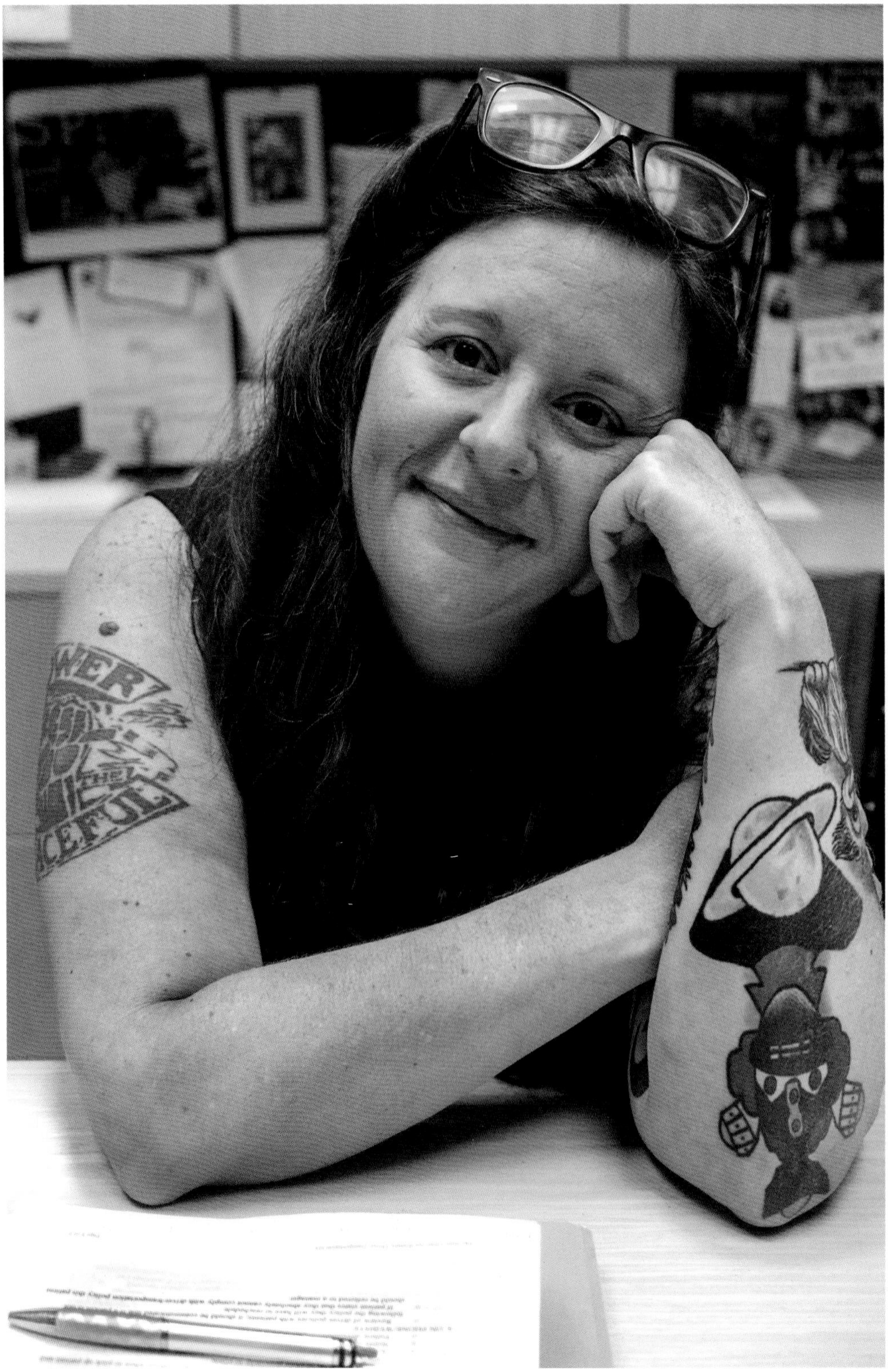

ALISON DREITH

Alison Dreith

MY MOM HAD always said I was the child who was always fighting for the little guy. I grew up in Alton, Illinois, a small town just ten or fifteen minutes down the road from here. It's in the larger St. Louis area, but still very rural. My parents were kind of nonpolitical, even though I knew they voted. My mom was a schoolteacher and a union member. My dad was a drug rep. My family is very proud of me.

I've spent the past ten years of my life doing abortion advocacy work on the reproductive rights side. It started in college, when one of my professors thought interning at Planned Parenthood would be a good fit for me. Getting that internship changed my life drastically, leading to where I am now: deputy director of the Hope Clinic in Granite City, Illinois. This clinic has been here for forty-five years.

PEOPLE ALWAYS ASK ME WHY I GOT AN ABORTION. THE ANSWER IS THAT MY HUSBAND AND I NEVER WANTED TO HAVE CHILDREN. THAT IS A GOOD REASON AND THAT'S ENOUGH OF A REASON.

I've had an abortion myself. It was in 2016, when my husband and I had been married for about a year and a half.

It was probably the most privileged abortion in the history of abortions. I was the executive director at NARAL Missouri at the time, so I knew the laws in both Missouri where I live, and across the river in Illinois, and how to maneuver between those laws. I knew all of the abortion providers in the area and had their cell phone numbers in my phone, so I could call them directly for support or for an appointment. I had the financial means to pay for the abortion. And I had the support of my husband and my community. I had everything at my disposal, which I feel all patients should have when they want to make this decision for themselves.

People always ask me why I got an abortion. The answer is that my husband and I never wanted to have children. That is a good reason and that's enough of a reason. We're all complicated people. We have multiple identities and complicated lives. Even though my great and perfect reason of not wanting to have children is enough, it's also so much more than that. Reasons can change on any given day depending how the wind blows, and that's okay too.

I knew my abortion story wasn't the story of most people. I had my abortion in Illinois. I wanted my abortion when I wanted it. I didn't want my state government to shame me. In Missouri I would have had two separate appointments, with a seventy-two-hour waiting period. In Illinois there is no seventy-two-hour waiting period, there is no state-mandated consent that has inaccurate information in it. I just wanted to access my basic reproductive health care.

Here at Hope Clinic in Illinois, 55 percent of our patients are Missourians who choose to come here so they don't have to face additional burdens and restrictions. We see patients from all over the country, particularly Indiana, Ohio, Kentucky, and Oklahoma.

And so in that way, my story is very much the same. I want to bring that privileged experience here, to help other patients as smoothly as possible. I also want to make sure independent abortion clinics' doors stay open.

In 2019, the Illinois General Assembly passed the Reproductive Health Act, one of the most sweeping pro-choice pieces of policy this country has seen. It mandates that Medicaid and private insurance can pay for abortions. Those reimbursement rates really tend to be low, so we're working closely with our allies within the state to make sure that those reimbursement rates are at levels that allow independent clinics and providers to keep their doors open. We're not a nonprofit. We don't solicit donations. We don't get government or state funding.

The first barrier to coming to our clinic is cost. The procedure can start at about $500 and go up into the thousands. We're connected to a couple of abortion funds to help people financially. For low-wage workers, another barrier is not being able to take a sick day and still get paid. Taking that time off work could be a huge loss in their paycheck.

Getting to our clinic is another barrier. We're in an industrial part of southern Illinois, but still in the St. Louis metropolitan area. There is no adequate public transportation. It's off of a main highway, but you have to navigate a town that may have been booming fifty years ago, but is now really rundown. For some people, finding a loved one they can trust to be able to drive them can be an issue. A lot of patients are already parents, and because children aren't allowed in the clinic, making sure they have childcare can be an issue.

To address those issues, we work closely with Midwest Access Coalition. It has lists of hundreds of volunteers across the Midwest who have signed up and are vetted to drive people or offer maybe a spare bedroom in their house, whatever is needed to get people to their procedure.

We used to talk about abortion as safe, rare, and legal. We've learned over thirty or more years that the "rare" part really shamed patients. Abortion is not rare at all. It's one in four women.

We have protesters at Hope Clinic every day. Today we had about two hundred of them, with a police escort. It's hard for me to keep my cool because it's so frustrating to see that patients coming for basic health care have to experience this.

Some of the protesters outside of the clinic come out of the goodness of their heart. They believe they're doing the Christian thing. They sit in their lawn chairs and pray. They're silent and they don't harass people. Others park their RVs outside and offer fake sonograms. They lie and purposely deceive patients about how far along they are in gestation to trick them into not being able to access abortion. There's a woman demonstrator outside with her RV who has had three abortions herself. She never talks about those abortions, but we know about them.

The biggest thing for me is that there's room for everybody in this reproductive rights movement. All tactics and strategies are valued and important, but at the core of it is remembering why we do this work: We are here to help patients and the providers who help them access basic reproductive health care. Just like in the disability rights movement, we need to put people first, patients and providers first.

In our own movement we used to talk about abortion as safe, rare, and legal. We've learned over thirty or more years that the "rare" part really shamed patients. Abortion is not rare at all. It's one in four women.

We need to keep reiterating that abortion is not just about fetal anomalies or tragic family stories. It's not just about not being able to afford the procedure or not wanting to parent. All of those are valid, real reasons. But sometimes it's also about so much more. I just want people to keep sharing and being honest with themselves and with the world. We try to de-stigmatize abortion so other patients are able to access the health care that we've been able to, and to hold space for the people who aren't there yet. We've made the world a really hard place to access health care. I want to just remind folks to help each other come along together.

Sheila Desai

I GREW UP in the suburbs of New York City. My parents are both immigrants from India. They came over in the '70s with the generation that was very professionalized: My dad was an architect and my mom was a pathologist. My sister was born in India but I was born in this country. We were one of the few Indian families, and one of the few families of color, in the area. So, we spent many of our weekends going to Jersey, or Jackson Heights, or other parts of Queens, where there were more people that looked like us.

Even though it was just the four of us, our extended families are huge. Growing up, family was central; it was the grounding force. There was also an immigrant mentality. Outside the home it was very much about assimilating, and inside of the home it was like, how can we hang onto the values of where we came from?

When I talk to my peers who grew up at a similar time, with a similar sort of culture and values, we often laugh about how you navigate all of these cultural aspects of your life. There's like a cultural piece of you that none of your school friends know about. It's a huge part of who you are, but it's not something that you bring to the larger world.

When I moved out of my parent's home, it was to go to college. That was when I started to explore a lot of the things that I care about a lot now. It was the first time I was exposed to the idea of abortion and reproductive health, and things that I carry very much in my life. My training is in public health and I work at the Guttmacher Institute, a reproductive health research and policy organization, where I do research related to abortion

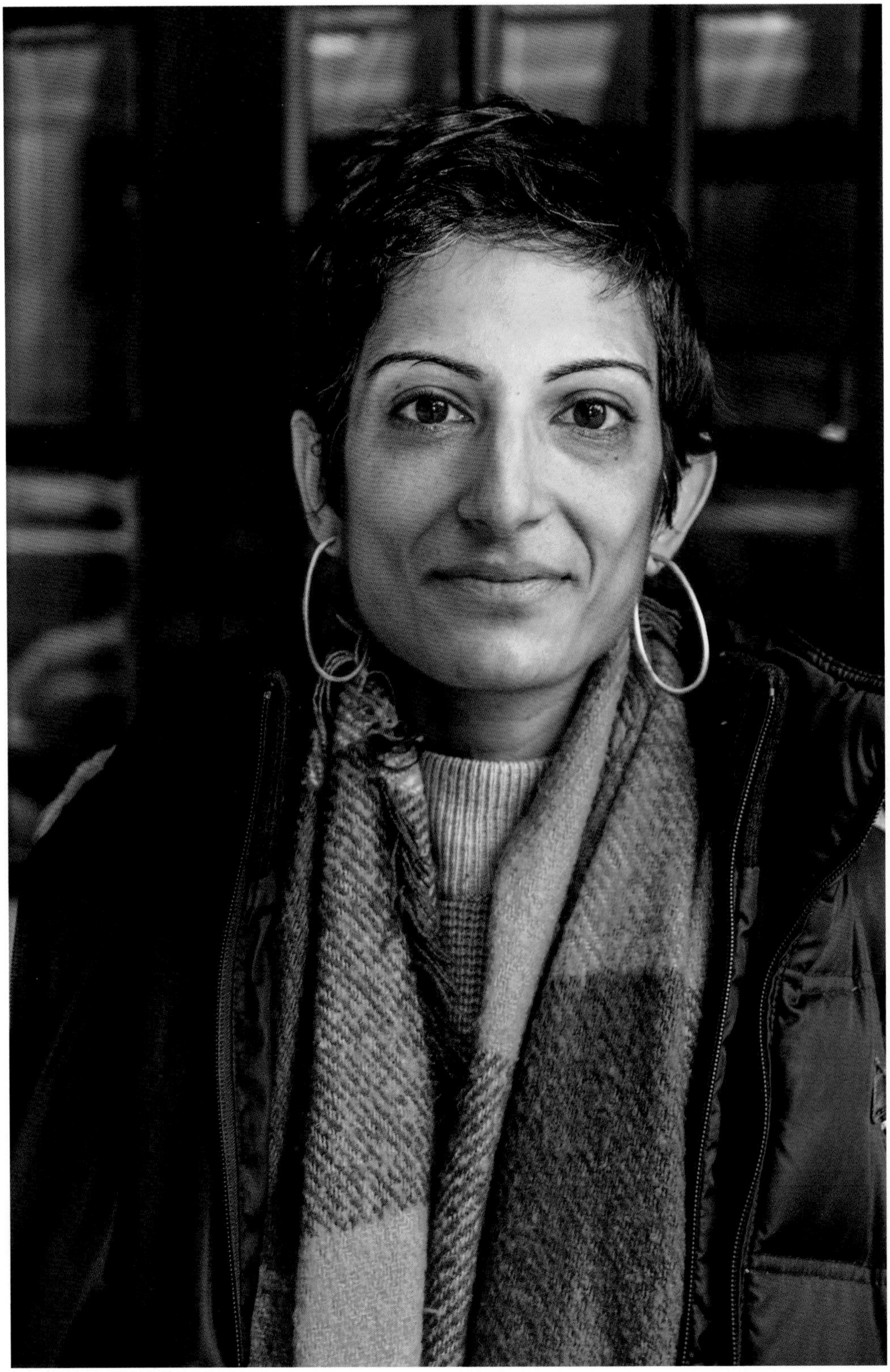

SHEILA DESAI

access and adolescent reproductive health. I'm also on the board of the New York Abortion Access Fund, which helps folks afford the cost of their abortion.

In my early 20s, I had finished college and was living in a small town in India, working at a maternal health clinic. Women would come for everything from contraceptive care to delivering their baby to bringing their baby for checkups. When I found out that I was pregnant, I knew immediately that I didn't want to be pregnant. This tiny town where I was working was socially conservative, although probably no more conservative than a lot of places in the US. You don't talk about sex, you don't have sex before you get married, and you certainly aren't getting pregnant before you get married.

What was really ironic was that I was working with providers, with midwives. I knew what an abortion was. I knew the different ways to have an abortion. But I also knew that I just wanted to talk with someone about what I should do, how I should do it. The stigma and the shame were just overwhelming. There was the fear of what the backlash would be if I spoke to somebody. There was this feeling of what are they going to think of me? Are they going to kick me out? I also did not talk to the guy involved.

I self-managed my abortion. I essentially took the drugs I thought would cause a medication abortion. Some of those drugs are available at pharmacies, but I didn't know that at the time. So through other means, I got the drugs and I took them. It was isolating and it was frightening.

I bled for a very, very long time. I remember thinking I should tell someone, but I was still way too scared to bring it up. More than six weeks later, I ended up going back to New York for family reasons. I was still bleeding, but at least in New York I felt I could do things a little more anonymously.

Then my mom found out that I had tried to self-manage my abortion. I made up a story about having a really unusual period. My mother worked in a lab, so she offered to do my blood work to just make sure things were okay. Without really thinking what that could mean, I agreed. One of my mom's lab colleagues brought her my lab results and congratulated her. Yes, I tested positive for pregnancy; the self-managed abortion in India had not done the job.

My mom's very pragmatic. She's also a scientist, and so for her, it became a question of solving a problem. She wasn't there to blame me. I remember shaking because I felt like I was going to let my mom down or make her feel ashamed. My mom isn't a very emotional person, but in that moment, she just put her hands on me and was like, "It's okay. Just tell me what's going on." And I explained that I had tried to give myself an abortion and it hadn't worked. Without blinking an eye, my mom said, "Okay. Let's figure out what needs to happen."

She didn't ask me any questions. In fact, seeing how freaked out I was, she, in such a surprising turn of events, started to share her own various reproductive experiences. She was just trying to normalize this. We took me to Planned Parenthood for the procedure.

The thing I remember the most is what happened after the abortion. I started to learn more about these kinds of experiences: abortions, contraception issues, sterilizations, miscarriages. It was really amazing to learn I was not alone, and at the same time I realized that we've all been keeping this quiet.

Growing up in a predominately South Asian community, sex wasn't really talked about. And if we weren't talking about sex, we weren't talking about any of the things that can come from it. Abortion wasn't framed in a positive light. Abortion wasn't a reproductive health outcome that was done by choice. It was framed as something you would do because you were very sick during the pregnancy or something was wrong with the fetus. It wasn't something that you would choose just because it was right for your life in that moment.

In the part of India where my family grew up . . . the tradition of oral storytelling dates back forever. Being able to share my abortion story is a meaningful way to carry forth that tradition . . . I feel like I stand on my mom's shoulders, and the shoulders of my ancestors in sharing this story.

About ten years ago, I told my story for the first time in public in front of a small audience. Sharing the story was emotional. I was later approached to share my story further, but it felt like my story was being made into a commodity, which I did not want.

Fast forward to a couple years ago while I was involved with the New York Abortion Access Fund as an intern, when the Purvi Patel case was in the news. She lived in Indiana and was trying to manage her own miscarriage, when she went to the ER to get care for her bleeding. She was prosecuted for attempted feticide and was incarcerated.

I remember so many stereotypes being assigned to her as a South Asian woman. And I realized that is the danger of a single story, or of no story. It gives people free rein to assign all kinds of assumptions and expectations to an individual person and to a group of people.

I decided it was time to try again to put my story out there, even if it's just for my own community.

Sharing stories is a really powerful way of potentially shifting how people think about abortion. If my sharing can change folks' minds, that's amazing. But for me, it's really about my community. I think about how I had nobody to look to who looked like me or who I could trust when I had my abortion. That was really isolating.

Should my nieces and nephews be in a similar situation, I think about what it would mean to them to know I had had an abortion. Or that others in our community have had a variety of reproductive health experiences. Knowing that would have made me feel so much more comfortable in my own skin. If my sharing could do that for my niece and nephew or the generations to come, I feel like that in itself feels like reason enough to share my story.

In the part of India where my family grew up . . . the tradition of oral storytelling dates back forever. Being able to share my abortion story is a meaningful way to carry forth that tradition. The way, and the form in which my mom shared her story, is probably the way and the form in which my ancestors shared their stories. When my mom shared her story, it gave me the power to share my story, and gave me the initial clarity around why it felt important to share my story.

I feel like I stand on my mom's shoulders, and the shoulders of my ancestors in sharing this story. I hope to do it in a way that sort of brings even more truth or even more power to that truth. When I can share my story with my niece, it won't be like, "And don't share this with anyone else." Maybe it will be shared loudly and proudly.

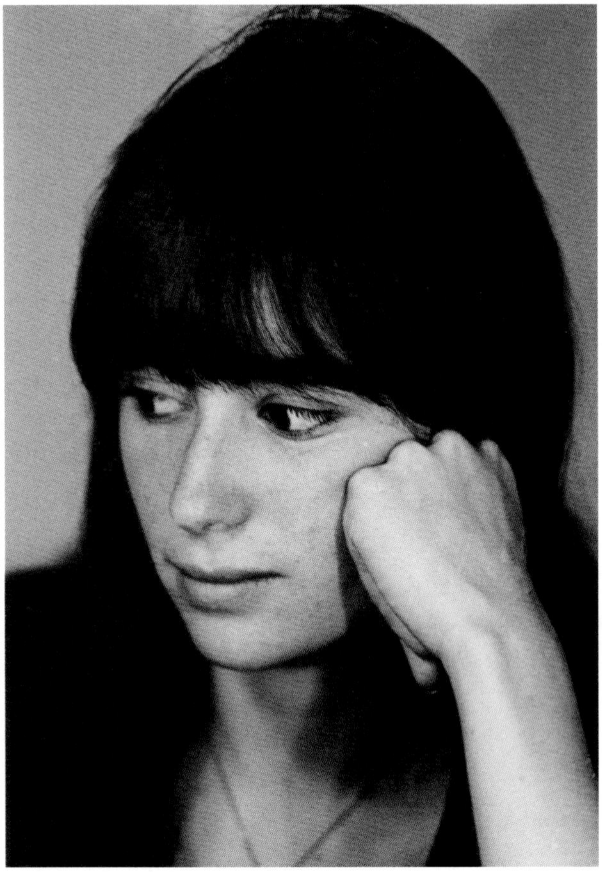
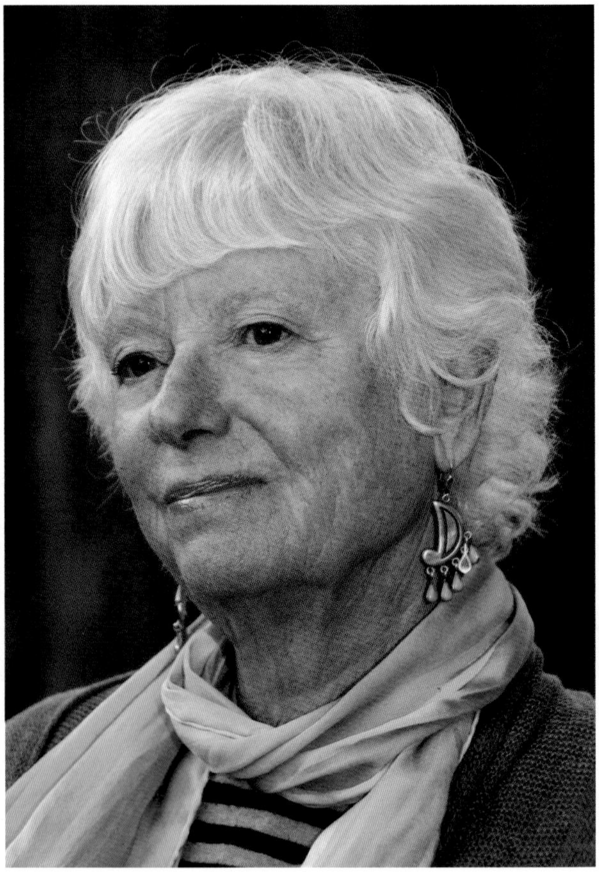

MARY WINEGARDEN

Mary Winegarden

I'M A BABY boomer, now in my early seventies. When I had my illegal abortion at age 22, I was in my first year of graduate school at the University of Chicago.

Understanding the historical context—especially now, with serious threats to our reproductive rights—is essential to this story. Four years earlier, in the fall of 1964 when I was a first-year student at the U. of C., the birth control pill had just become widely available. During Orientation—"O-Week"—between taking placement exams, finding our way around the leafy campus and initiating lifelong friendships, many of us young women stopped at the Student Health Center to get a prescription for the newly approved pill. The sexual revolution had arrived, with birth control pills being passed out like candy. Which was wonderful—a great breakthrough for my generation—but serious medical problems had yet to emerge.

Several years later, I was hit by a car while riding my bike to campus, and fractured my left foot. Even worse, I developed a blood clot in that leg (under the cast). I was rushed to Billings Hospital, where they gave me blood thinners and saved my life. If not treated in time, I could have died.

Medical researchers had discovered that the early pill (which included a too-high dosage of estrogen) caused blot clots and life-threatening strokes. I was immediately taken off the pill and given a diaphragm. But I wasn't told that it takes a while after being on the pill for one's cycle to normalize, that women could become especially fertile months later. I was using the diaphragm but was in a new relationship and not being as careful as I should have been.

So I found myself pregnant, in the middle of my first year as a graduate student in Comparative Literature. It was 1969, pre-Roe v. Wade, and I was shaken. Though I was absolutely in love with my boyfriend, an older grad student, I knew we would not stay together. I luckily—wisely—recognized that having a child with him was a really bad idea. So I didn't go through a lot of turmoil about what to do, fully determined to find a way to terminate the pregnancy. I was on a path that did not include having a baby at this point in my life, even though I knew I wanted children in the future.

As an anti-war activist, I'd already gone to several meetings on campus of the newly formed Women's Liberation Group, an offshoot of SDS—the women's movement having evolved from the radical politics of the larger protest movement. I believe this was the beginning of the "Jane Collective," the Abortion Counseling Service of Women's Liberation, an underground program which operated in Chicago from 1969 to 1973. The code word was "Jane" when you telephoned. The collective put me in touch with several doctors in Chicago who were known to perform illegal abortions that were reputedly safe. Their names were unknown to me—their anonymity was crucial.

However, I did have to find the $300 fee, an enormous obstacle at the time, as I was living on a graduate student's stipend. My beloved older sister generously agreed to send me half, promising not to tell our parents. I think I borrowed the other $150 from a friend, or maybe from my boyfriend, who agreed with my decision.

So arrangements were made by phone to meet at a street corner in downtown Chicago on a wintry Saturday in early March. I was told to wear a white carnation pinned to my peacoat so I would be recognizable. My boyfriend accompanied me to the street corner in the Loop where we awaited the car with two doctors who identified themselves only as "Dr. Tom and Dr. Harry"—as planned. I suppose I had blind faith that this was going to be okay, that I would be safe.

My boyfriend wasn't allowed to come with me. When I climbed into the back of the car, the men said to me, "We are going to go to a location that you can't know about so we have to blindfold you." My "blind faith" was now literal.

Astonishing as it now seems, I was nervous and scared but not terrified. I knew these doctors were affiliated with Women's Liberation; they seemed friendly enough, their faces bland and unmemorable. I must have not allowed myself to feel the terror that rises in me now when I think of all that could have happened.

Being blindfolded added to my nausea during the endless drive. When we got out, we were parked at a motel that looked to be in the suburbs though I had no idea where we were. I walked into the motel without the blindfold as one of the docs checked us in, then to an upstairs room, where they gave me an injection, a mild anesthetic. I remember very few details of the procedure—a D & C, which was mildly painful but over quickly. But I do remember one odd detail: the bathtub was running the whole time and I was really puzzled: Why was the bath water running? I didn't think to ask. Only much later did I realize that the running water was used to mask any sounds; if I were to cry out or yell, this would be risky.

The doctors were careful, giving me antibiotics to take for a week in case of infection. I had instructions about what to do, what to look for: excessive bleeding, pain, burning, signs of infection, and told simply to rest.

But just before I got dressed, one of the docs said to me, "Do you know how to do a breast exam on yourself?" I guess I was kind of stunned and said no, I didn't. And he proceeded to show me, but was actually feeling me up, fondling my breasts. That was as far as it went, but I was so shocked, so numbed by the trauma, that I simply did not have the resources to cope with what was happening at the time. Of course, I should have said, "Stop! What the hell are you doing?" But I was vulnerable, still under partial anesthesia. I was humiliated by this violation, but never told anybody about it. Anyone, ever—until now. Then we got into the car and they drove me back, blindfolded again, to the same street corner where my boyfriend was waiting.

I WASN'T EXACTLY ASHAMED, BUT THE ILLEGAL, SECRETIVE NATURE OF THE ABORTION KEPT ME FROM SHARING THE STORY WITH FRIENDS. I NEVER TOLD THEM ABOUT THE BLINDFOLD, THE FEAR, AND MOLESTATION.

The very next night we went to a dinner party at a friend's apartment in Hyde Park, but I don't remember discussing my abortion at all. I wasn't exactly ashamed, but the illegal, secretive nature of the abortion kept me from sharing the story with friends. I never told them about the blindfold, the fear, and molestation.

And I repressed the memory for a very long time. Yet compared to many "back-alley" abortions, it did not go badly. I did not get an infection, and two decades later had three successful, healthy pregnancies.

Several months after the abortion, I took a radical turn in my life when I decided to leave graduate school and head to Europe. The decision to leave Chicago had nothing to do with my abortion. It was just that I was less invested in academia and frustrated with the political scene. At this point, SDS was splintering, with some people joining the Weather Underground and advocating the use of violence, a stance I didn't share. I dropped out of grad school, left the country that summer, and ended up first in Paris, then in London, with a close college friend.

I stayed for four years—a heady time to be in counter-cultural London. I worked in several jobs that first year, then found both home and work and my future husband with an arts collective in North London called Inter-Action—a community theater company that performed original plays on the streets for free while running art and drama projects for working-class kids on deserted building sites in Kentish Town. Though not promoting a directly political agenda, we believed we could change people's lives through the arts.

I returned to the States on January 23, 1973—the day after Roe v. Wade. That was just serendipity, but it felt very affirming to return then. Things had changed, especially with the flowering of the women's movement.

I gaze at photographs of the 22-year-old girl I was at the time of my abortion and I find her mysterious, almost unknowable. But this young woman made a brave decision that I stand by today. It was very clear to me that I should not have a child with that partner at that time.

I've always had a fierce maternal instinct; I've loved giving birth and raising a family. Eventually I returned to graduate school and then taught English at San Francisco State University for several decades.

A lifelong feminist, I remain passionate about a woman's right to choose. My three grown children respect this, knowing that I had an abortion long ago, though I have never told them the full story. My family and two darling toddler grandsons are at the center of my life, along with poetry and political activism. And that's the vital importance of reproductive choice—we must continue to make these crucial decisions for ourselves.

Younger generations need to know what it was like before Roe v. Wade. Those of us who suffered illegal abortions—many much worse than mine—need to tell our stories.

Anne Marie Backstrom

I WAS ADOPTED at birth from Helena, Montana. My adoptive mother was infertile. It was never a secret in my family that I was adopted. It was kind of celebrated as this altruistic choice that I hadn't been aborted. My adoptive parents were part of an evangelical Christian sect called Quiverfull. It is an extremely patriarchal sect and the idea is that you fill your quiver full of arrows for God by having children.

In my family, unfortunately, religion and faith were used as vehicles of fear, shame, and intimidation. The faith that I grew up in was punitive. It was shame-based, and it was really scary. My growing up was nothing to write home about. I faced sexual abuse in my family. I knew that I was different from my family at really a young age.

My adoptive family was pretty deeply homophobic and very open about it. I knew from a pretty young age that while little girls were having crushes on boys, that I had crushes on other girls. When I played with my Barbies, sometimes, they married a boy and sometimes, they married each other. When I was about 12 years old, I came out as queer, as bisexual to my adoptive father. He was pretty horrified. That same year, I was sent to a Christian camp that had a heavy emphasis on conversion and changing people like me.

I have always had relationships with other women and it is just very natural for me. It wasn't until I met my ex-husband that I was like, "Oh, I'm going to date this man and maybe make a family." My partner today is also a heterosexual gendered man, but he's never questioned my sexuality and the validity of it. It's been a wonderful journey to grow up in this really oppressive world and to move to living a life where I can celebrate myself and the people of my life love and accept me.

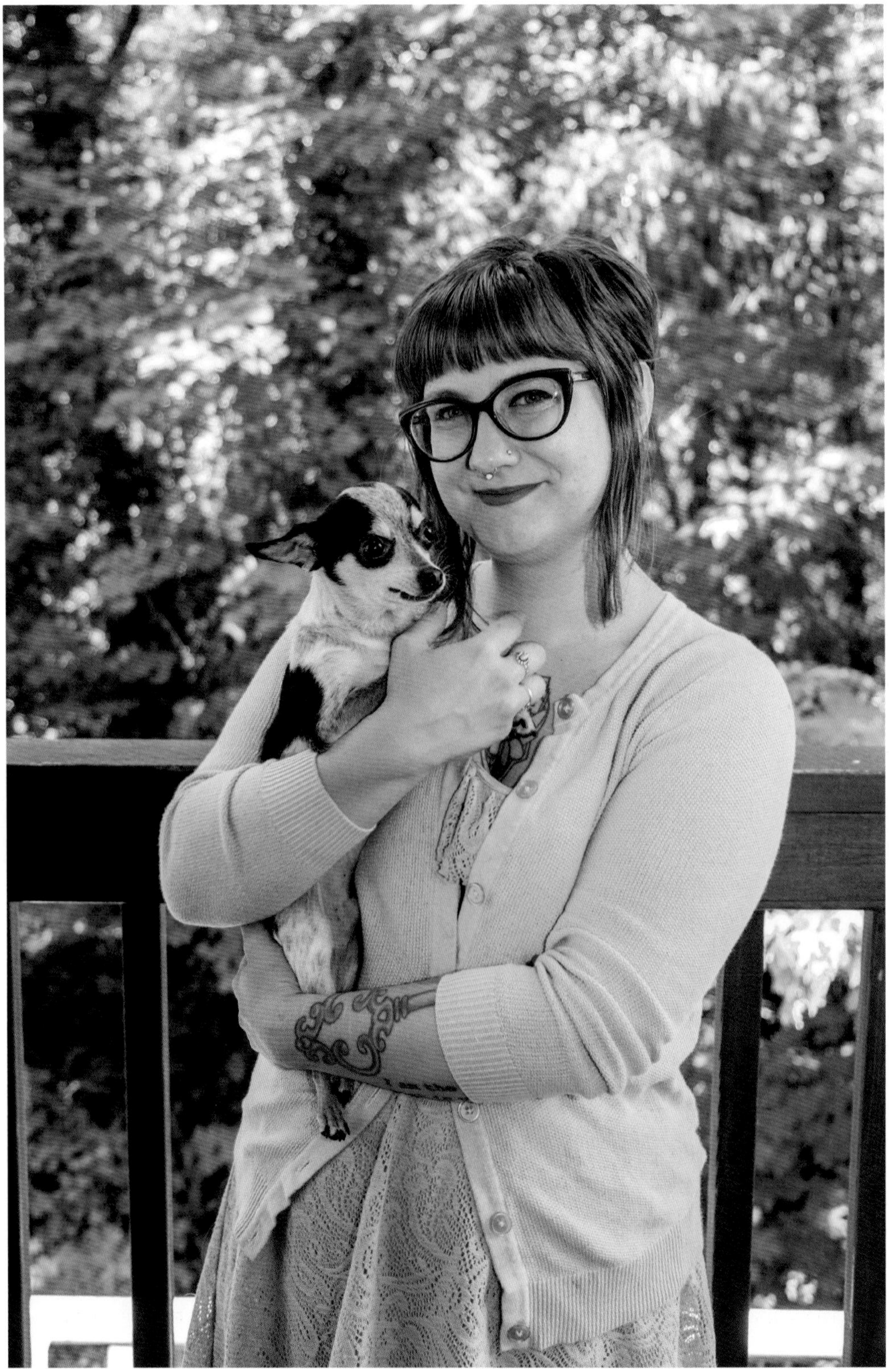

ANNE MARIE BACKSTROM

My abortion story is a little bit messy. I got married shortly after my 18th birthday and had a baby. After the birth of my daughter, I experienced really intense postpartum depression that developed into postpartum psychosis. I had a form of depression that turned into hallucinations and delusions, very similar to kind of a more classic form of psychosis like schizophrenia. I ended up being hospitalized the last almost three months of my daughter's first year of life.

My ex-husband and I really made an effort to make our marriage work. But then he abruptly left. Maybe three weeks later I found out that I was pregnant again. My daughter was a little over a year and a half my husband and I were in the process of getting a divorce. I remember taking a pregnancy test in a Target bathroom with my toddler with me, and my heart just fell. When I told my husband I was pregnant, he was so angry. We weren't living together. Our marriage had ended.

MY HUSBAND AND I WERE IN THE PROCESS OF GETTING A DIVORCE. I REMEMBER TAKING A PREGNANCY TEST IN A TARGET BATHROOM WITH MY TODDLER WITH ME, AND MY HEART JUST FELL.

Growing up religious, I put a lot of stock into my own worth as a wife and a mother. I was always one of those women who was pro-choice, but not for me. My husband, soon to be ex, did not want me to keep the pregnancy. Instead of holding me in this compassion of like, "What do we do?" it was "How dare you get pregnant!"

Growing up, I got the message that there are women who parent their children and there are parents who give their children up for adoption and there are horrible, evil women who murder their babies in the womb. That kind of rhetoric really stuck with me. This was really forefront in my mind when I was figuring out what to do about my pregnancy. I had already kind of loosened my grip on religion, but I had a lot of fear about what my family would think.

I used to not talk about my own abortion because my story is not perfect. It includes spousal abuse and a lot of intimidation. When I tell my story and say that I didn't want an abortion, but I did it anyway to make my then-husband happy, people ask if I regret the decision. No, I'm really glad I went through with this choice. But the biggest piece of my story is I wish it had been my choice.

I know that because of that decision I was able to go back to college, finish my degree, and build a life, meet a wonderful man who's my partner now. So much of that is because

I live in a state where I had access to a medical procedure so I didn't have to have another child in the messiest part of my life.

I didn't tell anyone about my abortion. Shortly afterwards, I got myself into therapy and found people I could talk to, but at the time, I felt very isolated. I just don't want anyone to ever feel that alone. Looking back, I deeply wish that I had had other people in my corner telling me, "Hey, this is your choice. Your body."

My daughter is my best friend. She's the best thing that ever happened to me. Being a young mom is the best thing that I've ever done. She's growing up in a family where she has safety and choice. My daughter gets to be herself in a way that women in my own family never did. What I want her to know is that no matter what society says, no matter what men in her life say, that she has full control and that she has a mom she can come to and be open with. It breaks my heart thinking that I never told my mom at the time that I had an abortion. I needed medical care after the abortion and I couldn't pick up the phone and call my mom.

It is really important for me to hold space for the fact that my abortion story sucks, but also, that it's okay. Both things are true. Yeah.

My biological mother lives out in Arizona. I met her about seven years ago when I was 21. She was 17 when I was born. She told me my older biological sister was barely 11 months at the time and my birth mother was overwhelmed. As someone who had a child at 19, I have a lot of compassion for my birth mother.

My birth mother is pretty fiercely pro-choice. She confided in me that she considered abortion when she got pregnant with me. I asked her because I grew up in this world where women who choose adoption are considered saints; adoption is like the holy grail of being a good person. That idea has never settled with me. Adoption is a choice, but it's not this like virtuous amazing thing. She told me it wasn't this like huge altruistic thing. She was further along than she thought, so she carried the pregnancy. She has no judgment for people who make that choice because putting her baby up for adoption was really hard.

It is really important for me to hold space for the fact that my abortion story sucks, but also, that it's okay. Both things are true. Yeah.

Amanda Williams

THE QUESTION OF my identity has very much been a part of my life. My mother is an immigrant from Mexico and my father came to Texas from upstate New York. I move through this world with brown skin, yet I've had the privilege that comes from having a white father, the last name Williams, access to education and middle-class family and all those things. I never knew that I had to pick one identity or the other. Our society can put people in boxes. But really, there's a lot of complexity and nuance. When you don't feel like you live in that either/or, it can feel a little bit isolating.

I KNEW I WAS A FEMINIST, BUT HAVING AN ABORTION WAS THE FIRST TIME MY OWN EXPERIENCE CATALYZED THIS FIRE INSIDE ME.

It's equally important to also understand my connection to immigration. I wouldn't exist if my mother hadn't crossed the border when she did. At the time she was undocumented and became a naturalized citizen. My mom put herself through school and lived in poverty for most of her life, working very hard to get her education. Knowing that she raised me and put her career first and knowing about her experience living as an immigrant Mexican woman, working her way through the system, helped politicize me.

I had an abortion when I was 19 and a freshman in college. Although I had been a student organizer and I was politicized around the idea of abortion access, having an abortion at that moment in my journey was really huge for me. I knew I was a feminist, but having an abortion was the first time my own experience catalyzed this fire inside me. It really led me to want to pursue abortion rights work and reproductive justice more broadly in a very, very serious way.

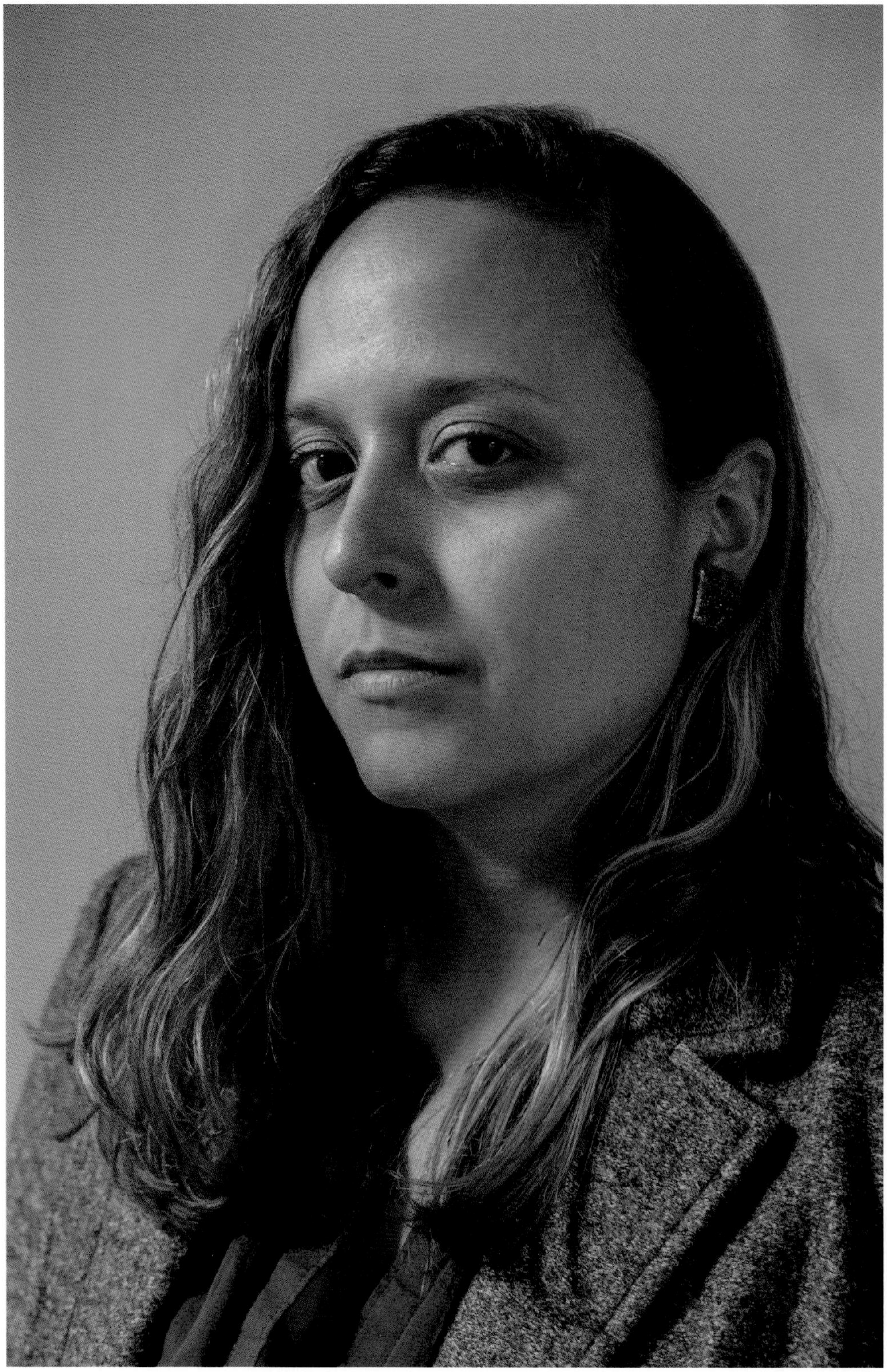

AMANDA WILLIAMS

When I had my abortion, I was in an unhealthy relationship. There was a lot of emotional abuse and some coercion, which of course I didn't have the language for while it was happening. Once I got pregnant, I knew I didn't want to be pregnant, that was just not an option. The decision-making process was fairly clear. It was very much a "yes and how" decision.

Even though my political position was pro-choice, up until then abortion never affected me personally. But suddenly, it was my life. You really look closely at who in your life can support you through this. I was very selective about who I chose to speak with. I went to a couple of close friends and my partner at the time, although things were a mess with him due to mental health issues.

I felt very much alone, like no one could really understand. I wasn't emotionally prepared to have the conversations in the deep ways that I think we should all be allowed to have. I wanted to talk about what it feels like to need an abortion, how to find the necessary support. I couldn't open up emotionally at the time because I was so scared.

I didn't tell my parents, even though I knew my mom would support me. I didn't go to them for money either. Instead, my partner at the time and I went to his family for money.

The pregnancy was fairly early. Although I was eligible for a medication abortion, I declined. I wanted to do the surgical abortion because the likelihood of it being effective was higher. There was no question. I wanted it over with fast, and I wanted to be sure.

I decided not to go to Planned Parenthood Gulf Coast in Houston, where I had volunteered as a clinic escort. I was afraid that people would recognize me. To this day, that decision shocks me. These are the last people who would have judged me. I think that just shows how internalized stigma can really be. So I went to the Houston Women's Clinic.

After the abortion procedure you're not pregnant anymore, so your hormones obviously are a little bit imbalanced. A lot of things are happening, which is another nuance I think we don't talk about and accept. Of course, my partner and I got into a fight about something. We got back to my apartment, and he left. I was alone, just kind of miserable.

I had the abortion early in the morning, and my mom had arranged for me to meet my aunt and her partner for dinner that evening. I remember thinking I absolutely could not skip that dinner. My mom came over to pick me up. At this point, I was a wreck. I was cramping. I just looked at her in the face, and I started crying.

It was just an instant. I just knew I couldn't lie to her. I also felt like she would've known if I hadn't said anything. I was drowsy, and the drugs were wearing off. I was an emotional mess. I just looked at her, and said, "Mom, I had an abortion today." She breathed, and she just said, "*Ay, mija*. I wish you would've told me. I would've gone with you." Instantly, I felt relieved.

Today, I am the executive director of Lilith, an abortion fund serving the central and southern regions of Texas. We provide funding to women to help them access and pay for abortion services. Most of the people we help are women of color, Black women, Latinas. A lot are poor women in rural communities without clinics in their towns. They have various backgrounds, working class, students. The majority of our clients are parenting two or more children. They are Spanish speakers, immigrants from all over, including undocumented people. The one thing they have in common, as far as we can tell, is they can't afford the cost of their abortion. They're struggling to come up with money for bills, for rent, for food on the table.

For the immigrants among our callers, there's this overwhelming fear of potential deportation or perhaps there's a lack of general information. This idea of "we have no rights."

The direct services, the connection and communication we have with our callers is very illuminating of the struggles and the conditions that prevent people from creating the families that they want in order to feel safe and healthy. It involves understanding economic justice and environmental justice, understanding issues with housing, with jobs, with parenting, other forms of health care.

For the immigrants among our callers, there's this overwhelming fear of potential deportation or perhaps there's a lack of general information. This idea of "we have no rights." There's a lot of hostility, especially close to the border. We also understand the lack of cultural competency when they do get to a doctor.

What keeps us going is those voices on the other end of the phone. My life revolves around keeping our hotline open, securing the funds needed to support people who are just trying to control their own lives, making sure we're doing that in a way that feels right and just. Despite Texas being a red state, there's true resistance here, and it's been here for a long time. Just being able to lift that up in any avenue is important, especially when we're talking about stories.

Storytelling is a tradition that should be treated with integrity and respect, as a way of honoring everyone's process and journey. With stories comes human connection. We can't just make abortion a political bargaining chip. It has to be about people first. I think that, unless we're centering those voices, those experiences, there's nothing to connect to. People have to see themselves in stories. That's why I share my story. It's our truth. Those experiences and the emotions and the struggles are very human. We have to ensure that our humanity is recognized, is centered, and that we're leading from a place of love and honesty. That's our strength as humans, and I think anyone can relate to that if they listen.

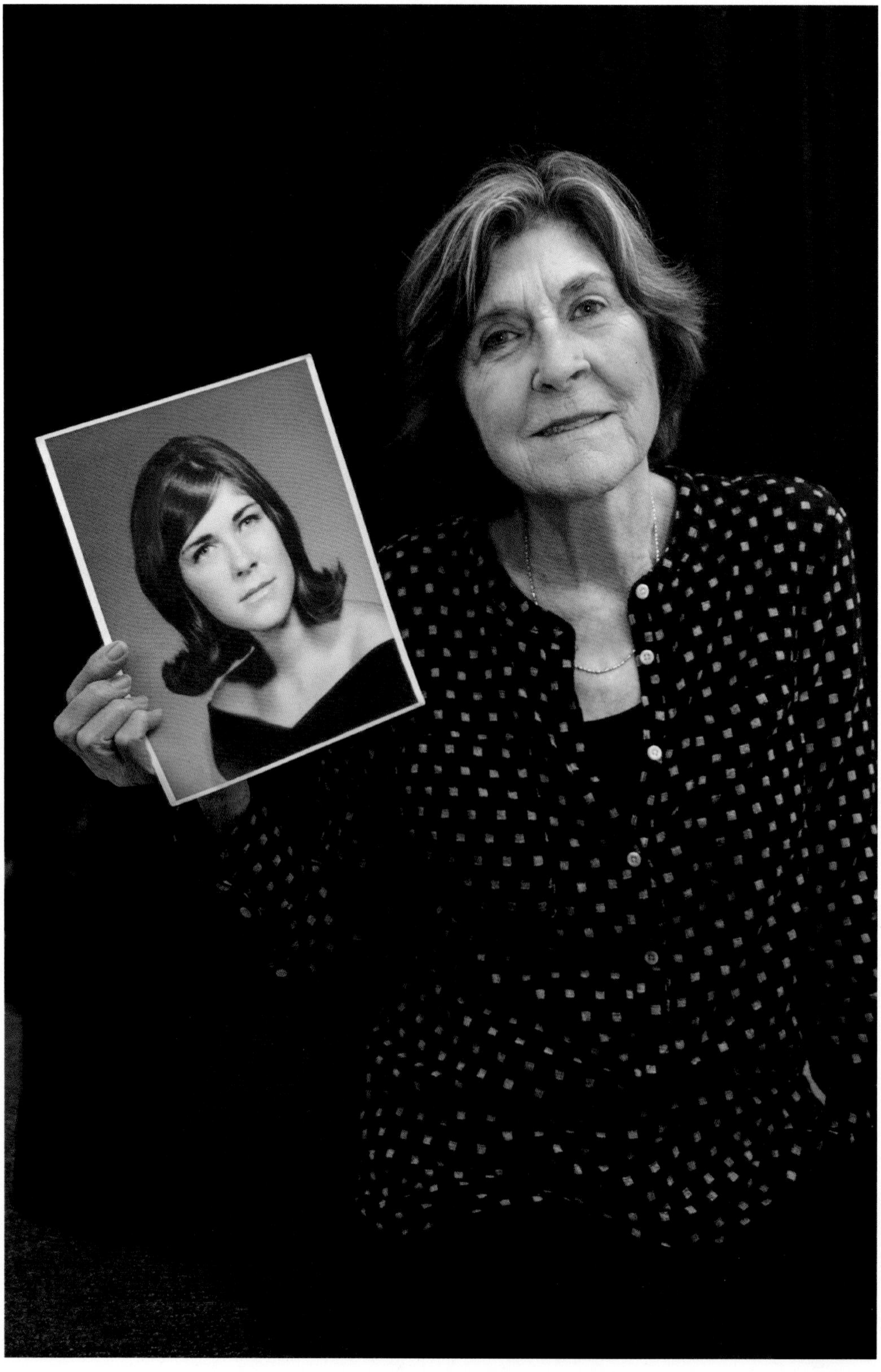

SUSAN BOSTROM-WONG

Susan Bostrom-Wong

I DON'T FEEL shame about my abortion. It's a woman's story and I'm a feminist. I think having abortion stories out in the world is important for other women so that they don't feel alone with it. I hope that sharing abortion stories will help normalize something that is our right: to own our own bodies, to make decisions about our own bodies.

I've always been very open about my story. I shared it with my close women friends and my daughter when she started being sexual, and definitely with my husband before we got married. I never told my parents. That's interesting.

I was 23 or 24, one year out of university. I had been a school teacher and had decided I wanted an adventure. So I moved to Hawaii because I had a good friend there, whom I had traveled in Europe with when I was 20. She was living and going to school there and I thought that sounded like paradise. In Hawaii, I very quickly met a man whom I fell madly in love with. We started a sexual relationship. For quite a while I had been on birth control pills, which my mother helped me get from my local doctor in Michigan, where I was from. But I ran out of birth control pills. I started using other kinds of birth control: foam and gel and condoms sometimes but not always, and thinking it was going to be fine. I guess I wasn't thinking very clearly. Six months into the relationship, I found myself pregnant. It was November 1967.

I was so young. I panicked. I was like, I'm not ready to be a mother, it is not the right time in my life. I called a friend in Michigan who had helped another friend who needed an abortion. He gave me the name of a doctor in Washington, D.C.. I got on the phone and I called the office. The doctor agreed to do an abortion. It would cost me $450 and I had to bring cash. He gave me an appointment.

I flew alone to Washington. My boyfriend wasn't in a position to go with me; he was in the Coast Guard. I don't remember how I found the money for the ticket and the abortion.

I had called an old friend who lived in Washington D.C. to tell him I was coming and this is why, and can I stay with you? He said yes, generously. The next morning, I went to the doctor's office all by myself. There were other young women in the waiting area. I waited for my turn. I hadn't a clue as to what to expect. But I thought, well this is safe because he is a real doctor with a real office with an examining table. Then he proceeded to do a D & C with no anesthesia. I was probably ten or twelve weeks pregnant. It was pretty horrifying, how painful it was.

It was a little crude because he demanded that I give him the cash before he did the surgery. It was pretty scary, but I think I was in some kind of altered state of denial and fear to let myself go through all that without completely freaking out.

I remember very clearly that he handed me a bottle of antibiotics and said "Start taking these right away," and then dismissed me. I didn't have friendly, warm feelings toward this doctor. He was not sympathetic. He was just in there doing a job that took twenty or thirty minutes and he wanted his money. The only thing I felt about it was that at least I didn't ruin my chances for future pregnancies.

When I left the office, I was bleeding heavily. So my friend went to a pharmacy and bought me a big box of Kotex. We went back to his apartment and I spent the night. The next day I got on a plane and flew back to San Francisco.

Back in San Francisco, I just jumped back into my life and started moving forward. Even though my boyfriend and I had decided to terminate the pregnancy, we nonetheless decided to get married at City Hall. All the emotional upheaval, the intimacy, and connection related to the pregnancy may have accelerated our relationship. But I think we would have gotten married anyway.

After the abortion I think I went into both relief and some kind of denial about what I'd gone through. I always assumed we would have a child when we were a little bit older. We stayed married for seven years, but then he fell in love with another woman and we divorced. I was 29 at the time.

I always wanted children. When I met my current husband I was very clear with him that this was part of my life plan. He wasn't pulled toward fatherhood in quite the desperate way that I was. He didn't care one way or the other. We did have a child together, a daughter who is now 35, married, and the mother of a 7-month-old daughter. When our daughter was in high school, I took her with me to my OBGYN when I had my annual Pap smear. She watched my doctor do it. We talked about how at some point you are going to get one too. And the doctor said to her, "Well you're not ready now but when you are sexually active, you'll come in and this is what we'll do." So there was always a permission giving. When she was sexually active, she knew immediately what to do. She went to the health service and got birth control. She had also asked her boyfriend to go get tested for AIDS before they had sex.

For thirty years, I practiced as a Jungian psychoanalyst. Part of my training was doing my own analysis. I worked on my own life issues for many years and the grief around that child. I always imagined it was a boy and I have thought about what it would be like if I now had a 50-year-old child. The little soul of that baby was in my life, and it's never left me. Maybe the fantasy that it was a boy, I don't know if that's like an intuition or it's because of the loss of the marriage, the male figure.

THE LITTLE SOUL OF THAT BABY WAS IN MY LIFE, AND IT'S NEVER LEFT ME . . . I THINK THERE ARE SOME LOSSES THAT YOU NEVER GET OVER 100 PERCENT. PERIOD. YOU MOVE ON AND YOU DEAL WITH IT . . . I LEFT IT BEHIND AND MOVED ON TOO. THAT'S HOW LIFE IS.

Did I breeze through it? I think what I did was to repress the trauma in order to move forward. That's what I did. I didn't grow up under the most wonderful circumstances so I think I was used to bucking up and marching on and being strong. But no, I've grieved it many times.

I just found the photo of me at age 22 to bring to this interview. At this moment, I feel like I'm on the edge of tears and grief. That's not a bad thing. I feel the sadness and I think there are some losses that you never get over 100 percent. Period. You move on and you deal with it, but you don't get over it. I left it behind and moved on too. That's how life is. I didn't stop growing or living my life or finding joy. But there's a wound. That wound doesn't just disappear, if you're willing to acknowledge it.

Looking back, I wouldn't have done anything differently. The only thing is I wish I had been on the legal side of the time, after Roe v. Wade in 1973.

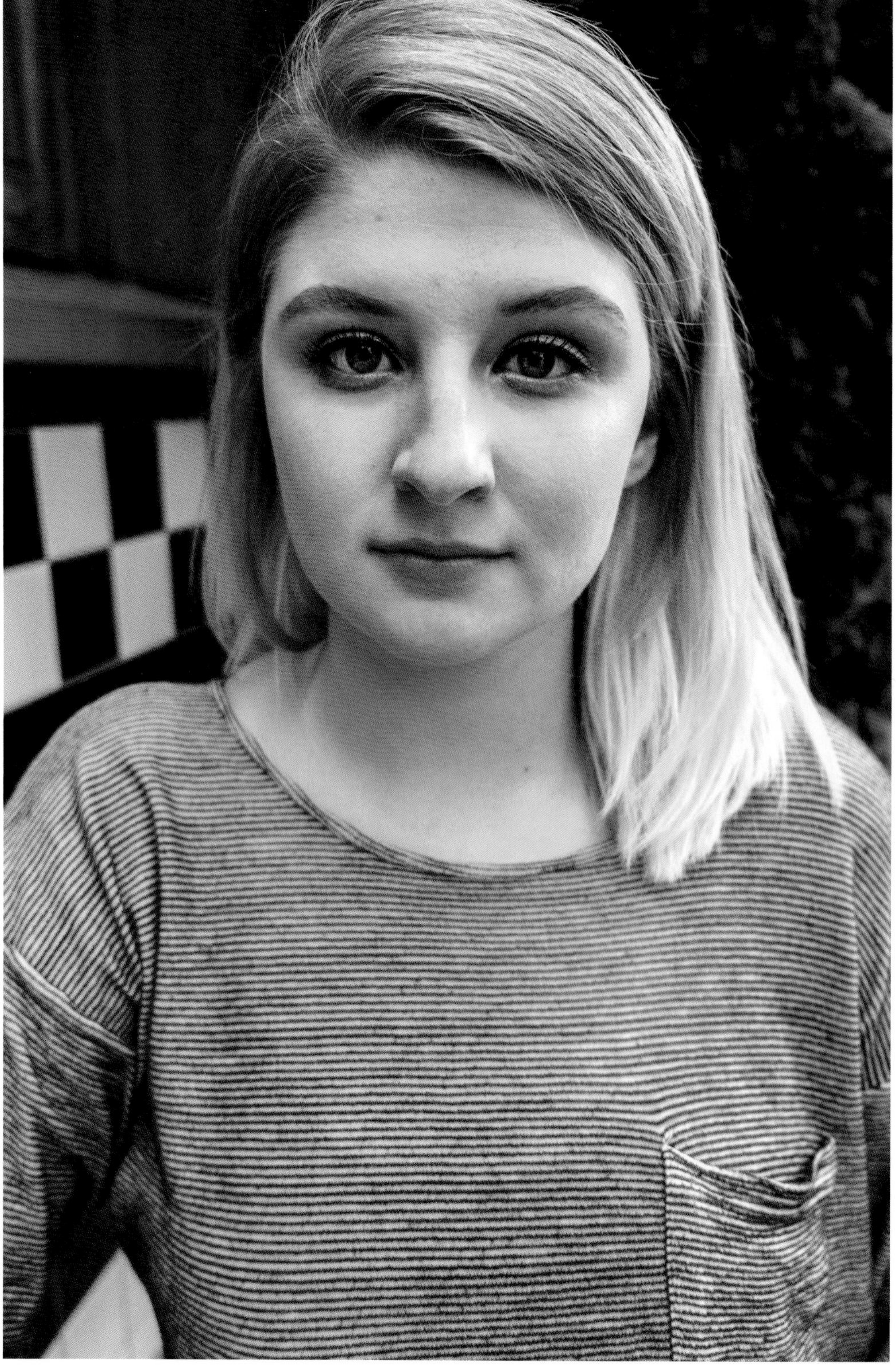

BETH VIAL

Beth Vial

I GREW UP in Portland, Oregon. My parents worked really hard for my sister and me. My dad, up until a certain point in my life, was always working nights and my mom was always working days, so it was like ships passing in the night. They showed me that it's not always easy to raise a family, but they definitely showed me that family is important and that it's worth it.

When I was 19, I was diagnosed with polycystic ovarian syndrome. There's a whole slew of symptoms, like missed or absent periods. The one thing the endocrinologist drilled into me when I was diagnosed was that I would be infertile. I would need intervention to be able to conceive. I was on the pill as a hormone supplement, but it was contraception. At that age, starting a family wasn't on my mind.

By the time I was 22, I was in a long-distance kind of relationship. I was still on my parents' insurance but some clerical glitch meant that I couldn't get my prescription filled, which is why I went off the pill. Because we had been having a monogamous relationship for quite some time, and I'd been told I was infertile, it didn't occur to us to use further contraception.

At the time, my sister had a fibroid removed from her uterus. When I started to have symptoms similar to hers, I kept telling myself that since I can't be pregnant, it's probably a fibroid like hers. I finally took a home pregnancy test for peace of mind. I got what would end up being a false negative. A doctor I went to see did another pregnancy test. It came back positive. From a sonogram, they guessed I was about four months along. I started crying. My partner and I had just broken up, like three or four weeks before.

The doctor said she would have her staff look into things and get back to me. They turned out to be religious. They referred me to a crisis pregnancy center.

This fake clinic made me go to two different sessions. My ex came with me to the first, an hour-long counseling. They wouldn't let him in the room. They made me take another pregnancy test, even though I was confirmed pregnant. Finally, they told me there was no one qualified, like a nurse, to do the required ultrasound. They sent me to a different clinic on a different side of town on a different day.

I had to go through it all again. I specifically asked not to see the ultrasound but they just projected it on this giant screen, which was upsetting. They were just saying really macabre, kind of cruel things. Finally, they told me I was sixteen weeks pregnant.

I gathered my things and left. I didn't feel good in my heart with the information they'd given me and the way they had treated me. I decided to go to our local major hospital in Portland. Another week went by and I finally got a true answer at the hospital. They were very respectful. They took their pictures. They didn't put anything up on the screen. Then the doctor came in and told me that I was not sixteen weeks, but twenty-six weeks.

Some doctors who didn't even know me, didn't speak to me, didn't know what I looked like, got to choose my fate. I was just an idea.

I cried a lot hearing that news. They did a blood test for fetal anomalies. They checked my vitals to make sure everything was okay. In Oregon, thanks to the Reproductive Health Equity Act, there's a whole lot of access to abortion regardless of gestational age, income, or immigration status. But in this hospital, because I was so far along my doctor would need the approval of a department review board.

Ultimately, I did not get board approval. Only my doctor and one other of the five on the panel voted to approve my abortion. Too many of the doctors didn't feel comfortable with my case. Some doctors who didn't even know me, didn't speak to me, didn't know what I looked like, got to choose my fate. I was just an idea.

I had only a week and a half to find a doctor anywhere in the US who would help me. The doctor I was working with told me about a clinic in New Mexico that does later term abortion. That clinic told me if I could get there by my twenty-eighth week, they would help me. I was coming up on twenty-seven.

At that point, I told my parents, because I needed help. They were quiet, listening, and processing and they just said, “We'll help you.” They stepped back and let me do what I needed to do and they were supportive along the way.

When I found out that the clinic was going to charge $9,500 for the abortion at twenty-six and a half weeks, or $10,500 at twenty-eight weeks, it was a huge challenge. I mean, I work a full-time job, but I'm 22 and I have like $2,000 in savings.

The clinic told me about abortion funds. Between the Religious Coalition for Reproductive Choice in New Mexico, the Northwest Abortion Access Fund, and the National Abortion Federation, I was able to raise $2,000. Finally, the clinic has a really great financing plan.

When I told my sister what was going on, she asked me to come over. One of her best friends approached me and said she went through a similar situation. And she's like, “A family member helped me and I've talked to her. We'd like to pay your deposit.” At that point I just lost it. I've never accepted money like that from anyone before or even ever held $6,000 in my hands. I was blown away. I offered to pay it back and she was just like, “No, this is what people do for each other. It's a gift.” I had never experienced such kindness and generosity in my life. I didn't know people like that still existed.

It all came together very quickly. I left for New Mexico on a Sunday. They saw me on Monday. It was a five-day-long procedure. It was a DNX, dilation and digoxin, a drug that they injected through my cervix to stop the fetal heartbeat. Then I spent the next three days dilating my cervix, basically inducing labor. It took a total of twenty hours of labor.

Of course, they do counseling ahead of time to make sure this is what you want and it's the right choice for you. It was such a positive experience. Their care is so all-encompassing and they really know what they're doing.

The decision to have the abortion wasn't the hard part. It was all the excess stress around it. I was there a whole week and then took two more weeks off work to heal. Then I had to go back to my life as if nothing had happened. Honestly, from the time I found out I was pregnant to the time I got to the clinic and started my abortion, was two weeks.

I saw in the paper that the two abortion funds that had helped me had merged and they were having a kick-off party in town. I decided to go. At the event, I signed up to volunteer—like how can I not want to give back? Later, they asked me to apply to be on their board. As of now, I've been on the board of the Northwest Abortion Access Fund for two years.

That's where I learned about We Testify. I flew out to Boston for a retreat where I met a bunch of other young people, like ages 17 through 25, who had experienced abortions. That helped me learn how to tell my story and find empowerment in it. I learned that however your abortion panned out, and whatever your course afterwards, it is OK and it is valid and no one can take that from you.

Prior to my training at We Testify, I was pretty soft-spoken and had a really hard time speaking in public. I failed speech class in high school because I had such a bad stutter. Now, when I'm speaking in front of crowds of over three hundred people, I don't stutter once. I can look back on my life and see the immense growth I've done in the last two years of my life.

Before I went to We Testify I had so much shame. I was just embarrassed and quiet before but then I found it to be like, "No. This is my experience. This is what I went through."

Hannah Thalenberg

I MOVED TO Texas in 2008, when the economic recession was a stark reminder that America's prosperity is reserved for very few people. The Texas Legislature was enacting an onslaught of restrictions on access to reproductive health care, in particular abortion. The intersection of these two trends made it clear to me that reproductive decisions couldn't be separated from people's economic realities.

Also, I come from Brazil, where abortion is illegal—meaning that if somebody can afford it, they can access the care that they need, while people in marginalized communities can't safely exercise that same bodily autonomy. Seeing Texas move toward this reality was really alarming. That's how I got involved in reproductive rights activism during my undergraduate career.

Now, I work for a state political advocacy organization that uses outreach, education, and policy to ensure that all people can decide whether, when, and how to have children, free from stigma and political interference.

My own abortion story took place four years ago. I found out I was pregnant one week before my 24th birthday. I was a recent college graduate renting an apartment on my own for the first time, waiting tables and supporting my partner. When I found out I was pregnant, there was no doubt in my mind that I would have an abortion. I might want children in the future, but certainly not then, not in that situation. It was quite a straightforward decision. At the time, however, House Bill 2 had just come into effect in Texas, imposing such burdensome requirements on clinics that many were forced to

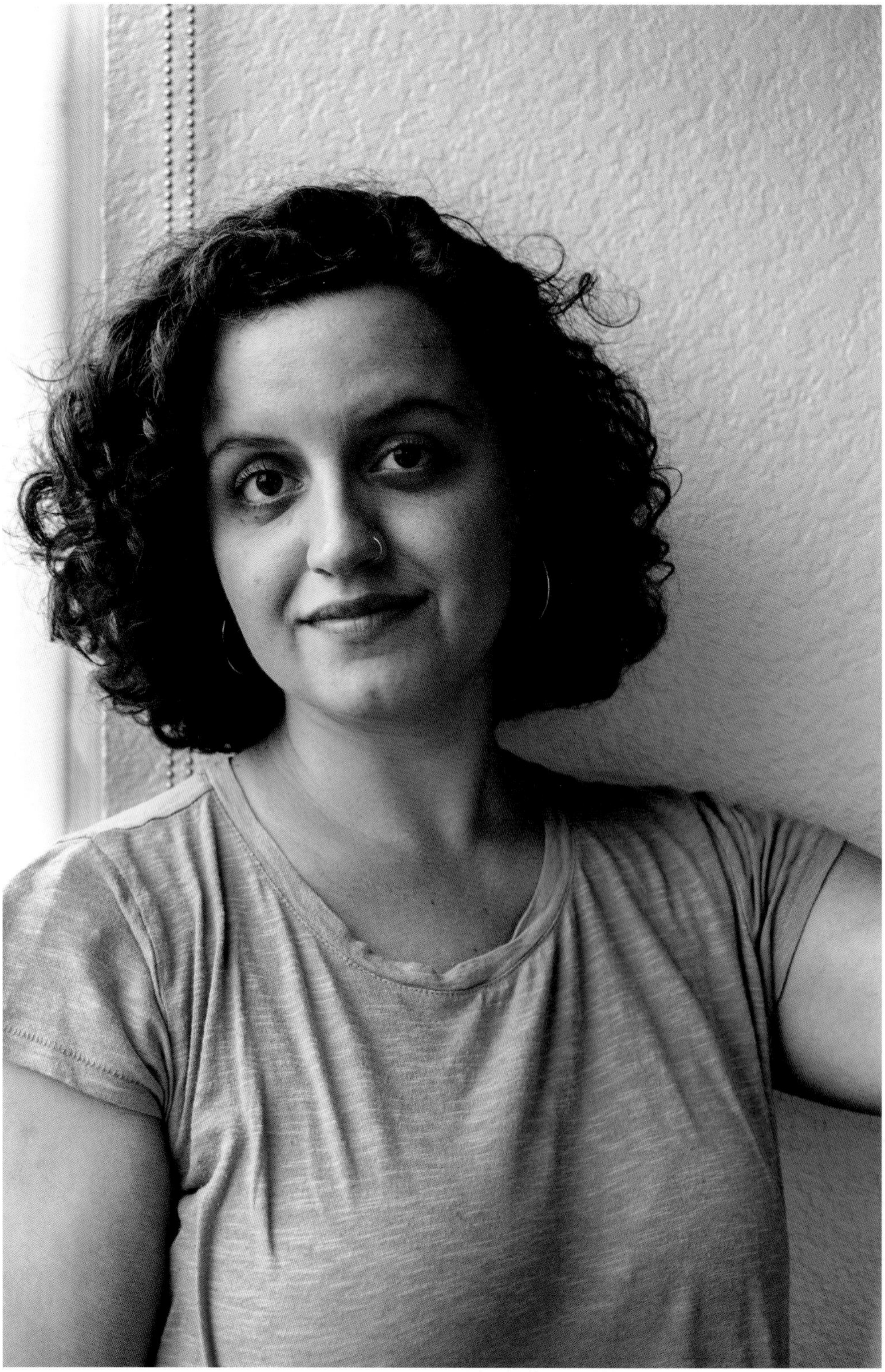

HANNAH THALENBERG

close. I was terrified. I knew that although my local clinics were still open, their volume of patients was going to be a lot higher. I was preparing to race against the clock. But it turned out to be easy.

I found out I was pregnant on a Saturday, called the clinic as soon as it opened on Monday, and I was extremely surprised when they told me I could come in for my first appointment on Tuesday, and they could schedule my procedure as soon as Wednesday. Wednesday happened to be my day off. Perfect.

Then came the calculations. How was I going to pay for this? Because I was only six weeks pregnant, it would have cost $350 to $500. That would use up all of my savings and I was figuring out how many extra shifts I would have to pick up at work to make up for it. But I was surprised to find out that the insurance I had through my stepfather's employment covered the procedure. I did not ask questions. I gave them my insurance card. In the end l only had a $50 co-pay. I could not believe it.

I opted for surgical abortion. It was a tense experience in the sense that I didn't have support. My partner was completely against the abortion. I didn't want to tell my parents: not my mother because she's completely opposed to abortion under any circumstance; not my dad, although I'm sure he would've been supportive, and would have helped cover the cost if I needed it. But he's a doctor with a penchant for teachable moments, and I didn't want a lecture on how I needed to be better about taking contraceptives.

The one close friend I had in Houston was out of town for a conference, so I had nobody to talk to. My partner at least was respectful enough to drive me to the clinic and back, although he was angry at not having input into the decision. My biggest fear the morning of the procedure was that there would be protestors at the clinic, and my partner would freak out, not let me out of the car, but turn around and take me away. Fortunately, that was not the case. He just dropped me off, picked me up, and left me alone in my apartment. With time, he proved to be an emotionally abusive partner. Our relationship dragged on longer than it should have, but at least it wasn't because of a child.

I don't remember a whole lot from that day because I was spaced out on meds. I remember the nurses being such a welcoming, compassionate presence. I didn't opt for sedation, but I popped a whole lot of pills. In the room with comfy chairs, soft lighting, and blankets where we waited for the medications to take effect, I found myself in a fleeting community with the five or six women who were sharing that space. For some of us it was our first time. Others had had abortions before, so they were talking about what their experiences had been.

I appreciated having that connection and remember hugging the nurse who walked me out of the clinic to the car very tightly. That's because outside of the clinic, I was going it alone. On one hand, I was totally certain of my decision and felt certain that I could do this on my own.

Treating my abortion as anything more than a normal medical procedure would just feed into the stigma that surrounded it, right? That afternoon I was just coming off the painkillers, and I remember being angry because I knew that my ability to get an abortion so quickly and easily rested on privilege. I had access to the information. I could afford the procedure. I lived fifteen minutes away from the clinic. I had somebody to take me there. I didn't even have to take time off work. I knew all of this was not the norm. I want everybody who wants an abortion to be able to have an experience as safe and timely and affordable and compassionate as mine.

AFTER A LONELY ABORTION EXPERIENCE, LATER SHARING MY STORY WITH PEOPLE I TRUSTED IS WHAT HEALED A TRAUMA I DIDN'T KNOW HAD BEEN THERE.

Before I had my abortion, I had been volunteering as a clinic escort, doing advocacy days, keeping up with all the news and protesting at the Capitol, so I was already in this struggle. My personal experience grounded my activism and moved me to learn about the reproductive justice framework and focus on dismantling barriers to abortion access.

Looking back, I realize how much I needed a network of support around me at the time. It would have been there had I chosen to reach out. After a lonely abortion experience, later sharing my story with people I trusted is what healed a trauma I didn't know had been there.

From clinic protestors to tweets, there's always someone speaking out against abortion. But even people who are in favor of abortion can implicitly paint it in a negative way. For example, when someone says they want abortion to be "safe, legal, and rare," that last part implies that abortion is undesirable. We want abortion to be safe and legal and available whenever and as often as anyone needs it. This also touches on the stigma against people who have multiple abortions—this judgment that they should have known better after the first time. No. Every pregnancy is different, every abortion is different, and every abortion is valid.

Accessing abortion can be tricky. In my state, abortion clinics are vastly outnumbered by crisis pregnancy centers, fake clinics whose main purpose is to manipulate pregnant people into not obtaining abortions through lies, delay tactics, and other shady practices. Finding a real clinic is a struggle.

Paying for abortion care is another major challenge. Abortion funds are crucial resources. We have quite a few wonderful funds throughout Texas that empower people who need to terminate their pregnancies through direct financial assistance. But they are always strained. We can't expect grassroots organizations to fill a gap that should be covered by the government.

I BELIEVE SHARING OUR STORIES IS KEY TO ELICITING COMPASSION TO BRING ABOUT CHANGE. I FEEL HONORED TO CONTRIBUTE MINE.

Finally, there's the logistics, starting with the fact that any abortion is necessarily a multi-day affair. Texas requires all patients to have an ultrasound and receive a state-mandated script full of false information and emotionally charged language about abortion at least twenty-four hours before the procedure or administration of the abortion pill. Regardless of what our beliefs regarding abortion are, we can't make that decision for anyone else. Once somebody has made the decision to have an abortion, how do we want the experience to be? Do we want them to feel safe and supported?

I believe sharing our stories is key to eliciting compassion to bring about change. I feel honored to contribute mine.

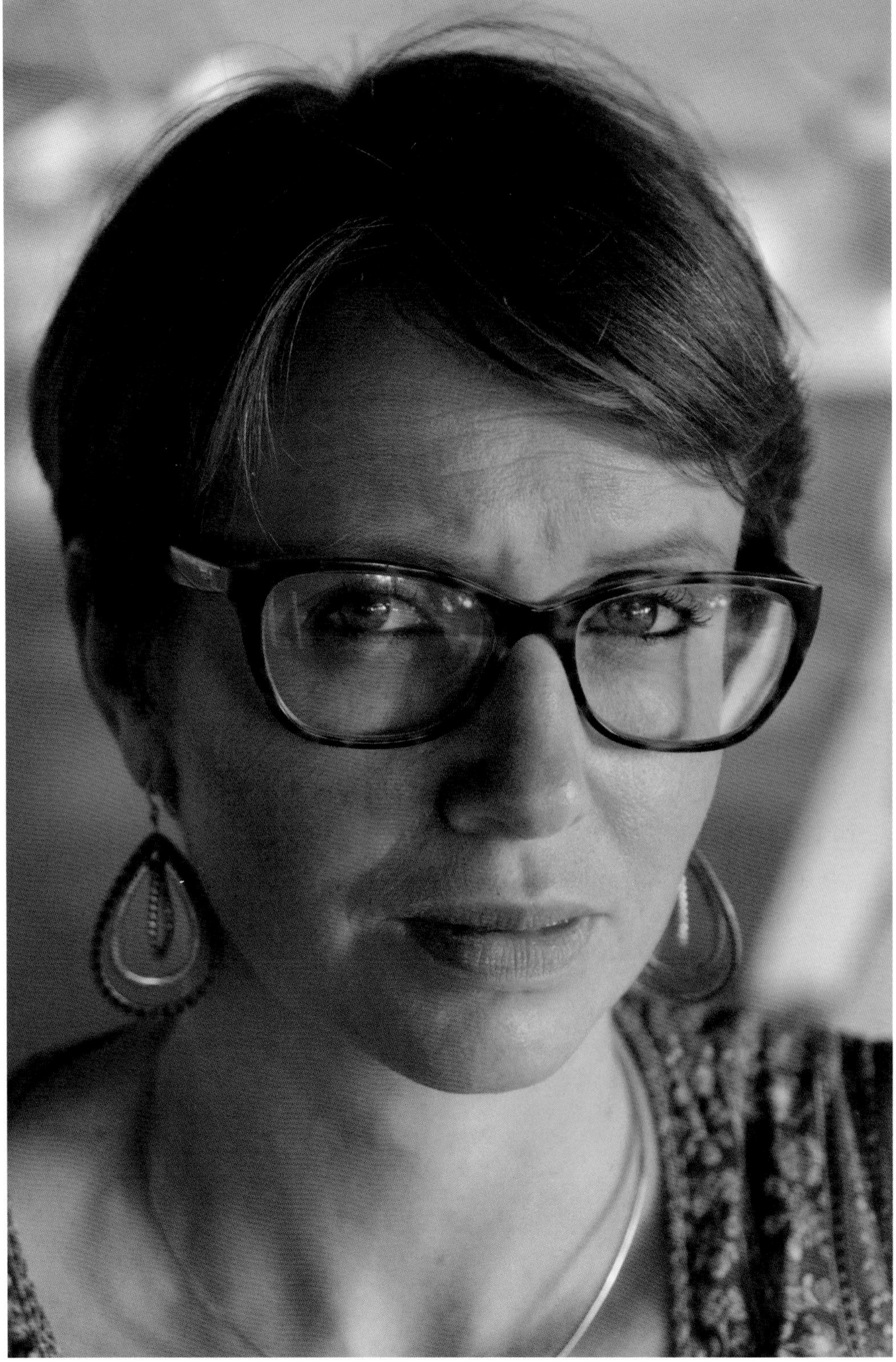

AMIE METTE

Amie Mette

GROWING UP, I remember my mother talked to me about sex for the first time when she became pregnant with my brother. I was probably in kindergarten. My mom doesn't sugarcoat things, so when I asked how the baby came to be, she told me. And then I remember when my second brother was conceived, I was like, "You did that again?"

I had my abortion when I was 30, five years ago. I was a single mom at the time, with two young kids. The father of these two children, he and I haven't been together for a decade now.

But we are co-parenting very well together. When you're in your 20s, you're still figuring out who you are as a person. By the time we hit 30, we kind of figured ourselves out a little bit more.

After going through that very rough breakup, I had reconnected with an ex-boyfriend from my teens and had an unfortunate night with him that culminated in my pregnancy even though I was on birth control and I took Plan B. I was not thrilled to be pregnant. I could barely provide for two children, let alone a third. I was not in a good place. I get very sick when I'm pregnant, so pregnancy would not have gone well at that time in my life. And, honestly, I am bipolar and I have CPTSD or Complex Post Traumatic Stress Syndrome.

I was working three jobs at the time of my abortion. One of my jobs was at a diner. The people at that job to this day are almost family. I had told one of my managers at the diner that I was pregnant. His wife was a nurse, and she told me about the Hope Clinic in Granite City, Illinois.

Missouri has some very strict abortion laws, which would've required me to take off from work for a few days. There's the initial appointment and then you have to wait three days, and then go back.

That's why I decided to go to the clinic in Illinois. I had an appointment within the week. I told my mom and my stepdad about my abortion. My mom was supportive of my decision. I believe she feels that's a decision between me and God. Like it's not really up to anyone to judge me. But she is a Union Baptist, and I think it was very painful for her when I had my abortion.

My stepdad went with me. It was about a three- or four-drive. When I showed up at the clinic, HBO was there making a documentary about abortion. I was really fed up at that point in my life, so they caught me right. I was 100 percent fine with being in their documentary. I needed that abortion and the people demonstrating outside the clinic were really pissing me off.

The people who worked at the clinic were very compassionate, and they took care of me really well. I had a medication abortion, the pill. Then three weeks later I went back for my follow-up appointment.

The documentary, *Abortion: Stories Women Tell*, by Tracy Droz Tragos, was premiered at the Tribeca Film Festival in New York. I went to New York for the event along with some of the others in the film. I felt empowered even being in the documentary. I thought, "Here I am going through this and no one really speaks out. This is a chance to speak out." At Tribeca, the director didn't just bring in the pro-choice side, she brought in the pro-life side. I got to stand up there and debate these women.

I remember someone said all women feel shame after they have an abortion, so I got to stand up there and say, "I don't feel ashamed to have an abortion at all." I was not holding back.

After the documentary's screening, that's when the news articles starting coming out. It was unreal to see my face everywhere. I know I was in the *Los Angeles Times* and the *New York Times* and then my Facebook feed.

I'd say the most backlash from being public about my abortion I received is online. I've lost some family relationships and some friendships for being in the documentary. Some people who saw the publicity around the documentary made remarks and some people have just disappeared and made it very clear how they feel about abortion. I can't say that

I didn't expect that going in. I don't regret being in the documentary and I don't regret having my abortion, but I do feel sad over those relationships from time to time, but I can't change my reality, you know what I mean? Even though a lot of people in my town don't agree with me about abortion, and I glean that from their Facebook feeds, everyone here is pretty polite and cordial. I can't say I've changed anyone's mind. But I think seeing the documentary really helped them understand that abortion is not black or white. Most people just think a woman doesn't want a baby. They don't really consider the nuances that come along with making the decision to have an abortion. So I think that some of my conversations, while I haven't necessarily changed anyone's stance on abortion, I've at least helped them understand that we don't just get abortions because we don't want a kid. There are so many other factors that go into the decision.

Everyone makes that decision for their own private reasons, and they might not be reasons that you understand. I think having empathy for these women is probably the number-one thing, instead of just seeing abortion as a topic in a Bible or a topic on a news page, something for you to glance over and get angry about. I want people to really stop to consider why women get abortions.

I feel like I grew a lot emotionally after the abortion. In a lot of ways that abortion was my metaphorical rock bottom.

Another thing people need to understand about abortion is that it's not a pleasant experience for anyone, and it can affect you emotionally. Even though I don't regret having my abortion, I still get sad about it from time to time and I still wonder what could have been.

Since the documentary, my life has changed quite a bit. I think it was a real wake-up call for me that I really needed to get it together. I really needed a more stable life for myself and my children.

Around the time of my abortion, I met a man who I ended up marrying. We have 2-year-old twins now. We bought a house that was big enough for six people, and I stay at home while my husband goes to work. I also run a business from my house, making cold-processed soap andother body products. With some of the profits, I support domestic violent shelters and crisis centers. You wouldn't believe the dirty looks I get when I take my soaps to these tiny towns once they read on the back of my label that I support domestic violence shelters.

I feel like I grew a lot emotionally after the abortion. In a lot of ways that abortion was my metaphorical rock bottom. I kind of realized there were a lot of people in my life who needed to go, they just weren't very good—I don't want to say influences—but they weren't very good to have around. And it got me thinking about the jobs I was doing. I remember I was bartending and I was still cramping and bleeding from my abortion, and I wasn't making enough money to support my kids on what I was making during that time.

I'VE HAD A LOT OF INTERACTION WITH PEOPLE WHO ARE PRO-LIFE, AND I TRY TO ALWAYS MEET THEM WITH COMPASSION AND TRY TO UNDERSTAND WHERE THEY'RE COMING FROM.

I've had a lot of interaction with people who are pro-life, and I try to always meet them with compassion and try to understand where they're coming from. I think a lot of it is not being able to break away from how you were raised.

I see two different sides of a spectrum of empathy. The pro-life people are empathetic to what they consider a child, and it's really hard for them to look past that. People who are pro-choice who are less empathetic to an embryo and more empathetic to a living, breathing woman. I feel like I'm just starting to have better conversations in that arena with people who have different views than I do.

Ariana Menefee

IT'S KIND OF cliché but my children are a part of me. They need me. They give me purpose. They are everything to me.

I had my daughter when I was 26, so she's 4 years old now. She changed my life completely. Her name is Phoenix. Rebirth. Resurrection. She's one reason why I'm an activist and an advocate for abortion. I want a world where my daughter can be happy being herself, loving herself, growing and nurturing herself. And have the right tools to do so. I also have three sons, ages 15, 10, and 2.

My mother and my father are living, but we aren't close at all. I was lucky to have my grandmother and grandfather. They definitely are my saviors and my siblings' saviors. Everybody was always telling them to give us up for adoption. They took us and were determined to keep us together and they did.

IT'S KIND OF CLICHÉ BUT MY CHILDREN ARE A PART OF ME. THEY NEED ME. THEY GIVE ME PURPOSE. THEY ARE EVERYTHING TO ME.

My grandmother always taught me to be about my business. I had an error in my life, as we were partying all the time. That just aggravated her so much. She would get on me for not taking care of what I was supposed to. Now that I am trying to keep my life together, I see exactly what she was talking about.

My grandmother told me that Martin Luther King said, "If you're going to be a street sweeper, you be the best damn street sweeper anybody has ever seen. And always respect others. You never know when you're entertaining an angel."

I had a few abortions in the past. When I had the first one, I was 17. At the time, I already had a son who was born when I was 16. I knew at that point that I did not want

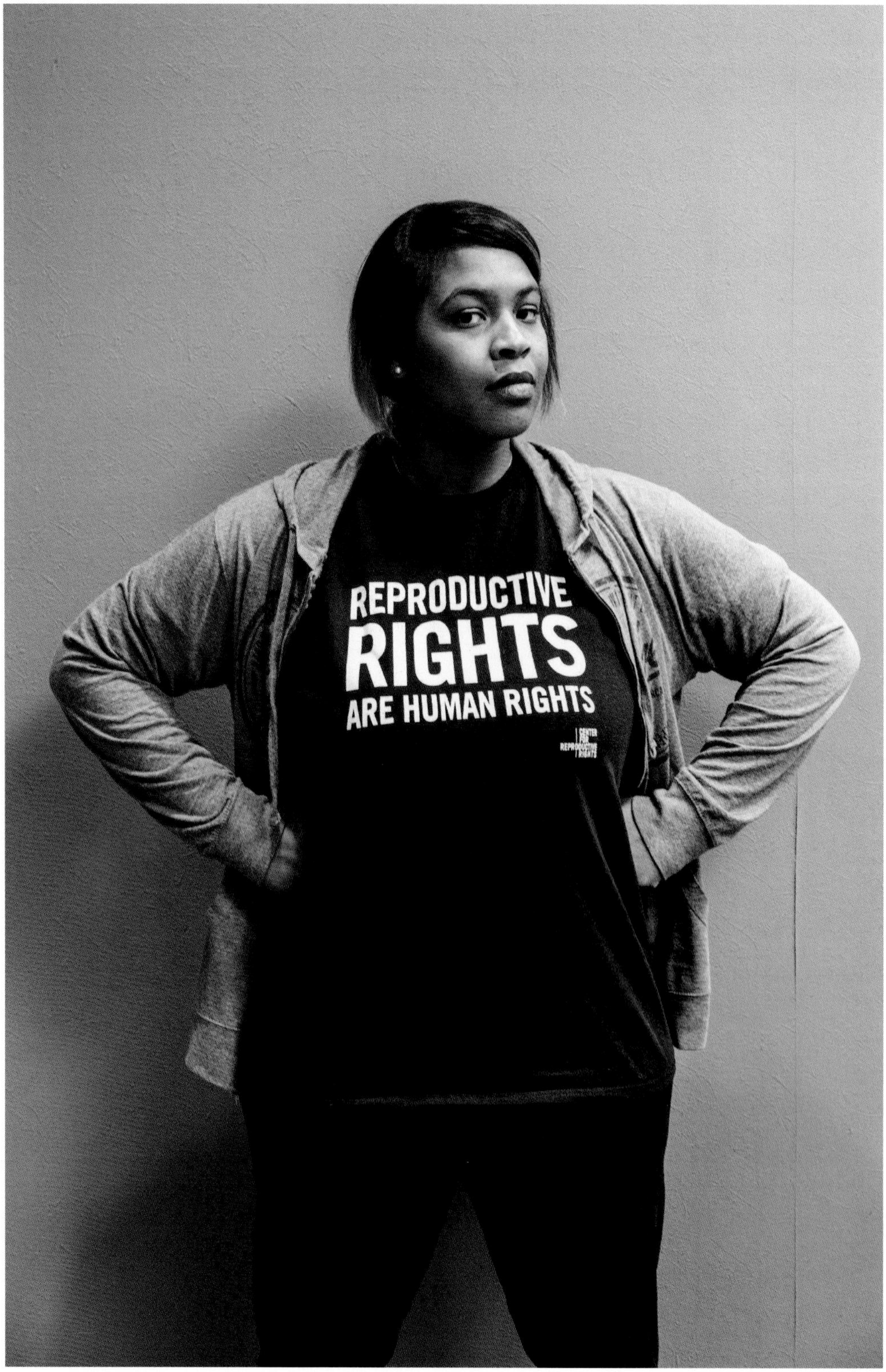

ARIANA MENEFEE

to have more children out of wedlock. My last abortion was last year. The abortions were really heavy on me. I was very regretful. I was beating myself up a lot over the years. But I did manage to get over it.

I just didn't have the education or the guidance to make the right decisions. When I was 15 and got pregnant with my son, I told my grandmother I didn't want an abortion. I wanted to keep my baby. And my grandmother told me, "You can keep the baby." So I kept the baby, who is now my eldest son.

When I had my baby we kind of stopped going to church because of the side-eyes, the whispering, the talking. In the Black community, the church is prominent. We shun each other, as opposed to being open and trying to deal with our issues. I felt bad for my grandmother because she loved that church. And I always held guilt about that because she still pays her tithes there, but she just doesn't go.

My grandmother helped me get my first abortion because I was a minor. I remember another abortion I had, I stripped to earn the money. I did several parties in a weekend just to add up my money enough to get that abortion. That's how important it was to get the abortion.

I've dealt with a lot of regret over the years. I just wish I could do my twenties over again. I was reckless with my life. I was reckless with my body. I was not there for my children like I should have been. The regret just goes on and on. And it has a lot to do with the abortions, because after the first abortion is when I kind of gave up. I just gave up with my faith and where I was trying to go. I'm still a very spiritual person. So I feel things deeply. My abortions stuck with me.

And that's why I'm fighting now, because my daughter is going to have to make these decisions. She may get pregnant, she may not. She may have to have an abortion, she may not. Who knows? I just want her to see the things that happened to me, the decisions I made. I would like my daughter to live in a world where society does not tear her down and beat her up for being her, and for making the decisions that she's going to have to make. If we take away the right to get an abortion, to birth control and things of that nature, we take away a person's control over their life. Everybody should have control over their life.

I've sat my boys down, taught them about the birds and the bees, sex. I'm not giving them condoms, but I am teaching them about what can happen. My oldest is 15. I was 15 when I had him. I mean, life is life. We can't avoid obstacles.

I want a world for my children where we care about each other and each other's feelings. Too much of the time we look at other people's mistakes and decisions, and we dwell on them. We label people. I don't want any labels. I want people to just be people. Everybody is a person. We all are here. We all love each other. We all care. We're going to build each other up.

I've come a long way from homelessness and drug addiction. The only thing that took me out of those things was my kids. I cried for my kids every day in the shelter. I stopped all drugs for my kids. When I could have lost my children, I gave up everything. And I'd do it again. My kids are my life.

I was helped by this transition program. I had just had two babies back-to-back, and I was moving forward, out of an abusive relationship. And still to this day, we have a group on Facebook and we keep in contact. When you get into a room with eleven other women that come from totally different backgrounds, and we all are at a transition point with totally different circumstances, it changes your view on how you trust people and other women, as well. Those ladies were just wonderful. When somebody would miss a day or be sick, we would call and make sure and take them stuff. Just a sisterhood.

If we take away the right to get an abortion, to birth control and things of that nature, we take away a person's control over their life. Everybody should have control over their life.

I had a choice when I wanted to be a parent, and when I needed to not be a parent. It's just a matter of people accepting themselves and their decisions and trusting themselves that they are making the right decision, because as I said before, I dealt with so much regret when people didn't even know I had an abortion. I was beating myself up in other people's voices.

I have people reaching out to me about advice on where to get an abortion and how to move forward. You know I support people. If I can help another 16- or 17-year-old girl, just one, that will be my life dream. I don't want it to just be my daughter. Every young girl needs a support system at that point in their life because times are hard, and that's a pretty big decision to make. I just want women to know you got somebody here for you. These girls need to know they have somebody. Don't turn to the street. Always try to talk to somebody. Let your voice be heard. Don't bottle your feelings up, don't try to go it alone, because that's what's going to hurt you the most.

Glossary

Abortion: The ending of a pregnancy before an embryo or fetus can survive outside the body. An abortion without intervention is often referred to as a miscarriage or a spontaneous abortion. An abortion can also be brought on, or induced, with medications, herbs, trauma, or a medical procedure to open the cervix and remove the contents in the uterus. The medical profession has determined that inducing an abortion with approved medications (see medication abortion) or a procedure done under clean and controlled circumstances is safe and effective.

Aspiration abortion: A procedure that ends pregnancy by emptying the uterus with a plastic curette and suction using a manual syringe (also called a manual vacuum aspiration, or MVA) or with machine-operated suction (also called an electric vacuum aspiration, or EVA).

Cervix: The lower end of the uterus, with a small opening connecting the uterus to the vagina.

Dilators: Metal, plastic, or osmotic rods used to open the cervix. Osmotic dilators are either made of seaweed fiber or hydrogel, which absorb the moisture of the cervix.

Dilation and curettage (D & C): A catch-all description of an abortion. Technically, it involves dilating the cervix and scraping the lining of the uterus with a curette—a surgical instrument with a narrow loop at the top. A metal curette has been replaced with a plastic one and manual or electric suction is used to remove tissue from the uterus (i.e., an aspiration abortion).

Dilation and evacuation (D&E): A surgical procedure in which the cervix is opened and the content of the uterus (pregnancy) is removed with forceps. This procedure is done after the first trimester.

Embryo: The name for the group of cells that forms after the sperm and egg have fertilized. It is called an embryo for eight weeks after fertilization (or ten weeks from the first day of the last menstrual period). After this point in time, the embryo is called a fetus.

Fetus: The term for a developing embryo after ten weeks of pregnancy.

Fetal anomaly: Refers to structural changes of a fetus caused by chromosomes, drugs, or environmental factors that could be incompatible with life, or can lead to severe limitations and/or physical function.

Fetal indication: A medical reason for an abortion based on an estimation of risk for a developmental abnormality or genetic disorder.

Gestational age: The length of a pregnancy. Can be measured from the first day of the last menstrual period or by ultrasound.

"Late-term abortion": A non-medical term that refers to a rare procedure to end a pregnancy after twenty-four weeks of pregnancy, which represent 1 percent of all abortions in the United States.

Medication abortion/abortion pill: Usually refers to the two most common medicines to end a pregnancy: mifepristone (also known as Mifeprex or RU-486) and misoprostol. Misoprotol can be used alone, although it is somewhat less effective than mifepristone and misoprostol used together.

Morning after pill: Emergency contraception (EC) that can be used within 120 hours (five days) of unprotected vaginal intercourse to decrease the chance of pregnancy. EC is available either over the counter (Plan B) or by prescription (Ella).

"Partial birth abortion": A non-medical term that has been used for political purposes and often refers to an abortion procedure called **dilation and extraction (D&X)**, in which the pregnancy is removed intact.

Self-managed abortion: This refers to inducing an abortion outside of the clinical setting, without direct oversight from a medical provider.

Suction/vacuum abortion: See aspiration abortion.

Surgical abortion: An umbrella term used to describe all methods of emptying the uterus of a pregnancy (uterine evacuation) using suction or instruments.

Trimester: Nine months of pregnancy are commonly divided into three trimesters including: 1) the first trimester from week one to end of week twelve; 2) the second trimester from week thirteen to the end of week twenty-six; and 3) the third trimester from week twenty-seven to the end of the pregnancy.

Viability: The point at which a fetus has the potential to survive outside the woman's body based on the fetus's developmental progress and may vary by pregnancy between twenty-four (very rare) and twenty-eight weeks of gestation.

Acknowledgments

SO MANY PEOPLE generously shared their time, introductions, knowledge, experience, and support. I would have not been able to carry out this project without them.

I am particularly grateful to Daniel Grossman, MD, ANSIRH Group (Advancing New Standards in Reproductive Health). University of California, San Francisco, for his good counsel, for writing the introduction to this book, and most of all, for his dedication to reproductive health care.

My thanks to Jennie and Dave Anderson, Bean and Trish Anderson, Jon Anderson, Albert Adams, Susan Adams, Sue Adams, Nancy Adler, PhD, professor and director, Center for Health and Community, University of California, San Francisco; Aspen Baker, founder, Exhale; Renee Bracey-Sherman, founder, We Testify; Claire Brindis, PhD, professor and director, Philip R. Lee Institute for Health Policy Studies, University of California, San Francisco; Lynn Bunim, Charlotte Burchard, Kate Cockrill, Amy Cohen, Caroline Crawford, Andrew W. Epstein, Paula Fracchia, Debra Hauser, president, Advocates for Youth; The Hope Clinic, Granite City, IL; Carole Joffee, PhD, Fran Moreland Johns, Margaret Johnston, Abortion Conversation Projects; Jennifer Karlin, MD, Katherine Kennedy, Katrina Kimport, PhD, Uta Landy, PhD, founder and National Director, Ryan Residency Training and Fellowship in Family Planning; Ann Lazarus, Arthur Martin, Lydia Mendoza, Henry Little, Sanjai Moses, Alissa Perrucci, Women's Option Center, Zuckerberg San Francisco General Hospital; Michelle Samplin-Salgado, Cathy Schreiber, Shelley Sella MD, Harvey Solomon, the Southwestern Women's Options, Albuquerque, NM; Nicole

Stewart, founder, *Out from Under the Rug*; Kina Sullivan, Rebecca Susser, Sandra Treacy, Deirdre Visser, Curator, California Institute of Integral Studies; Keith Walsh, Sue Wollack, Reverend Joann Lee, Calvary Presbyterian Church, San Francisco, CA.

Special thanks to Paul A. Epstein, whose insights, patience, and support were the best gifts of all, to Bill Aron and Kathy Richland Pick, my exceptional photography buddies; Diane Fraser, whose keen editing skills enhanced the project; and to advisors Lori Horne and Barbara Kimport, whose generous counsel helped with the most daunting task of all: finding funds to support the project.

My appreciation to Dagmar Dolby, whose seed grant helped launch this project, and to the following donors: Abortion Conversation Projects, Sue & Bruce Adams, Susan & Al Adams, Doris & Harvey Adelstein, Nancy Adler & Arnie Milstein, Jennie & Dave Anderson, Anonymous, Jennifer & Frank Block, Sherry Brown, Charlotte Burchard & Bahman Sheikh-ol-Eslami, Julie Cheever & Fred Altshuler, Virginia Coe, Andrew Epstein, Arlene Epstein, Paul A. Epstein, Sylvia Ettenberg Memorial Fund, Barbara Finkle, Anne Finkelman, Carla Fracchia, Gary & Paula Fracchia, Pratima Gupta, Jane & Kevin Hart, Ann Hatch, Lori Horne, Daria Joseph, Barbara & David Kimport, Sue Korsower & Ira Priesman, Kay & John Ladd, Vivian & Richard Levitt, Carol A. Levy, Myles Lippe, Molley & Richard Lowry, Kathy Lynaugh & George Hamilton, Lucky & Bill Marmon, Alice McGuire, Jackie McMahan, Barbara Meislin, Alan Mendelson, Beth Matusoff Merfish, Daniel Coleman, and daughters Etta and Flora; Sherry & Gerald Merfish, Brett Matusoff Merfish and Christina Canales Gorczynski, Gail Murphy, Kathleen Murray & Arthur Perkins, Lynne & Bob Myers, Daphna & Shamy Noily, Jan O'Brien & Craig Hartman, Kris & Owen O'Donnell, Frances & Richard Penn, Naomi & Greg Pesky, Wendy & Alan Pesky, Kathy Richland Pick, Sally & Toby Rosenblatt, Abby & Gene Schnair, Anna & Mark Siegler, Holly & Bill Shepard, Alice Schaffer Smith, Sarah Smith, Marion & Irwin Spirn, Gretchen & Rocky Stone, Michele & Richard Stratton, Rebecca & Phil Susser, Marsha Torkelson, Barbara Tversky, Rae Victor, Bonnie Willdorf, Ronald C. Wong & the late Susan B. Jordan, Janet and Art Wong, Maxine Zhukov.

My biggest thanks of all go to the thoughtful, articulate, and courageous individuals who shared their stories with me. Clearly, they are the substance and spirit of this book and made it all possible.